P9-DBJ-451

Readers tell us that EATER'S CHOICE really works...

"Using the 10% saturated fat diet in your book I lowered my lipids from 347 mg/dL to 204 mg/dL. . . . The magnitude of the results was both rewarding and surprising."

Joe D. Burek, D.V.M., Doylestown, Pennsylvania

"I started on the 3% saturated fat regime and lowered my cholesterol from 249 to 145 without exercise and lost the 20 pounds I wanted to lose in the process. . . . Thank you for writing such a simple, easy-to-understand book."

Cary Lichtenstein, Chicago, Illinois

"Thank you for your wonderful book. . . . I have had a cholesterol problem for 3 years and have been unable to decrease it. After only 2 weeks on your food plan, my cholesterol dove from 220 to 199."

Mildred Kani, Kenner, Louisiana

"Thought you'd like to know that between your great recipes and sat-fat/cholesterol information and my husband's will power, he went from 340 to 220 in 4 months. We couldn't have done it without you!"

Adrienne Breen, Chicago, Illinois

and gives them the facts they need...

"Bravo! Your book provides everything one should know in order to outwit the heart attacker."

Mundy Torok, Dover, New Jersey

"Your book is a revelation — what I've been looking for for years. Now for the first time I have facts and figures, and it's simple for me to stay within our fat budget. It's very exciting to know what to do."

Bernadette Stubbs, San Jose, California

"I am proud to say that after 3 weeks and 5 days my total cholesterol went from 301 to 209. Thank you for your book, which made counting the sat-fats easy and fun."

Gary Crouch, San Antonio, Texas

EATER'S CHOICE is recommended by experts . . .

"I've recommended your book to all my patients needing cholesterol-control diets. I've given it numerous times as a gift — even since Christmas."

Mary H. Belenky, R.D., Arnold, Maryland

"Among all the cholesterol books from the technical/professional point of view, yours is the best."

Richard N. Podell, M.D., M.P.H., New Providence, New Jersey

"I loved your book! I am a nurse and work for a cardiologist. We have recommended your book to many of our patients."

Debbie Ouillette, Pinconning, Michigan

"I am the Health Educator for our Health Department. I have found your book to be an excellent, clear, and *practical* resource."

Eric Triffin, West Haven, Connecticut

and provides delicious eating!

"My compliments to the chef!"

Marcia Dunn, Pittsburgh, Pennsylvania

"A whole new way of living with food."

Carol Beatty, Montpelier, Vermont

"One of our patients came in for a check-up — cholesterol 301. I suggested *Eater's Choice*. Last week his cholesterol was 171. . . . He and his wife feel like they are eating gourmet meals all the time."

Naomi Shaiken, New York, New York

"The recipes are fantastic! No boredom here. I have not tried one that we haven't liked. Yours is the first book I turn to when trying to decide what to cook for company."

Debbie Bailey, Pittsburgh, Pennsylvania

"My husband had a 410 cholesterol count, and the diet sheets his doctor gave him totally confused me. I got *Eater's Choice*, and at the end of 6 weeks his chol was 198! . . . As an Iowa farm girl I learned to cook using all the 'good' things — lots of butter, eggs, cream, and meat. This gives you an idea of what a total change it has been for me. . . . Best of all, my husband tells anyone who listens how well he eats, how good the meals are, and how pleased he is."

Jean M. Gray, Scottsdale, Arizona

EATER'S CHOICE

A FOOD LOVER'S GUIDE TO LOWER CHOLESTEROL

Dr. Ron Goor and
Nancy Goor

Illustrations by Nancy Goor

Fourth Edition

HOUGHTON MIFFLIN COMPANY
Boston New York

Copyright © 1987, 1989, 1992, 1995
by Ronald S. Goor and Nancy Goor

All rights reserved

For information about permission to reproduce
selections from this book, write to Permissions,
Houghton Mifflin Company, 215 Park Avenue
South, New York, New York 10003.

Library of Congress Cataloging-in-Publication Data
Goor, Ron.
   Eater's choice : a food lover's guide to lower
cholesterol / Ron Goor and Nancy Goor ;
illustrations by Nancy Goor. — 4th ed.
       p.   cm.
   Includes bibliographical references and index.
   ISBN 0-395-70813-3
   1. Low-cholesterol diet.   2. Low-cholesterol
diet — Recipes.   I. Goor, Nancy.   II. Title.
RM237.75.G66   1995   94-23187
613.2'6 — dc20   CIP

Printed in the United States of America

AGM 10 9 8 7 6 5

Book design by Joyce C. Weston

Eater's Choice® and Choose to Lose® are registered
trademarks of Ronald S. and Nancy M. Goor.

To the staff and participants of the
Coronary Primary Prevention Trial, whose
dedication and perseverance helped prove
that lowering blood cholesterol reduces
the risk of heart attack.

And to Charles Suther,
whose encouragement helped make
this book possible.

Acknowledgments

The authors wish to thank the many people who have contributed to the development of this book: Annette Arbel, Mary Evelyn Bedenbaugh, Robert Betting, Buffie Brownstein, Judy Chiostri, Karen Feinstein, Leslie Goodman-Malamuth, Charles and Jeanette Goor, Alex and Dan Goor, Ilene Gutman, Anita Hamel, Mary Hanke, Barbara Hilberg, Arlene Howard, Dr. Donald Hunninghake, Grace Hyslop, Eleanor Iverson, Sally and Carl Jones, Ann Jons, Esther Krashes, Dr. John LaRosa, Suzanne Lieblich, Bonnie Liebman, Morton Liftin, Eva MacLowry, Berengere and Jean-François Maquet, Sherri McKissick, Joy Mara, Alyssa Mezebish, Martin and Helen Miller, Ted Mummery, Linda Nelson, Nancy Ocshner, Dr. James and Ruth Phang, Muriel Rabin, Helen Rosenfeld, Isabelle Schoenfeld, Dr. Helmut Schrott, Judith Sheard, Lian Tsao, Philip Wagenaar, and Linda York.

CONTENTS

A NOTE ON THE FOURTH EDITION

IN THE TWO YEARS since the third revision of *Eater's Choice* was published, interest in cholesterol has remained strong. New cholesterol guidelines for adults stress the importance of HDL and LDL levels in addition to total cholesterol levels in determining risk. Scientific evidence supporting the benefit of lowering cholesterol continues to accumulate. Consumers have become more sat-fat savvy. Tropical oils have almost completely disappeared from our food supply, only to be replaced by equally heart-risky trans fats in hydrogenated vegetable oils. There has been an explosion of new low-fat and nonfat food products. However, the most dramatic change in the supermarkets has been the introduction of the new food labels mandated by the Food and Drug Administration. These labels go a long way toward reducing the hype and misleading claims of food manufacturers and toward providing universal food labeling and standardization of food labels.

To keep *Eater's Choice* current and responsive to your needs, we have made numerous changes and additions. The all-new section on food labels will show you how to use the new labels to choose foods and stay within your Sat-Fat Budget. You will be happy to know that the Food Tables have been completely updated based on the new food label information. Many more commercial brand-name foods are listed. We have also included Italian and Mexican restaurant food in addition to Chinese restaurant food and updated and expanded the fast-food section. To help you make more informed food choices, we have included figures for total fat in addition to saturated fat. The Food Tables Index following the Food Tables has been updated and will help you find specific foods in the Food Tables.

Writing *Choose to Lose* has made us extremely aware of total fat as well as saturated fat. As a result, we reduced the total fat calories of many of the *Eater's Choice* recipes for the Third Edition and have reduced them even more for this new edition. To help those following *Choose to Lose*, we have added the total fat calories of all the *Eater's Choice* recipes to the nutrition analysis at the end of each recipe. In addition, a list of the total fat calories of all the *Eater's Choice* recipes in this edition is found in the Appendices to help you compare the fat content of all the recipes.

We would like to thank you for your wonderful letters. When you write that you have lowered your cholesterol from 280 to 190 or that you have lost 25 pounds or that your friends adore Apricot Chicken Divine or that your doctor recommended the book to you or you recommended *Eater's Choice* to your doctor (!) or that your whole family is eating more healthfully, we feel very, very good. Thank you!

Our goals for this edition remain unchanged: we want you to understand how foods affect blood cholesterol and the risk of heart disease and, more specifically, how to evaluate your own diet and learn how to make heart-healthy food choices. High cholesterol is one of the few medical conditions that **you** can control simply and without sacrifice. Having a Sat-Fat Budget allows you to fit in your high-sat-fat favorites as well as judge the sat-fat "cost" of all foods. The 290 recipes in *Eater's Choice* allow you to experience the true pleasure of eating delicious food while lowering your cholesterol. Good luck!

FOREWORD

MODERN MEDICINE deserves much credit for improving the health and longevity of Americans by reducing the incidence of many infectious diseases and other causes of death of the past. However, as Americans live longer, diseases of a somewhat different nature — chronic diseases — are taking a relatively larger toll. Just when many people reach the peaks of their careers or a much deserved retirement, their lives may be devastated by heart disease or cancer. Heart disease alone accounts for 50 percent of the deaths in the United States. It is a major cause of disability and a major drain on our emotional and financial resources, both national and personal.

Heart disease is the result of multiple risk factors associated with our high living standard: rich foods, smoking, lack of exercise. In other words, the American way of life may be dangerous to our health. But I am convinced that lifestyles can be changed; in fact, they are changing. Scientific evidence has proven that quitting smoking reduces the incidence of lung cancer and heart disease. Lowering blood pressure reduces the incidence of stroke and heart disease. It is gratifying to see the decline of these diseases in the segments of the population that have made changes. As a consequence, mortality from heart disease has declined by 30 percent and that from stroke by 45 percent in the past twenty years.

While an individual cannot be given a guarantee, these trends show that the adoption of a sensible lifestyle can prevent the development of diseases that threaten both the length and quality of life.

Now a major national public health campaign is being launched against a third, equally potent risk factor for heart disease: high blood cholesterol. Recent evidence has shown that lowering high levels of blood cholesterol will indeed reduce the risk of heart disease. Blood cholesterol levels can be lowered by eating less saturated fat and cholesterol.

The first step is consciousness raising. We need to become aware of the hazards of elevated blood cholesterol levels. To discover if you are at increased risk for heart disease, know your blood cholesterol number. High blood cholesterol is a silent killer. There are no symptoms to warn you until the disease is fully developed, and by then it is often too late. Sudden death can be the first symptom.

If your blood cholesterol is too high, take steps to lower it with the help of your physician. It is up to you, however, to take control over this risk factor. Learn what can be done about it, make the necessary changes, and stick to them.

One of the changes to lower blood cholesterol recommended by the American Heart Association is to reduce total fat intake to 30 percent of daily caloric intake, saturated fat intake to 10 percent, and cholesterol intake to no more than 300 mg per day. Many people find this advice hard to apply. What does it mean in practical terms? How much of which foods should you eat to consume 10 percent of calories from saturated fat?

I have found that *Eater's Choice* addresses these questions in an easy, effective way. *Eater's Choice* discusses the saturated fat content of foods along with a comprehensive discussion of various risk factors of heart disease. Armed with this knowledge, you can figure out exactly what you should be eating to follow the American Heart Association guidelines. The *Eater's Choice* approach to lowering blood cholesterol works because *you* choose the foods you eat.

Eater's Choice is a valuable tool for physicians and other health professionals. Because it uses a quantitative assessment, both you and your physician know exactly what changes you must make in your eating pattern to achieve a healthy blood cholesterol level. Most important, *Eater's Choice* gives those at risk the facts and skills they need to modify their own diet in order to lower their cholesterol. I have found that people who assume responsibility for their own problems are more likely to devise solutions they can live with and thus achieve results that will be lasting.

Eater's Choice will help you discover that a healthy way of eating can also be delicious and satisfying. Far from being a sacrifice, eating heart-healthy foods makes the good life worth living. This book should become a handbook for the making of a modern public health campaign designed to improve the quality of life for all Americans.

— *Julius Richmond, M.D.*
Former Surgeon General of the United States and Assistant Secretary of Health, Department of Health and Human Services

Professor of Health Policy Research and Education, Harvard University

INTRODUCTION

LIKE MILLIONS of other Americans, I come from a family with a history of heart disease. My father had his first of three heart attacks when he was only thirty-one. I was three years old at the time. I grew up with heart disease. It was there, but I didn't take it too seriously.

When I was thirty-one, my blood cholesterol level was measured for the first time. It was 311 mg/dL, the doctor told me — an abnormally high level that put me at very high risk for heart disease, especially with my family history. He sent me to the National Institutes of Health (NIH) to be screened for participation in a clinical trial. The trial was designed to test the effect of lowering blood cholesterol on the risk of heart disease.

At NIH, physicians explained the degree of risk associated with my blood cholesterol level and the nature of the experiment. The experiment included coronary angiography. This test involves inserting a tube through a leg artery up to the heart. A dye is injected so that the amount of blockage of the coronary arteries can be visualized. The mortality rate for the test was only 1 in 100, I was assured.

Learning about the risks of the experiment as well as the risk associated with my elevated blood cholesterol level scared the hell out of me. Although I was excluded from participating in the study (my blood cholesterol level dropped below the cut-off point for entry into the study when I went on the mild study diet), this experience may well have saved my life.

For the first time, I began to realize the seriousness of high blood cholesterol. I was a heart attack just waiting to happen. But equally important, I got a taste of what it is like to be a patient, to have tests done on me and to think of myself as sick. This was hard to take. After all, I was a young man of thirty-one, and I felt great.

This experience taught me two lifesaving lessons. First, although I felt fit and vigorous, I was actually at high risk for heart disease because of my high blood cholesterol level. And with my family history, it could not be ignored. Second, I could lower my blood cholesterol level simply by changing what I ate.

It was too bad it took me all those years to realize the wisdom of my parents' advice about the foods I ate. They were always recommending a low-cholesterol, low-fat diet. I resented their insistence when there seemed to be little relevance to my health. My father was the one who was sick, not I.

How foolish I was. Coronary heart disease is a slow, insidious disease that begins in childhood and develops without symptoms over decades. Then, all of a sudden, boom — a heart attack that may be fatal and, if not, will certainly change your life.

My NIH experience changed my life. I wanted to do something professionally about cholesterol and heart disease. I took my wife and young sons to Boston and added a master of public health degree to my Ph.D. in biochemistry. I then returned to Bethesda, where I got a job as the National Coordinator of the Coronary Primary Prevention Trial at the National Heart, Lung, and Blood Institute of the National Institutes of Health. As I will explain later, this trial was developed to test the hypothesis that lowering your blood cholesterol really does lower your risk of heart disease.

I was involved with this trial for seven years, from its beginning to its end. After it was successfully completed, I took a new job in the Heart Institute as Coordinator of the National Cholesterol Education Program. I wanted to get the word out to the public, physicians, and dietitians about blood cholesterol, diet, and heart disease.

After a year and a half, I became convinced that the way to reach the public was for my wife and me to write a book — this book, which is filled with the information I have gained as a professional in this field. This is not just an academic subject for me. I have lowered my blood cholesterol from 311 mg/dL to 200 mg/dL merely by changing the foods I eat. My two young sons consider heart-healthy eating the natural way to eat. They are not even aware that they are reducing their risk of coronary heart disease and developing healthy habits for the future; they just enjoy eating good food.

Changing my eating habits has been an easy, inexpensive, and pleasant way for me to lower my risk of heart disease. That is what this book is all about. I want to tell *you* how to do it.

— *Dr. Ron Goor*

ONE

EATER'S CHOICE

FOR YOU

THIS BOOK was written for you, whether you are an average, healthy American, a recipient of a triple coronary artery bypass or an angioplast, or a survivor of four heart attacks. If you are in good health, it will give you the knowledge and skills to help you stay healthy and improve your chances of avoiding heart disease and possibly some common forms of cancer. And if you already have heart disease, this book will give you the tools to help you slow down further progression of your condition or even reverse it.

THE INSIDIOUS DISEASE

It may be difficult for you to worry about heart disease if you are healthy, active, and in the prime of life. But here are some alarming statistics that should jar you out of your complacency.

- Fifty percent of Americans die of heart disease.
- Heart disease is the leading cause of death in the United States, outnumbering deaths from cancer and accidents combined.
- Three Americans suffer heart attacks every minute.
- One American dies from a heart attack every minute.
- The first symptom for half the victims of heart disease is death.
- More than 500,000 Americans die from heart attacks each year.
- More than 650,000 Americans are hospitalized for heart attacks each year.
- More than 5 million Americans have angina or other symptoms of heart disease. Many of these people lead highly restricted, painful, and fearful lives.

Choose Not to Be a Part of These Grim Statistics. These statistics are a national shame. They need not be true. Heart disease is

4

not a natural consequence of aging. The epidemic of heart disease is a product of the way we live. By changing our lifestyles, we can make an impact on our health.

In fact, it is already happening. Coronary heart disease has declined by 30 percent in the past twenty years and stroke has decreased even more. Many experts believe that the lifestyle changes Americans are making are reducing the incidence of heart disease. Americans are consuming less cholesterol and saturated fat and have lower blood cholesterol levels. They are smoking fewer cigarettes. They have lowered their blood pressure. They are exercising more.

The lifestyle changes you and your family make can also make a difference. You can increase the chances that you and your family will escape coronary heart disease by the way you choose to live.

But you must act now. The first symptom of half of those who die of heart attacks is death itself. All the improvements in emergency coronary care are of no help in such cases. This high rate of sudden death places an important premium on *prevention*. No one but you can make the necessary decisions that affect your heart disease risk.

Three Major Risks

How do you know if you are at increased risk for coronary heart disease? You are at increased risk if you

- smoke,
- have high blood pressure (over 140/90),
- have elevated blood cholesterol (over 200 mg/dL).*

These are the three major risk factors for coronary heart disease that you can control.

One Plus One Equals Four. The presence of any one of the risk factors (high blood cholesterol, cigarette smoking, or high blood pressure) *doubles* your risk of coronary heart disease. Having two of these risk factors *quadruples* the risk. Thus, if you smoke and have high blood pressure, your risk is enhanced fourfold. And if you smoke, have high blood cholesterol, and have high blood pressure, your risk increases *eightfold* (see Figure 1). It certainly makes you think. We hope it will make you stop smoking, seek advice on con-

---

*Milligrams of cholesterol per deciliter of blood

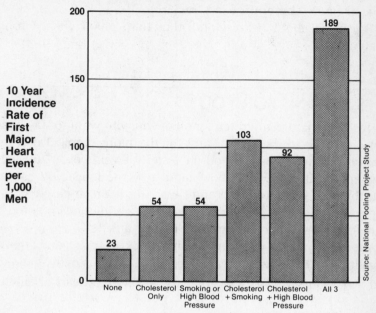

Risk of Coronary Heart Disease Increases with Additional Risk Factors

10 Year Incidence Rate of First Major Heart Event per 1,000 Men

Risk Factor Status at Entry

Source: National Pooling Project Study

Figure 1: Risk Factors for Coronary Heart Disease The three major risk factors — blood cholesterol, blood pressure, and smoking — have additive effects on the incidence rate of coronary heart disease.

Adapted with permission from the Journal of Chronic Diseases, *vol. 31, Pooling Project Research Group, "Relationship of Blood Pressure, Serum Cholesterol, Smoking Habit, Relative Weight, and ECG Abnormalities to Incidence of Major Coronary Events: Final Report of the Pooling Project." Copyright 1978, Pergamon Press, Ltd., and with permission of the American Heart Association, Inc.*

trolling your high blood pressure, and continue reading this book to find out how to lower your blood cholesterol.

What do all these risks mean and how do they apply to you and your life decisions? Perhaps this analogy will help you understand: Suppose that life is like playing Russian roulette. In this game of Russian roulette, you have a partially loaded gun pointed at your head. Obviously, the more chambers that contain bullets, the higher the chance that you will die.

Think of risk factors as the bullets in the chamber of the gun. The more risk factors for coronary heart disease you have, the greater are the chances you will have a heart attack and, perhaps, die. The question is: Do you want to play with one chamber loaded or two or three or four? **The choice is yours!**

(For more about risk factors other than blood cholesterol, see Chapter 9.)

THIS BOOK IS FOR YOU

This book has been written for all of you who want to stay healthy and enjoy life to the fullest, and for the more than 50 percent of American adults whose blood cholesterol level is over 200 mg/dL. This book will help you understand how the foods you eat affect your blood cholesterol level and thus your heart disease risk. Most important, it will teach you the necessary eating and cooking skills to reduce your chance of suffering a heart attack.

Act Now. Don't wait for a heart attack to grab your attention. The clogging of your arteries is happening NOW, slowly, but surely, and it won't wait for you to decide to change your ways. It's not too late (and never too soon) to take action to reduce the risk of heart disease for yourself, your spouse, and your children.

A Special Note to Those Who Already Have Heart Disease

Especially if you already have angina or have had a coronary bypass operation or a heart attack, you can benefit from this book. As we will explain in Chapter 3, you can slow or stop the progression of the life-threatening blockage of the coronary arteries and, in some cases, even reverse it.

A Special Note to the Total Population

This book is for everyone. The *Eater's Choice* low-fat eating plan and recipes are not just for people who are worried about coronary heart disease. The National Cancer Institute recommends a diet low in fat and high in fiber to help prevent some common cancers, such as colon and breast cancers. A similar low-fat diet is also recommended for diabetics. For those concerned with their looks as well as their health, eating foods low in fat is one of the best ways to lose weight and stay trim. You'll feel better, too. As Dr. Richmond points out in the Foreword, "Far from being a sacrifice, eating heart-healthy foods makes the good life worth living." So, no matter who you are, take this book to heart.

Remember:

1. Heart disease is the leading cause of death in the United States.
2. Three major risk factors for coronary heart disease are high blood cholesterol, high blood pressure, and cigarette smoking.
3. *You* can control the three major risk factors of heart disease.

2 IT'S YOUR HEART — KEEP IT TICKING

Y OU GO to the doctor for a physical. You're feeling great. You're not *too* heavy — well, just a few pounds; a bit soft and blubbery around the middle. But, you've never felt better. You get a little breathless walking up steps, but other than that, you feel like a twenty-year-old. Your doctor sits you down. His expression is serious. "You are in good physical condition," he tells you, "but your blood cholesterol is 245." "So?" you ask. "So," he answers, "you're a good candidate for a heart attack. The higher your blood cholesterol, the higher your risk of heart disease."

You feel a queasy sensation in your stomach. Your head begins to spin. "What is blood cholesterol?" you ask. "How does it affect my heart?" You've read about cholesterol in the newspapers. You remember something about HDL, or good cholesterol, and triglycerides, but it never really sank in. Now you're ready to listen. You *need* to understand it. It's *your* heart. It's *your* life.

THE HEART AND HEART DISEASE

The heart is a muscle that pumps blood throughout the body to deliver nutrients to all the body's cells and to remove waste materials. Just how much work the heart does is mind-boggling. Even while you rest or sleep, the heart beats between 70 and 80 times each minute and pumps nearly 5 quarts of blood. That adds up to about 100,000 beats and about 1800 gallons of blood pumped each day.

During vigorous exercise, the heart can increase its output nearly fivefold. Blood is kept moving through the extensive network of arteries, capillaries, and veins by the pumping heart at such a rate that

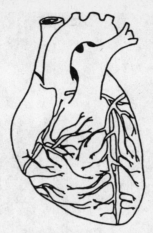

Figure 2: The Heart and Coronary Arteries *The coronary arteries and the network of vessels branching off from them come down over the top of the heart like a crown (corona) and supply the heart muscle with oxygenated blood. Drawing by Judy Beavers.*

blood can make the trip from the heart to the big toe and back in less than one minute.

In order to do all this work, the heart muscle needs a constant supply of nutrient-rich, oxygenated blood. This is supplied by the coronary arteries that branch off from the aorta (see Figure 2).

What Is Atherosclerosis? The underlying cause of coronary heart disease is a process called atherosclerosis. Atherosclerosis is the clogging of the coronary arteries with fatty, fibrous, cholesterol-laden deposits (called atheromata or plaques). These deposits thicken the artery wall, thus narrowing the channel through which the blood flows. Plaques are caused by an excess of cholesterol in the blood (see Figure 3).

When Does Atherosclerosis Begin? In countries where people eat foods high in saturated fat, plaques begin to develop in childhood. Plaque formation progresses at different rates in different people, depending on their ability to metabolize fat. (Both high blood pressure and smoking speed up the rate of atherosclerosis.) Over the course of the first three to four decades of life, plaque deposits gradually increase and the openings of the coronary arteries gradually narrow (see Figure 4).

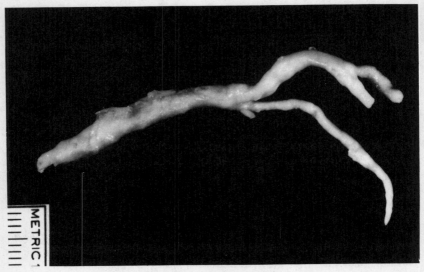

Figure 3: Plaque Removed from a Coronary Artery   *This plaque acquired the shape of the coronary artery that it completely blocked. Photo by Maggie Moore, laboratory of Dr. William C. Roberts, NHLBI.*

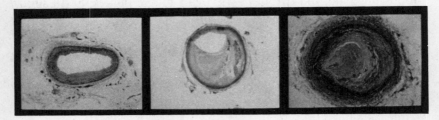

Figure 4: Progression of Blocking of a Coronary Artery   *The progressive blocking of a coronary artery by the accumulation of plaque is shown in these three cross-sections.*

During this time there are usually no symptoms. You feel good. You are active, in your prime, enjoying the good life. Then suddenly, or so it seems, the inevitable occurs. An artery that feeds blood to the heart muscle becomes 75 percent or more blocked with plaque.

What Is Angina? If you are lucky, the first symptom of coronary heart disease may be angina pectoris. This mildest and earliest symptom is brief chest pain, usually experienced upon exertion. Angina occurs because not enough blood can get through the blocked arteries to supply oxygen to the heart muscle cells. Cells deprived of oxygen for only a few minutes can recover if you rest, thereby reducing

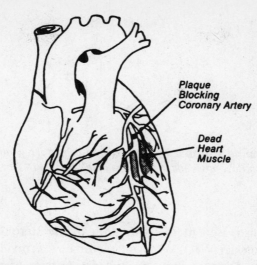

Figure 5: Damage to the Heart Muscle After a Heart Attack   *The shaded area shows the extent of dead heart muscle resulting from the blockage of a coronary artery. Drawing by Judy Beavers.*

the demand on the heart. If the oxygen supply is cut off for longer periods, permanent damage to the heart may result.

The First Symptom May Be Your Last. If you are not so lucky, a small blood clot may become lodged in the narrowed artery and completely block the flow of blood to part of the heart. This part of the heart muscle dies. Result: **heart attack or sudden death** (see Figure 5).

WHAT IS CHOLESTEROL AND WHY DO WE HAVE IT?

Let's backtrack. The doctor says your blood cholesterol is too high. What does heart disease have to do with cholesterol?

Cholesterol is an odorless, white, powdery substance (see Figure 6). It is like a fat in that it does not mix with water. We are concerned with cholesterol because in excess it forms plaque, which clogs the coronary arteries and causes heart disease.

Cholesterol also has many beneficial and vital functions. It is a necessary ingredient of the cell walls of *all* animals, including humans. Cholesterol in the cell wall helps make your skin waterproof and also slows down water loss by evaporation from the body. Cho-

Cholesterol

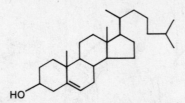

HO

Figure 6: Chemical Structure of Cholesterol *Cholesterol is a fatlike substance with a sterol ring structure. It is found in foods and in the VLDL, LDL, and HDL lipoproteins in the blood.*

lesterol is also used in the formation of the steroid and sex hormones. Cholesterol acts as an insulator in the myelin sheath that surrounds nerves and allows normal transmission of nerve impulses.

Cholesterol is transported in the blood stream together with fats. It is in this capacity that cholesterol becomes implicated in heart disease.

FAT FACTS

In your blood right now are various kinds of particles carrying fat around to do useful work or get stored for later use. Everyone has his or her own balance of the various kinds of particles, depending on diet, heredity, and physical activity. Because we now know one kind of particle is good and another bad, it is worth knowing which is which.

Lipoproteins

Fats* in your body (and in foods) generally occur as *triglycerides*. They are transported in blood, which consists mainly of water. They are broken down and their energy released by enzymes,** which function in a water medium. However, fats do not mix with water. So fats are packaged into particles to keep them from separating out

---

*Fats are one of the five major classes of nutrients; the other four are proteins, carbohydrates, minerals, and vitamins.
**Enzymes are proteins that speed up chemical reactions without themselves being changed.

from the water in the blood. These particles, which also contain proteins and cholesterol, are called *lipoproteins* (*lipo* means fat). Four of the major types of lipoproteins are very low density lipoproteins (VLDL), low density lipoproteins (LDL), high density lipoproteins (HDL), and chylomicrons.

VLDL Lipoproteins. The liver uses excess carbohydrates and fats from the foods you eat to make triglycerides (fats). These triglycerides are packaged into VLDL (very low density lipoprotein) particles for distribution from the liver to the rest of the body. VLDL particles contain large amounts of triglycerides and lesser amounts of cholesterol, protein, and other fats. VLDL particles are produced and released into the blood stream in large quantities after meals.

LDL Lipoproteins: The Bad Cholesterol. As the VLDL particles circulate through the blood stream, triglycerides are removed from the particles and enter cells, where they are used as a source of energy. The fat-depleted VLDL particles are called LDL (low density lipoprotein) particles. The cholesterol and protein that remain constitute a large part of the LDL particles.

LDL particles remain in the blood stream for different periods of time in different people. The longer the LDL particles remain in the blood stream, the greater the chance they will become oxidized and taken up by cells called monocytes. Monocytes that have become engorged with LDL-cholesterol lodge in the coronary artery wall. As more and more LDL is oxidized, taken up by monocytes, and lodged in the artery walls, the artery channel becomes more and more narrow. You know the result. When blood can no longer flow through a coronary artery, the part of the heart supplied by that artery dies. Result: heart attack.

Thus, the higher the LDL level in the blood, the more cholesterol is available to clog the coronary arteries and the higher is the risk of developing atherosclerosis and coronary heart disease. The cholesterol in LDL deserves its name of "bad cholesterol."

In some people, LDL particles are quickly removed from the blood stream by special LDL receptors on cell surfaces. Once inside the cells, cholesterol from the LDL particles is broken down. When these fortunate people with a normal or high number of LDL receptors have their blood cholesterol measured, their LDL is very low.

Other people have reduced numbers of fully functioning LDL receptors (the genetic constitution and diet of the individual determines the number and activity of the LDL receptors). In these people, LDL particles remain in the blood stream longer, producing a higher LDL level in the blood. Since LDL particles are so rich in cholesterol, a high LDL level results in a high blood cholesterol level.

HDL Lipoproteins: The Good Cholesterol. HDL (high density lipoprotein) particles are the smallest of the lipoprotein particles. HDL removes cholesterol from LDL particles and cells and transports it to the liver. Here most of the cholesterol is broken down into bile acids and excreted into the small intestine. Some of the cholesterol is reprocessed into new VLDL particles.

By removing cholesterol from LDL, HDL prevents cholesterol from accumulating in the coronary arteries and thus protects against the development of heart disease. The higher the HDL level, the more cholesterol is removed from the blood stream and the lower is the risk of heart attack. The lower the HDL level, the less cholesterol is removed from the blood stream, and the greater is the risk of heart disease.

Cholesterol. While cholesterol is not a lipoprotein, it is contained in all the lipoproteins. It is of particular interest because it is a major culprit in the formation of plaque.

Cholesterol in the blood is derived partly from cholesterol in the foods you eat and partly from cholesterol made in the liver and the intestine. Because cholesterol is so vital to the normal functioning of the body, all of the body's cholesterol needs can be met by cholesterol made in the liver. In addition, each cell in the body can make cholesterol. Even if you consumed no cholesterol at all (i.e., if you were a strict vegetarian), your body would manufacture enough cholesterol for proper growth and development. However, consumption of too much cholesterol can overload your system and end up as plaque in your coronary arteries.

Note: Cholesterol in foods is not the only, or even the most important, nutrient that affects your blood cholesterol level. The amount of saturated fat in foods is a more important factor in raising blood cholesterol levels, as we will see in Chapter 5.

What *Your* Cholesterol and Lipoprotein Values Mean

All this talk about lipoproteins and cholesterol is very abstract. You want to know about *your* lipoproteins and *your* cholesterol. What do the numbers that you receive from your doctor or from a blood cholesterol screening mean? Do your levels put you at increased risk for heart disease?

First, the total blood cholesterol reading is the sum of the cholesterol in your VLDL, LDL, and HDL particles. Thus, if your total blood cholesterol level is 250, the breakdown may look like this:

$$
\begin{array}{r}
45 \text{ mg/dL of HDL-cholesterol} \\
+ \quad 20 \text{ mg/dL of VLDL-cholesterol} \\
+ \, 185 \text{ mg/dL of LDL-cholesterol} \\
\hline
250 \text{ mg/dL of total cholesterol}
\end{array}
$$

HDL. Average HDL-cholesterol levels for adult males are about 45 mg/dL and about 55 mg/dL for adult females. Levels lower than average place you at increased risk. The lower they are, the greater your risk. Levels below 35 mg/dL should be a cause for concern. Levels above the average decrease your risk. The higher they are, the lower your risk.

If your HDL is low, you can raise it, but only within narrow limits. Regular aerobic exercise and losing weight if you are overweight will increase your HDL levels. On average, nonsmokers have higher HDL levels than smokers.

A low HDL-cholesterol level coupled with other heart disease risk factors, such as high blood pressure, smoking, or a family history of heart disease, significantly increases risk. You should see your physician and take vigorous steps to reduce these risk factors. You should lower your blood pressure, stop smoking, exercise regularly, and lose weight if you are overweight.

If your HDL-cholesterol is low, you should make a determined effort to lower your LDL-cholesterol. Give your HDL a break. If you eat too much saturated fat, you have an abundance of LDL particles circulating in your blood. To remove the cholesterol from the LDL in your blood, you need a lot of HDL particles. But you don't have a lot of HDL particles. So, the cholesterol in the LDL that the HDL cannot handle remains in the blood and is eventually deposited in your artery walls. However, if you eat less saturated fat, fewer LDL particles circulate in your blood. This gives your HDL a fighting chance. Your HDL particles, although limited in number, are able to remove cholesterol from the smaller amount of LDL particles in your blood so the LDL-cholesterol won't end up clogging your arteries.

Because of their sex hormones, most premenopausal women have higher levels of HDL than do men of the same age. During the thirty or so years that women are protected from developing atherosclerosis by high levels of HDL, many men are accumulating plaque at a fast rate. As a result, many men begin to experience heart disease at early ages (as early as their forties). This is not to imply that women are immune to heart disease. Once women reach menopause and lose their protective hormones, they too begin to develop plaque at a fast rate. Women's risk may rise as much as a thousandfold after menopause. In fact, heart disease is the leading cause of death in women, occurring fifteen to twenty years later than in men.

VLDL and Triglycerides. VLDL is not measured directly. It is calculated from your triglyceride level as follows:

$$VLDL = triglycerides \div 5.$$

Triglycerides can be measured only after a twelve-hour fast.

Average values of triglycerides are about 140–150 mg/dL for men and about 100–120 mg/dL for women. Triglycerides are considered a risk factor for heart disease at levels above 150 mg/dL, especially when coupled with an HDL level below 40 mg/dL. If your triglycerides are too high, restrict your intake of simple sugars (sweets) and alcohol (an important factor in raising triglycerides), exercise regularly, and lose weight if you are overweight. Eating less simple sugar, less fat, and more complex carbohydrates (grains, vegetables, and fruits) will help you lose weight and thus lower your triglycerides.

LDL. Average levels of LDL-cholesterol are about 135–145 mg/dL for men and about 120–135 mg/dL for women. About half of American adults have levels higher than these. Such levels are too high for long-term health and are the major reason heart disease is the leading cause of death in this country.

You can lower your LDL-cholesterol levels by changing the foods you eat and by losing weight. Specifically, eating foods low in saturated fats and cholesterol lowers your LDL. Eating less saturated fat increases the number of LDL receptors, thus allowing for increased removal of LDL (bad) cholesterol from the blood. Eating less cholesterol reduces the amount of cholesterol available to be made into lipoproteins in the liver and released into the blood.

The majority of total blood cholesterol is carried in the LDL. Since the total blood cholesterol level is a reflection of the LDL level, it is usually sufficient to monitor only total blood cholesterol. In the rest of this book, we will refer only to total blood cholesterol. But you should know that when you reduce your total blood cholesterol by changing the foods you eat, you are primarily lowering your LDL level and thus your risk of heart disease.

LIPOPROTEINS AND YOUR RISK OF HEART DISEASE

LIPOPROTEIN	RISK INCREASES IF:	TO REDUCE YOUR RISK:
HDL	Low	Exercise regularly Stop smoking Lose weight if overweight
VLDL (Triglycerides)	High	Restrict alcohol Exercise regularly Lose weight if overweight Eat less simple sugar (sweets) Eat less fat and saturated fat
LDL	High	Eat less saturated fat Eat less cholesterol Lose weight if overweight

Lipoprotein Ratios

Your doctor, health professional, or lab report may have expressed your cholesterol numbers in the form of a ratio. The ratio of total cholesterol to HDL-cholesterol, or the ratio of LDL-cholesterol to HDL-cholesterol, is a shorthand measure of heart disease risk which has been reduced to one number. Ratios take into account the fact that total cholesterol by itself does not tell the full story of your risk. Remember, the higher your LDL level, the higher your risk of coronary heart disease. The higher your HDL level, the lower your risk.

The following example shows how completely different lipoprotein ratios may produce the same total cholesterol level.

	Fred	Ted
LDL-cholesterol	120 mg/dL	165 mg/dL
HDL-cholesterol	65 mg/dL	30 mg/dL
VLDL-cholesterol	35 mg/dL	25 mg/dL
Total cholesterol	220 mg/dL	220 mg/dL
Total/HDL ratio	3.4	7.3
LDL/HDL ratio	1.8	5.5

In this example, Fred is at much lower risk than Ted despite the fact that both have the same total cholesterol level.

The Two Ratios. Two different ratios are commonly used. Be sure you know which is being used to describe your risk because the actual numerical values of the ratios are quite different.

1. **Total cholesterol/HDL-cholesterol ratio:** you are considered to be at lower risk if your ratio is below 5.0. Dr. William Castelli of the Framingham Study (see page 21) feels the ideal ratio is under 3.5.
2. **LDL-cholesterol/HDL-cholesterol ratio:** you are considered to be at lower risk if your ratio is below 3.0.

Ratios as Predictors. With total cholesterol levels between 200 and 240 mg/dL, the ratios are better predictors of your risk than either LDL or total cholesterol alone. However, if your total cholesterol is over 240 mg/dL, LDL alone is the best predictor of risk. Even if your HDL is high, making your ratio look good, it can never be high enough to protect you from such high LDL levels.

Likewise, if your total cholesterol level is very low, your ratio will not be a useful predictor of risk. Persons with very low total cholesterol levels, and thus low LDL levels, do not need high HDL levels to protect them. For example, HDL levels are low among rural Japanese, but so are LDL levels. Despite the resulting ratio, heart disease is rare in these people.

YOU CAN CHOOSE TO LOWER YOUR RISKS

Chylomicrons: Yet Another Lipoprotein

If you are sitting there chuckling because you gobble up Quarter Pounders and stuff Wendy's cheese potatoes down your gullet with abandon and still maintain a low total and LDL-cholesterol level, wipe the smile from your lips. New scientific studies show that even with low LDL-cholesterol levels, eating a diet high in fat and saturated fat puts you at risk for heart disease. Eating a low-fat, low-sat-fat diet is still the healthiest route for everyone.

Here's why. In addition to getting fat from the liver, cells get fat directly from the fat in the foods you eat. The fat that you eat is transported from the intestine to the rest of the body in chylomicron particles produced in the intestine. As the chylomicrons circulate through the blood stream, fat is removed and almost all — 97 percent — goes directly into your fat stores, those plump places around your waist, hips, and thighs. The fat-depleted chylomicrons become chylomicron remnants. Under normal conditions, chylomicron remnants are rapidly removed from the blood stream and broken down in the liver (good news). However, studies have shown that animals fed diets high in fat and saturated fat accumulate large amounts of chylomicron remnants in their blood. Because there are too many remnants for the body to dispose of quickly, they remain circulating in the blood for a period of time. Eventually they are oxidized and taken up by cells called monocytes which lodge in the artery wall, causing atherosclerosis, or narrowing of the coronary arteries (bad news). So even if your total or LDL-cholesterol levels always read low, eating a diet high in fat and saturated fat can clog your arteries and put you at high risk for heart disease.

The bottom line is that a diet low in fat and saturated fat is heart-healthy, no matter if your cholesterol is sky-high or 170 mg/dL. And that's what this book is all about. *Eater's Choice* gives you the most effective, inexpensive, safe, and palatable way to lower your risk: **change the foods you eat.** YOU can stop clogging your arteries simply by eating a low-fat and low-sat-fat diet. YOU can make a difference in your heart's destiny.

By the time you finish Chapter 10, you should be convinced that it really does matter what foods you pour into your body. If you bought a new car and wanted to keep it in tiptop operating condition, you would never fill it with dirty gas oozing big globs of grease that could collect in the pipelines and clog the fuel line. You would make sure you fed it the best gas available. Why not treat yourself as well as you treat your car?

Remember:

1. The heart is a living pump that must be constantly supplied with oxygen and nutrients via the coronary arteries.
2. Atherosclerosis is the process by which the coronary arteries are progressively blocked by cholesterol-rich deposits.
3. Heart attacks occur when a coronary artery becomes 75 percent or more blocked. A heart attack involves death of the part of

the heart muscle normally supplied by the blocked coronary artery.

4. Cholesterol in the blood is found in the lipoprotein particles involved in fat transport: VLDL, LDL, and HDL. Total blood cholesterol is the sum of the cholesterol in VLDL + LDL + HDL.

5. High levels of HDL cholesterol ("good" cholesterol) lower the risk of heart disease. You can raise your HDL by exercising regularly, losing weight if you are overweight, and stopping smoking.

6. High levels of LDL cholesterol ("bad" cholesterol) raise the risk of heart disease. You can lower your LDL and your risk of coronary heart disease by eating less saturated fat and cholesterol.

THE EVIDENCE   3

$\mathbf{A}$T THE END of the last chapter, we categorically stated that you could lower your blood cholesterol and thus stop clogging your arteries by changing your eating habits. Before you consider a major revamping of your old eating style, you may want proof that the change will indeed lower your blood cholesterol level and that lowering your blood cholesterol will reduce your risk of coronary heart disease.

Without drowning you in a sea of scientific data, we will merely touch on a few of the more important studies that show that:

1. elevated blood cholesterol is a risk factor for coronary heart disease;
2. blood cholesterol levels can be raised or lowered by the foods you eat;
3. lowering blood cholesterol reduces the risk of coronary heart disease.

EVIDENCE PART I: ELEVATED BLOOD CHOLESTEROL IS A RISK FACTOR FOR CORONARY HEART DISEASE

The Framingham Study

For almost forty years, investigators have been studying the health of the population of Framingham, Massachusetts, paying particular attention to risk factors for heart disease. Blood cholesterol levels have been measured and remeasured, heart attacks have been recorded. Even today, data on the original participants and their chil-

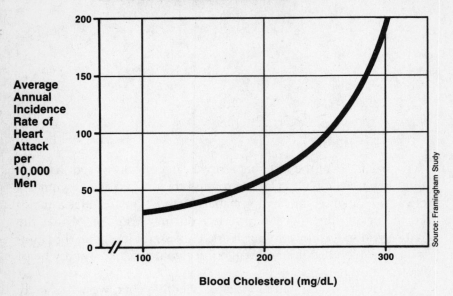

Risk of Coronary Heart Attack Rises as Blood Cholesterol Increases

Average Annual Incidence Rate of Heart Attack per 10,000 Men

Blood Cholesterol (mg/dL)

Source: Framingham Study

Figure 7: Coronary Heart Disease Risk and Blood Cholesterol *Risk of coronary heart disease rises with increasing blood cholesterol levels. Risk increases rapidly as blood cholesterol levels rise above 200 mg/dL.*

dren are being collected and analyzed. The results of this long-term population study are conclusive: **blood cholesterol levels predict the future incidence of heart attacks.**

The relationship between blood cholesterol levels and heart attacks is shown in a curve popularly known as the "Framingham risk curve" (see Figure 7). This curve is smooth and continuous. As blood cholesterol levels go up, risk of heart attack rises. At blood cholesterol levels above 200 mg/dL, risk rises rapidly. The risk is four times greater at a blood cholesterol level of 300 mg/dL than at a blood cholesterol level of about 200 mg/dL. (The Framingham risk curve could just as accurately be expressed in terms of LDL-cholesterol level instead of total blood cholesterol.) Although even the lowest blood cholesterol levels carry some risk of coronary heart disease, Dr. William Castelli, director of the Framingham Study, has stated that no one with a blood cholesterol level below 150 mg/dL has ever had a heart attack in Framingham.

EVIDENCE PART II: BLOOD CHOLESTEROL LEVELS CAN BE LOWERED (OR RAISED) BY DIET

Blood cholesterol levels are not set in concrete. They can be changed. To a large extent YOU can lower (or raise) your blood cholesterol level by what you eat. Here's the evidence to prove it.

International Comparisons

Comparing diets of countries with low and high coronary heart disease rates reveals a direct correlation between the amount of saturated fat in the diet and the blood cholesterol level and incidence of heart disease among the different populations.

The rates of coronary heart disease among countries varies almost tenfold from a low of 100 per 100,000 in Japan to a high of 900 per 100,000 in Finland. The Japanese eat little beef (a food high in saturated fat) and much fish (a food low in saturated fat and rich in polyunsaturated fat). The Finns, on the other hand, eat large amounts of cheese and whole milk products — foods high in saturated fat.

Countries with high average blood cholesterol levels and high rates of coronary heart disease have diets in which saturated fat accounts for over 15 percent of total calories. This includes the United States, Scotland, England, Finland, and Holland. Countries with very low blood cholesterol levels and very low coronary heart disease rates have diets in which saturated fats contribute less than 10 percent of total calories. Such countries include Japan and Greece.

Is the Evidence Valid? How can we be sure that these differences in coronary heart disease rates among countries are really due to dietary differences and not to genetic differences?

Japan to Hawaii: Changing Dietary Habits. An interesting study of Japanese migrants to Hawaii and San Francisco sheds light on this question. Japanese in Japan have one of the lowest rates of coronary heart disease. They have low blood cholesterol levels (the average blood cholesterol level was found to be less than 170 mg/dL) and eat a diet in which fat contributes only about 10 percent of total calories and saturated fat only about 3 percent. By Western standards, this is a very low fat diet.

The Japanese who have migrated to Hawaii have adopted some Western dietary habits. They eat a diet higher in fat and saturated fat than the typical Japanese diet but not as high as a typical American diet. The Japanese in Hawaii have higher blood cholesterol levels and higher rates of coronary heart disease than those in Japan but not as high as those in San Francisco.

Japan to Hawaii to San Francisco: Accumulating Bad Dietary Habits and Plaques. The Japanese who have migrated to San Francisco have gone even further in adopting American dietary habits, have blood cholesterol levels similar to native Americans, and, alas, have rates of coronary heart disease similar to Americans. Clearly, it is diet, and not genetics, that is raising the blood cholesterol levels and consequently the coronary heart disease rates of the migrants.

Japan Revisited: A Postscript. Alas. In the last few years, American fast food has been introduced to Japan and has become extremely popular. As you would expect, Japanese blood cholesterol levels are rising and the incidence of acute myocardial infarctions (heart attacks) has increased fivefold.

Vegetarians Provide Evidence. Most Seventh-Day Adventists are ovo-lacto vegetarians and thus eat some eggs and dairy products. Some, however, are strict vegetarians and eat no animal products at all. Others eat meat.

In general, those who are strict vegetarians have the lowest blood cholesterol levels. Ovo-lacto vegetarians (the majority of Adventists) have slightly higher blood cholesterol levels. Those who eat meat have the highest levels. *The vegetarian Adventists (including ovo-lacto vegetarians) have significantly lower heart disease rates than other Americans of the same age and sex.* It should be kept in mind that Adventists also do not drink coffee or alcohol or smoke tobacco.

Dietary Studies in Normal Volunteers. The strongest and most direct evidence that diet affects blood cholesterol levels comes from studies of normal volunteers whose intakes of saturated, polyunsaturated, and monounsaturated fats and cholesterol are varied under tightly controlled conditions on special hospital wards. These studies show that LDL cholesterol levels decrease when dietary saturated fat and cholesterol are decreased and when dietary polyunsaturated fat is increased. Removing saturated fat from the diet has two times the blood cholesterol–lowering impact as does adding an equal amount of polyunsaturated fat. Note: The best strategy for lowering cholesterol is to reduce saturated fat in your diet. The benefits can be tremendous — up to a 33 percent lowering of total blood cholesterol levels. For the relative merits of saturated versus poly-unsaturated fats, see the discussion on page 39.

How Your Heredity Fits In

At this point a question always seems to pop up. If blood cholesterol levels are affected by diet, why do people who eat exactly the same diet have different blood cholesterol levels?

Your blood cholesterol level is determined by how your genetic constitution affects the metabolism of the fats and cholesterol you eat. In other words, blood cholesterol level depends on an interaction between genetics and diet — that is, how sensitive you are to the amounts of saturated fats and cholesterol you eat.

We are a population with a great range of genetic constitutions affecting the control of blood cholesterol levels. Upon exposure to the typical high-fat, high-cholesterol American diet, these different genetic constitutions are expressed as widely divergent blood cholesterol levels. Thus, some people can eat large amounts of saturated fat and cholesterol and maintain a blood cholesterol level of 150 mg/dL. Other people on the same fatty diet maintain a blood cholesterol level of 350 mg/dL.

The Japanese in Japan show much less variability in blood cholesterol levels. However, the fact that there is much genetic variability in the Japanese population is revealed when they are exposed to a typical American diet of high saturated fat and cholesterol. Thus, one person with a blood cholesterol of 170 mg/dL in Japan may find it rise to 230 mg/dL on a San Francisco diet, while another may find it rise to 280 mg/dL, while yet another may find it rise only to 180 mg/dL.

EVIDENCE PART III: LOWERING BLOOD CHOLESTEROL REDUCES YOUR RISK OF CORONARY HEART DISEASE

The big question that remains is: Does lowering elevated blood cholesterol levels in humans reduce the risk of coronary heart disease? The answer is a resounding and definite YES.

The Coronary Primary Prevention Trial Gets Results

In 1973, the National Heart, Lung, and Blood Institute (one of the National Institutes of Health) began a ten-year study, the Coronary Primary Prevention Trial (CPPT), to test the lipid hypothesis: lowering blood cholesterol levels reduces the incidence of coronary heart disease.

The basic plan of the study was as follows. To test the lipid hypothesis, two groups of men with identical risks of coronary heart disease were selected. At the outset, both groups had identical average blood cholesterol levels of almost 300 mg/dL. Both groups followed a mild cholesterol-lowering diet. In addition, one group received a drug (cholestyramine) that lowered their blood cholesterol levels while the other group received a placebo that looked and tasted like the real drug but had no blood cholesterol—lowering effect. During the study, the only risk factor difference between the two groups was the lower blood cholesterol level of the drug-treated group.

CPPT Results: Lowering Blood Cholesterol Cuts Risk. At the end of the ten years, there was a definite difference in the incidence of coronary heart disease between the two groups. The group treated with the active drug had a lower average blood cholesterol level and a lower incidence of fatal and nonfatal heart attacks than the group that was not drug-treated.

Blood cholesterol levels in the drug-treated group were, on average, 9 percent lower than those in the placebo group. The incidence of fatal and nonfatal heart attacks in the treated group was 19 percent lower than in the placebo group. (There were reductions of a similar magnitude in new cases of angina, coronary bypass surgery, and electrocardiographic abnormalities in the treated group.)

This figures out to a fantastic ratio: for every 1 percent reduction in blood cholesterol, there was a 2 percent reduction in risk. Thus, participants who achieved a 25 percent reduction in blood cholesterol reduced their risk of heart attack by 50 percent.

These results may be applicable to you. For every 1 percent you reduce your blood cholesterol, your risk may be reduced by as much as 2 percent. Pretty good odds.

Another NIH Study Confirms CPPT Results. Another NIH study, which was conducted at the same time, also tested the lipid hypothesis. It produced results that could actually be seen in the coronary arteries. In this study, men and women were chosen with elevated blood cholesterol levels and atherosclerotic narrowing of their coronary arteries. They were randomly divided into two groups. Both groups followed a mild cholesterol-lowering diet. One treatment group received a blood cholesterol–lowering drug (cholestyramine) and the other a placebo.

At the beginning of the study, both groups underwent coronary angiography to evaluate the extent of atherosclerosis or narrowing of their coronary arteries. (Coronary angiography is a technique that uses an iodine-containing dye and x-ray pictures to allow visualization of the coronary arteries.) At the end of the study, five years later, the severity of atherosclerosis of the coronary arteries of both groups was once more assessed by coronary angiography.

The results were dramatic. Investigators could actually *see* that lowering LDL-cholesterol levels in the drug treatment group prevented the further narrowing of the coronary arteries.

In 1987 these results were confirmed. The Cholesterol-Lowering Atherosclerosis Study (CLAS) was an angiographic study of middle-aged men who had undergone coronary bypass surgery. Those men who were treated with a combination of drugs (colestipol and niacin) and diet had lower LDL levels, higher HDL levels, and, as a result of these changes, significantly less accumulation of atherosclerotic plaque than those not treated with a combination of drugs and diet. More exciting, 16.2 percent of the drug-and-diet-treated group experienced regression of atherosclerotic plaque.

Diet Versus Drug. You may wonder how we can assume that lowering blood cholesterol levels by diet is effective in reducing risk of coronary heart disease when the CPPT and the NIH and CLAS studies were drug studies.

Participants in the placebo group in the CPPT showed a range of reduction of LDL-cholesterol levels. These reductions were achieved by diet alone since these men received no active drug. Just as in the drug group, the greater the reduction in LDL-cholesterol by diet, the greater was the reduction in the incidence of coronary heart disease.

A follow-up study of the participants in the CLAS study who did not receive drugs showed the effect of diet on the development of new plaque-containing lesions in their coronary arteries. During the study, those whose fat intake averaged 27.5 percent of total calories developed **no new** plaque-containing lesions. But, those whose fat intake averaged 34 percent of total calories did develop new lesions. Those participants who reduced their LDL-cholesterol by an average of 7 percent developed *no new* lesions, while those who reduced their LDL levels by only 0.6 percent did develop new lesions.

Proof in the Pudding: Low-Fat Diet Causes Reversal. The most dramatic demonstration to date that a diet low in fat and saturated fat can actually reverse the narrowing of the coronary arteries comes from the Lifestyle Heart Trial. The trial consisted of 41 patients with angiographic evidence of coronary heart disease. The 22 participants in the experimental group consumed a very low fat diet (less than 10 percent of total calories), exercised regularly, and participated in a stress management program. Their total blood cholesterol levels were reduced by 24 percent and LDL levels by 37 percent. The 19 control subjects who followed no particular diet or exercise or stress program got no significant cholesterol reduction.

Angiographic analysis of the coronary arteries of the experimental group showed the following dramatic results: At the beginning of the study, the plaque in the coronary arteries was so thick it narrowed the openings to 60 percent of the original diameter. After only one year, plaque was reduced (regressed) so that the diameter opened up to 62.2 percent. In the control group, just the reverse was true. The plaque accumulated (progressed), closing the diameter even further, from 57.3 percent to 53.9 percent.

The results were even more dramatic when lesions that reduced the artery diameter by more than 50 percent were considered. After a year, plaque in the experimental group's arteries *regressed* so that the average diameter enlarged from 38.9 percent to 44.2 percent of the original opening and *progressed* in the control group, narrowing the opening from 38.3 percent to 35.6 percent of the original.

You may look at these results and think, 2.2 percent regression and 3.4 percent progression, or even 5.3 percent regression and 2.7 percent progression — what's the big deal? But you must remember that this study measured regression or progression after only *one* year. These percentages will be more impressive to you when you realize that reducing the diameter of your arteries 3.4 percent year after year will eventually narrow them to 25 percent or less of the original diameter. When the openings of coronary arteries are reduced this much, small blood clots floating through the blood stream can get caught in the narrowed artery and block the flow of nutrient-rich blood to the heart muscle. You know the result: heart attack.

On the other hand, just think how clear your arteries can become if the plaque that clogs them is reduced 2.2 percent or 5.3 percent, year after year.

These results are inspiring. But before you restrict yourself to a diet limited to 10 percent of total fat, be advised that it is unclear whether such a restrictive diet — mainly fruits, vegetables, greens, soybean products, egg white, and nonfat milk — is truly necessary to achieve regression. Regression was achieved in the CLAS study with a much less stringent diet.

The Benefits. In conclusion, definite regression can be expected in 16 to 47 percent of people, provided they lower their LDL level by 34 to 48 percent for 3 to 5 years. As proved in these studies, the main benefit of a diet low in saturated fat is that progression (continued narrowing of the coronary arteries) can be slowed, stopped, and in some cases reversed. Not a bad reward for just eating a lot of delicious low-fat food!

Remember:

1. The higher the blood cholesterol, the greater is the risk of developing coronary heart disease.
2. Blood cholesterol levels are determined in part by genetic factors and in part by the foods you eat.
3. Reductions of up to 33 percent in blood cholesterol level can be achieved by diet alone.
4. Reducing blood cholesterol levels lowers risk of fatal and nonfatal heart attack.

4 IS YOUR BLOOD CHOLESTEROL TOO HIGH?

THE CORONARY Primary Prevention Trial (CPPT) results were positive. **Lowering blood cholesterol (and LDL) prevented heart attacks.** The lipid hypothesis was proven.

What do these results mean to you personally? How high is *your* risk? How much do *you* have to lower your blood cholesterol to reduce your risk?

NATIONAL INSTITUTES OF HEALTH RECOMMENDATIONS

To provide guidelines to physicians and the public, the National Cholesterol Education Program of the National Institutes of Health (NIH) convened an Adult Treatment Panel. This distinguished panel of scientists and physicians reviewed all of the available scientific and medical data and, on June 15, 1993, made the following recommendations (see Appendices for a more complete summary of the Adult Treatment Guidelines, page 626):

- Know your blood cholesterol number.
- Keep your blood cholesterol below 200 mg/dL by diet (and drugs, if necessary).
- Diet is the first line of treatment to reduce blood cholesterol below 200 mg/dL and should be given a fair and rigorous trial for at least 6 months before even considering drugs. In fact, most adults can expect to lower their blood cholesterol below 200 mg/dL by diet alone.
- The presence of coronary heart disease or other risk factors for heart disease, such as male sex, family history of premature heart

attack (before age 55), cigarette smoking, high blood pressure, low HDL (below 35 mg/dL), diabetes, cerebrovascular or peripheral vascular disease, and severe obesity (30 percent or more overweight) indicate the need for more vigorous therapy.

NATIONAL INSTITUTES OF HEALTH ADULT TREATMENT PANEL RECOMMENDATIONS

BLOOD CHOLESTEROL LEVELS, MG/DL

CATEGORY	TOTAL CHOLESTEROL	HDL CHOLESTEROL	LDL CHOLESTEROL
Desirable	<200	≥35	<130
Borderline-high risk	200–239	<35	130–159
High risk	≥240	<35	≥160

What Is Normal Blood Cholesterol?

The NIH recommendations are very definite: keep your blood cholesterol level below 200 mg/dL. However, you may be (or may already have been) told by health professionals that a blood cholesterol much higher than 200 mg/dL is *normal*. These advisers are not trying to dig you an early grave. They are just confusing the two meanings of normal — normal in a statistical sense and normal meaning disease-free.

But you must understand what normal means in reference to your blood cholesterol so you will not be lulled into a false sense of security about your blood cholesterol level. Ask for numbers. Blindly accepting your blood cholesterol level as "normal" may be injurious to your long-term health.

"Normal" Statistically Speaking. Here's what "normal" means in a statistical sense. You begin with a curve (see Figure 8) which plots the percentages of Americans with different blood cholesterol levels. This curve looks like many other curves, for example, curves that plot the distributions of weights, heights, or blood pressures in a population. In all such curves, persons with normal values in a statistical sense are found in the middle 95 percent of the curve.

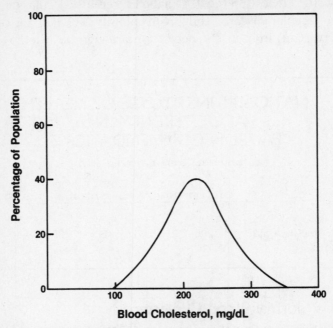

Current American Population Distribution

Figure 8: Current U.S. Distribution of Blood Cholesterol   *The average blood cholesterol level for adult Americans is about 215–220 mg/dL. Over 50 percent of American adults have blood cholesterol levels above 200 mg/dL.*

In Figure 8, normal blood cholesterol would include values that range from about 150 mg/dL to about 300 mg/dL.

Normal Is Not Necessarily Healthy. Just because values occur *often* in a population, this does not make them normal in the healthy sense. Blood cholesterol levels in the statistically normal range of 200 to 300 mg/dL are too high for long-term health. That is why there is an epidemic of heart disease in this country, why 550,000 people die of heart disease each year — one each minute — and why 5.4 million people have been diagnosed as having coronary heart disease.

As one physician so wisely explained, "We confuse normal with optimal. Normal in America is to have a heart attack in middle age, and we don't think that is good. We need new optimal levels. Somewhere around 180 to 200."

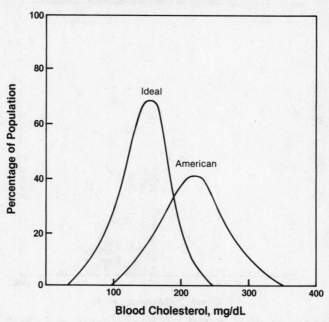

**Comparison of Ideal and Current
American Population Distributions**

*Figure 9: Comparison of Current U.S. Blood Cholesterol Distribution with an
Ideal Distribution   The ideal distribution of blood cholesterol levels exhibits lower
levels than the current U.S. distribution and has an average of about 150 mg/dL. Only
a small percentage of the ideal population has blood cholesterol levels above 200 mg/dL.*

A Truly Normal Distribution. If the current distribution of
blood cholesterol levels in the United States is not normal, what
would a distribution of truly normal blood cholesterol levels (i.e.,
levels not associated with disease) look like? In Figure 9, an "ideal"
distribution of normal blood cholesterol levels (i.e., levels associated
with little or no heart disease) is shown together with the distribution of current levels in the United States.

You can see that the entire ideal curve of normal blood cholesterol
levels is shifted to lower levels. It has an average level of 150 mg/dL
instead of 215–220 mg/dL. Only a small percentage of the ideal population has blood cholesterol levels above 200 mg/dL. In this ideal-
ized population, a blood cholesterol level of 230 mg/dL is highly elevated rather than normal. Where does your blood cholesterol fit on
this curve?

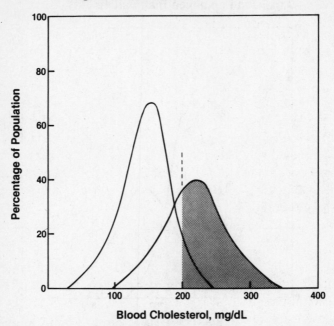

Average is *Not* "Normal"

*Figure 10: Average is **NOT Normal*** *The shading indicates blood cholesterol levels associated with increased risk of heart attack.*

Relating Risk to Blood Cholesterol Levels in Different Populations

In Figure 10, shading indicates cholesterol levels (above 200 mg/dL) associated with increased risk of heart attack. You can see several interesting facts.

First, very few people in the ideal population are at increased risk of heart attack due to elevated blood cholesterol levels. Heart disease would be relatively rare in this population. Those few people at highest risk have cholesterol levels slightly above 200 mg/dL, levels currently considered normal in the United States. A real-life example proves the point. The distribution of blood cholesterol levels among rural Japanese farmers and fishermen is essentially identical to the ideal distribution. Heart disease in Japan is indeed rare: one-tenth the rate in the United States.*

*As the Japanese diet becomes more Americanized, so will Japanese heart-health statistics. "Rare" will no longer describe the heart disease rate in Japan.

BYPASS PATIENTS — TAKE HEED

Bypass operations may eliminate the symptoms of heart disease, such as angina; but they do not cure the underlying atherosclerotic process, which goes on depositing fat in your coronary arteries. Bypass artery grafts have been found to accumulate plaque at a faster rate than the original arteries they replaced. They accumulate plaque at a faster rate the higher your blood cholesterol level. It is common for such grafts to close completely within three to five years. *This need not happen.* You can slow or even reverse the clogging of your bypass artery graft by changing what you eat and thereby lowering your blood cholesterol level.

Second, a study of these curves makes it clear that a large percentage of the current population of the United States is at increased risk of heart disease due to elevated blood cholesterol levels. Alas, heart disease is not at all rare in the United States. Over 50 percent of the population has blood cholesterol levels above 200 mg/dL, a level at which the risk curve begins to rise steeply. It is no coincidence that the NIH Adult Treatment Panel recommends that people with elevated blood cholesterol levels take action to reduce them to below 200 mg/dL.

While those people with very high blood cholesterol levels (say, above 280 mg/dL) are clearly at very high risk, they account for only a small percentage of the total population and thus for only a small percentage of the number of heart attacks. There are many more people with "normal" levels of about 225–235 mg/dL and they account for the great bulk of heart disease.

Now you can see why we recommend that you should insist on knowing your blood cholesterol level. Know your numbers. Don't settle for a statement that your cholesterol is normal.

AVERAGE BLOOD CHOLESTEROL OF HEART ATTACK PATIENTS

In fact, the average blood cholesterol level of patients admitted to coronary care units with heart attacks is about 225–235 mg/dL. The average blood cholesterol level of persons receiving coronary artery bypass grafts is also about 225–235 mg/dL. These levels are mistakenly considered normal by many health professionals. Pretty scary news, yes?

Because many of these patients do not have high blood pressure, do not smoke, and have no family history of premature heart disease, until recently they were considered to have no risk factors for heart disease. But today their blood cholesterol of, say, 225–235 mg/dL is understood to be a prime factor in the development of their disease.

AN ACTION PLAN FOR ALL AMERICANS: EAT LESS FAT

No matter whether you have been told that your blood cholesterol level is normal or that you are at borderline-high or high risk, if you want to reduce your risk of coronary heart disease you must get your blood cholesterol level down to below 200 mg/dL. The recommended method is to change the foods you eat.

The National Institutes of Health (NIH) and the American Heart Association (AHA) recommend that all Americans over the age of two years adopt a diet that reduces total dietary fat intake. (See Chapter 12 for a discussion of cholesterol and children. For more information about dietary fats and their effects on blood cholesterol levels, see the next chapter.) Total fat should be reduced to no more than 30 percent of total calories. The fat calories should be evenly distributed among the three types of fat as follows:

	FATS (% OF TOTAL CALORIES)				CHOLESTEROL (MG PER DAY)
	TOTAL	SAT.	MONO.	POLY.	
AHA and NIH recommend no more than	30	10	10	10	200–300
Current U.S. intake	40	17	16	7	470

You may find these recommendations complicated and difficult to follow. That is why we developed *Eater's Choice*. As we explain in the next chapter, *Eater's Choice* not only simplifies the AHA recommendations by focusing only on reducing saturated fat intake, but also provides a method for translating the abstract guidelines into actual food choices.

Eat Right and Your Blood Cholesterol Will Show It

Do not be discouraged if your blood cholesterol level is too high. The picture is not bleak. Most people can lower their blood cholesterol simply by changing the foods they eat. In fact, it takes only about three weeks to see a change in your blood cholesterol level. Of course, you must make enough changes in the foods you eat and stick with them for your blood cholesterol level to fall below the danger zone and stay there.

You may expect to achieve dramatic reductions of your blood cholesterol — reductions up to 30 percent, depending on your responsiveness to diet and how much you change the foods you eat. Reductions of 10 to 15 percent are common. Thus, if your starting blood cholesterol level is 270 mg/dL, you might be able to lower it by about 80 mg/dL (about a 30 percent decrease) to 190 mg/dL. If your starting blood cholesterol level is 240 mg/dL, you might be able to lower it by about 70 mg/dL (about a 30 percent decrease) to 170 mg/dL.

How much you can lower your blood cholesterol by changes in the foods you eat depends on the following factors:

- your original eating pattern;
- your heredity, which determines how responsive your blood cholesterol is to changes in your diet;
- how much you change the foods you eat.

The higher the amount of saturated fat and cholesterol in your original eating pattern and the higher your resulting blood cholesterol, the greater will be the fall in your blood cholesterol with a decreased intake of saturated fat and cholesterol.

Those Who Need It the Most Benefit the Most. As you can see, although the percentage decrease is the same for both, the person with the higher blood cholesterol level achieved a greater reduction (80 mg/dL decrease) in response to a blood cholesterol–lowering eating plan than did the person with a lower starting level (70 mg/dL decrease). Both will benefit from changes in what they eat, but persons with the highest risk can expect a larger absolute reduction. This should motivate those most in need of reducing their coronary heart disease risk.

Your Own Private Statistics. Enough of official edicts. You are already on your way to eradicating heart disease — even if it's only your own. The next chapters will help you apply all you have learned about blood cholesterol, foods, and heart disease to your own life. You will set personal blood cholesterol–lowering goals and learn how to meet those goals.

Remember:

1. A blood cholesterol level considered to be "normal" in the United States may be too high for long-term health. Over 50 percent of the adult American population has blood cholesterol levels above 200 mg/dL, the point at which risk begins to rise sharply.
2. All adults are advised to reduce their blood cholesterol below 200 mg/dL by adopting a diet that reduces total dietary fat intake.

EATER'S CHOICE: EATING FOR LIFE

5

YOU HAVE BEEN inundated with statistics, biochemical explanations, and evidence. Enough! Let's get started with practical advice to improve and lengthen your life. Let's get started with the *Eater's Choice* plan for lowering your blood cholesterol level.

Eater's Choice is the name given to this plan because it is an eating plan with choice — your choice. *Eater's Choice* gives you the knowledge to decide your own personal blood cholesterol goals and tailor your food choices to meet these goals.

Eater's Choice focuses on the saturated fat content of foods as the basis for making food choices. You determine the amount of saturated fat you should eat to lower your blood cholesterol and you keep track of how much saturated fat you are eating.

FATS

Total fat in a food is the sum of three kinds of fat: saturated fat, monounsaturated fat, and polyunsaturated fat. Each has a different effect on the blood cholesterol level. Foods contain mixtures of these different types of fat in different proportions (see Figure 11). No food contains pure saturated, monounsaturated, or polyunsaturated fat.

Saturated Fat. Saturated fat is called saturated because all the carbon atoms in the long fat molecule carry the maximum possible number of hydrogen atoms; that is, the carbon atoms are *saturated* with hydrogen atoms (see Figure 12). Saturated fat is generally solid at room temperature. Foods high in saturated fats are beef, lamb, veal, pork, and whole milk dairy products, including butter and cheese. Five kinds of vegetable fats are saturated: coconut oil, palm oil, palm kernel oil, cocoa butter (in chocolate), and hydrogenated

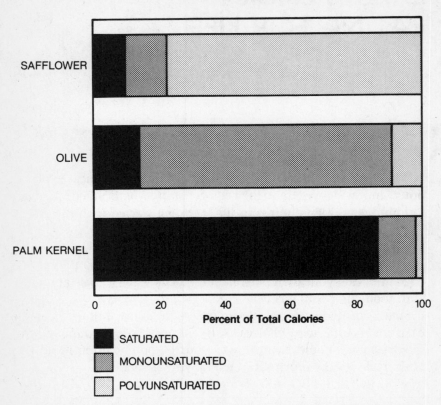

COMPOSITION OF FATS

SAFFLOWER

OLIVE

PALM KERNEL

Percent of Total Calories

SATURATED

MONOUNSATURATED

POLYUNSATURATED

Figure 11: Composition of Fats   *Total fat in a food is the sum of three kinds of fat: saturated fat, monounsaturated fat, and polyunsaturated fat. This graph shows that all fats are mixtures of the three types of fats. Safflower oil is called a polyunsaturated fat because it contains more polyunsaturated fat than either mono or saturated fat. Olive oil is called a monounsaturated fat because it contains mainly, but not exclusively, monounsaturated fat. Palm kernel oil is called a saturated fat because it contains predominantly saturated fat. Look closely to see that palm kernel oil contains a tiny amount of polyunsaturated fat.*

vegetable oil. In general, animal fats are high in saturated fats and plant fats are low. **Saturated fat raises LDL-cholesterol and total blood cholesterol levels.**

Monounsaturated Fat. Monounsaturated fat has one point of unsaturation; that is, there are two fewer hydrogen atoms than in a

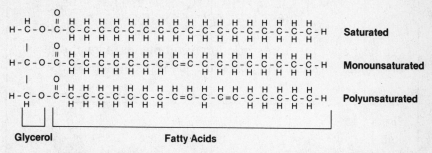

Figure 12: Chemical Structures of the Fats *Triglycerides are composed of three fatty acids attached to a glycerol molecule: In saturated fats all the carbon atoms (C) in the molecule carry the maximum possible number of hydrogen atoms (H). Monounsaturated fat has one point of unsaturation and thus can absorb two additional hydrogen atoms. Polyunsaturated fat has two or more points of unsaturation and thus can absorb four or more additional hydrogen atoms.*

fully saturated fat (see Figure 12). The richest source of mono-unsaturated fat is olive oil. Recent scientific evidence indicates that monounsaturated fat lowers total blood cholesterol by lowering LDL-cholesterol without lowering HDL-cholesterol. In addition, new studies show that olive oil prevents the oxidation of LDL particles. The oxidation of LDL particles promotes their uptake by monocytes. LDL-filled monocytes are deposited in coronary artery walls, causing the narrowing (atherosclerosis) that may eventually block blood from flowing to the heart muscle. By preventing the oxidation of LDL particles, olive oil helps retard the atherosclerotic process.

Polyunsaturated Fat. Polyunsaturated fat has two or more points of unsaturation; that is, there are four or more fewer hydrogen atoms than in a fully saturated fat (see Figure 12). Polyunsaturated fats are generally liquid at room temperature. In general, vegetable oils, except coconut, palm, palm kernel, and cocoa butter, are high in polyunsaturated fat. Polyunsaturated fat lowers blood LDL-cholesterol levels and, to a much lesser extent, HDL-cholesterol levels.

Because consumption of large quantities of polyunsaturated fats lowers HDL-cholesterol and has been implicated in the development of certain cancers in animals, we recommend limiting intake of poly-

CHOLESTEROL CONTENTS
OF SELECTED FOODS*

(The American Heart Association recommends that your intake of cholesterol should not exceed 200–300 mg each day.)

FOOD	PORTION	CHOLESTEROL, MG
Dairy		
Butter, regular	1 pat	11
Cheeses		
cottage, creamed	1 cup	31
2%	1 cup	19
low-fat	1 cup	10
natural and processed	1 oz	16–35
Egg yolk	1 large	213**
Milk		
whole	1 cup	33
2%	1 cup	18
skim	1 cup	5
Yogurt		
low-fat	8 oz	10–14
nonfat	8 oz	0–1
Meat, Fish, Poultry		
Cooked beef, veal, pork, chicken, turkey, fish	1 oz	18–25
Crab, cooked	1 oz	28
Kidney, beef, cooked	1 oz	200
Liver		
beef, cooked	1 oz	126
chicken, simmered	1 oz	180
Scallops, cooked	1 oz	15
Shrimp, cooked	1 oz	43
Plant Products		
Fruits		0
Grains		0
Vegetables		0
Vegetable oils		0

*Adapted from *Composition of Foods*, Handbook No. 8, U.S. Department of Agriculture.
**In previous editions of *Eater's Choice*, we reported the cholesterol content of an egg yolk as 274 mg. Based on updated lab measurements, the Egg Board has revised the cholesterol content of egg yolks to an average of 213 mg per yolk (range: 180–230 mg).

unsaturated fat to about 5–7 percent of total calories and when possible, choosing olive oil instead. (See the discussion of trans fats on page 81.)

Dietary Cholesterol. Dietary cholesterol raises LDL-cholesterol. Cholesterol is found *only* in animal products, such as beef, pork, poultry, fish, cheese and other whole milk dairy products, and eggs. Especially rich sources of cholesterol are egg yolks and organ meats, such as liver, pancreas, and brain. Cholesterol is *not* found in foods made from plants, such as vegetables, fruits, nuts, or seeds.

FOCUS ON SATURATED FAT, NOT CHOLESTEROL

Eater's Choice focuses on the saturated fat content of foods because, of the four dietary constituents that influence blood cholesterol levels (saturated fat, monounsaturated fat, polyunsaturated fat, and cholesterol), saturated fat is the most potent determinant of blood cholesterol levels. The more saturated fat you remove from your daily consumption, the more your LDL-cholesterol level will fall.

Monounsaturated fats, olive oil in particular, have a positive effect on heart disease by preventing the oxidation of LDL particles and thus limiting their uptake by monocytes and deposition in the artery walls. However, the consumption of too much fat of any variety is not healthy. Fats have more calories per unit weight than either proteins or carbohydrates. Fat contains 9 calories per gram while proteins and carbohydrates each have only 4 calories per gram. **Fats make you fat.** In addition, fats have been implicated as a risk factor for some common cancers, such as breast, colon, and prostate. (If you are interested in learning more about how fat affects your health and/or you are interested in reducing the fat from your body, read our book *Choose to Lose,* Houghton Mifflin, 1995.)

Eater's Choice focuses on the saturated fat and *not the cholesterol content of the foods you eat* for the following reasons. First, with only a few easy to remember exceptions, saturated fat and cholesterol occur in the same foods; they are fellow travelers. So, by avoiding foods high in saturated fat, you are also avoiding foods high in cholesterol. The exceptions are: egg yolks and organ meats (brain, pancreas, liver, kidneys), which are high in cholesterol but have only moderate amounts of saturated fat. On the other hand, coconut oil, palm oil, palm kernel oil, hydrogenated vegetable oil, and cocoa butter (in chocolate) are very high in saturated fat but have no cholesterol.

Second, the cholesterol you eat has much less effect on raising blood cholesterol levels than does saturated fat. Many people assume that all you have to do to lower your blood cholesterol level is to eat less cholesterol. Eggs are loaded with cholesterol. Eat fewer eggs and your blood cholesterol problem is licked, so the argument goes. However, contrary to popular belief, the amount of fats, especially *saturated fats*, that you eat has a much greater effect on your blood cholesterol level than does the amount of cholesterol you consume.

Of course, this does not mean that you should eat unlimited numbers of eggs or other high-cholesterol foods. Remember that the American Heart Association and the Adult Treatment Panel recommend a daily cholesterol intake of no more than 200–300 mg (one large egg yolk contains 213 mg). Avoid foods high in cholesterol. Think before you eat.

Third, keeping track of only saturated fat makes *Eater's Choice* a simple yet effective plan to follow. The simpler a plan is to follow, the more likely you are to follow it and the more likely you are to succeed in lowering your blood cholesterol level.

HOW TO REDUCE YOUR SATURATED FAT INTAKE

You can reduce your saturated fat intake in two ways:

1. Reduce the amount of fat you eat by substituting foods high in complex carbohydrates (starches) and fiber (such as rice, whole-grain pastas, breads, and cereals, vegetables, and fruits) for foods high in saturated fat. And replace high-fat foods with low-fat or nonfat foods, such as sour cream with low-fat yogurt. (See the Food Tables at the end of the book for the saturated fat contents of common foods.)
2. Substitute foods high in unsaturated fat (such as olive oil or margarine) for foods high in saturated fat (such as butter, lard, and beef tallow). Go light on margarine (see the discussion of trans fats on page 81).

The Total Diet Counts

As you establish your new eating plan, you must remember that to lower your blood cholesterol you will have to make changes in what you eat. **You will have to make enough changes to make a difference.** What is important are the amounts and types of fats you eat and not the actual foods that supply them. Individual foods either raise or lower your blood cholesterol level by the way they contribute to the daily total of total fat, saturated fat, polyunsaturated fat, and cholesterol.

But how many changes do you have to make to make a difference? How much is enough? *Eater's Choice* is a plan that allows you to determine how much is enough by keeping track of your saturated fat intake. How you set your daily Sat-Fat Budget will depend on how much you want to reduce your blood cholesterol level. Periodic monitoring of your blood cholesterol level will tell you if your change in food choices has made a sufficient difference in lowering it or if you must make more changes in your eating pattern.

You need not wait months to see if your heart-smart eating behavior has lowered your blood cholesterol level. It takes only about three weeks to achieve up to 30 percent lowering of your blood cholesterol if you have made the right food choices.

While the types and amounts of fats and not the foods that contain them are important to the health of your body, which foods contain the fats you eat are of utmost importance to you. Thus, 30 calories of saturated fat from bacon or from cheesecake may have identical effects on your blood cholesterol level but undoubtedly quite different effects on your palate and psyche. And that is why *Eater's Choice* is useful for you. You tailor your food choices to fit your saturated fat budget *and* your taste buds.

Cold Turkey: A Dish for Some. Before we delve into *Eater's Choice* we realize some of you may not want to take the trouble to monitor your sat-fat (saturated fat) intake. You may wish to restrict your diet totally to foods low in saturated fat: fish, white meat turkey or chicken without skin, loads of vegetables and fruits, bread (made without hydrogenated oils), oatmeal, rice, pasta, skim milk, low-fat yogurt and cottage cheese, tub margarine and olive, safflower, sunflower, or corn oil, etc.

Going cold turkey means completely eliminating all foods high in saturated fat. This includes red meats, such as beef, veal, lamb, pork, ham, and cold cuts, as well as whole milk dairy products, such as cheese, sour cream, cream, whole milk, 2% milk, butter, and ice cream, in addition to most commercial snacks and baked goods and other products made with palm oil, palm kernel oil, coconut oil, hydrogenated vegetable oil, cocoa butter, or lard.

If you want to try this approach, all the recipes in this cookbook are dishes you can eat with complete freedom. They are designed to be low in saturated fat *and* delicious.

Take It Easy: A Strategy for Others. If you feel there are too many foods that you cannot give up without sinking into a deep depression, that life would not be worth living without brie and crackers, *Eater's Choice* gives *you* control over your choices of food and still allows you to lower your blood cholesterol level.

Of course, you will not be able to eat *everything* you want in the amounts and as often as you want, but you will be able to eat that brie if you make enough low-fat choices in your diet to compensate for the added saturated fat. This is a flexible plan that you will change and modify until you reach your target low blood cholesterol level.

A STEP-BY-STEP GUIDE TO *EATER'S CHOICE*

First, if you have not already done so, have your physician measure your total blood cholesterol. (New technology is now available to measure blood cholesterol in mere minutes from a drop of blood taken from your finger. This revolutionary advance in blood analysis will make it possible to have your blood cholesterol measured at your workplace, health clinic, even shopping malls, as well as at your physician's office.) If your total blood cholesterol level is elevated, you should also know your levels of HDL, triglycerides, and LDL. (Remember: a twelve-hour fast is required before your blood is drawn to measure triglycerides and LDL.) See Chapter 2 for a discussion of all the lipoproteins in the blood.

Ask for numerical values. Make sure you know both your HDL and your LDL levels in addition to your total blood cholesterol. Remember, the lower your HDL level, the higher your risk and the greater the incentive to lower your LDL level.

NOTE: Cholesterol levels measured within three months after a heart attack, surgery, or other physical trauma may be abnormally low.

Set Your Blood Cholesterol Target

Set your own personal blood cholesterol goals. You know what your blood cholesterol level is. You know that you want it to be below 200 mg/dL. Recall from the Framingham risk curve (Chapter 3) that the lower your blood cholesterol level, the lower your risk of coronary heart disease.

Perhaps you want to lower your blood cholesterol level in stages. Perhaps it is now 260 mg/dL and you want to take it down to 230 mg/dL as the first step. Fine. You just have to tailor your eating to meet this goal. After a month, have your blood cholesterol level measured again. When you have achieved your goal of 230 mg/dL and feel comfortable with your new eating pattern, you are ready to make additional diet changes to lower your blood cholesterol to 200 mg/dL.

Know Your Desirable Body Weight

Because the amount of saturated fat allowed on the *Eater's Choice* plan is based on the number of calories you eat each day, you need to know how many calories you consume or should consume. If you are overweight, you should choose your desirable weight as a goal. You may already know your desirable weight. If not, Table 1 on page 48 lists desirable weights for men and women of different heights and body frame sizes.

To help keep your weight down, you should also exercise. (Be sure to consult your doctor about what exercises you can do safely.) Even just walking for twenty minutes or more each day will help you lose weight. (And you'll feel better too!) Losing weight if you are overweight will contribute to reducing your blood cholesterol

---

ON EXERCISE AND LOSING WEIGHT

Contrary to popular opinion, the main value of exercise is not burning calories, but building and preserving muscle. By exercising, you force your body to burn fat from the fat stores rather than protein from the muscle tissue. By engaging in regular aerobic exercise and eating a low-fat diet, you maximize depletion of your fat stores and thus ensure permanent weight loss.

Table 1: Desirable Weights for Adults Age 25 and Over*
(weight in pounds without clothing)

HEIGHT WITHOUT SHOES		FRAME		
(FEET)	(INCHES)	SMALL	MEDIUM	LARGE
Men				
5	1	112–120	118–129	126–141
5	2	115–123	121–133	129–144
5	3	118–126	124–136	132–148
5	4	121–129	127–139	135–152
5	5	124–133	130–143	138–156
5	6	128–137	134–147	142–161
5	7	132–141	138–152	147–166
5	8	136–145	142–156	151–170
5	9	140–150	146–160	155–174
5	10	144–154	150–165	159–179
5	11	148–158	154–170	164–184
6	0	152–162	158–175	168–189
6	1	156–167	162–180	173–194
6	2	160–171	167–185	178–199
6	3	164–175	172–190	182–204
Women				
4	8	92–98	96–107	104–119
4	9	94–101	98–110	106–122
4	10	96–104	101–113	109–125
4	11	99–107	104–116	112–128
5	0	102–110	107–119	115–131
5	1	105–113	110–122	118–134
5	2	108–116	113–126	121–138
5	3	111–119	116–130	125–142
5	4	114–123	120–135	129–146
5	5	118–127	124–139	133–150
5	6	122–131	128–143	137–154
5	7	126–135	132–147	141–158
5	8	130–140	136–151	145–163
5	9	134–144	140–155	149–168
5	10	138–148	144–159	153–173

*Courtesy of Metropolitan Life Insurance Company, New York, N.Y., 1959
For persons between 18 and 25 years of age, subtract 1 pound for each year under 25.

and LDL levels (and blood pressure), raising your HDL level, and reducing your risk of coronary heart disease morbidity and mortality. For more information about weight loss and exercise and a budget plan to lose weight, read *Choose to Lose: A Food Lover's Guide to Permanent Weight Loss,* by Dr. Ron Goor and Nancy Goor (Houghton Mifflin, 1995).

Determine Your Frame

In order to use the table of desirable weights (Table 1) you need to know if your body frame is small, medium, or large. You can determine this by placing your left thumb and middle finger around your right wrist. Squeeze your fingers as tightly as possible. If the thumb and finger overlap, you have a small frame. If they just touch, your frame size is medium. If they do not touch, then you have a large frame. This method is a bit crude, but accurate enough for our purpose. Find your desirable weight by sex, height, and frame size on the chart.

Know Your Ideal Daily Caloric Intake

In order to determine your daily caloric intake, you must know your approximate daily level of activity (daily energy expenditure) in addition to your desirable weight. To determine your level of activity, try to identify which of the following five descriptions most accurately describes your level of activity during the preceding week. Choose a lower level of activity if you are not sure which of two levels best describes your activity.

Activity Levels*

Very Sedentary. Limited activity, confined to a few rooms or a house. Slow walking, no running. Most major activities involve sitting.

Sedentary. Activities involve mostly walking or some sporadic slow running at a jogging speed of approximately ten minutes per mile. Recreational activities include bowling, fishing, target shooting, horseback riding, motorboating, snowmobiling, or other similar activities. Less than ten minutes of continuous running (faster than a jog) per week.

---

*From *The DINE System* by Dr. Darwin Dennison

Moderately Active. Activities include golf (eighteen holes), doubles tennis, sailing, pleasure swimming or skating, aerobic dancing, Jazzercise, downhill skiing, or other similar activities. Between ten and twenty minutes of continuous running at least three times per week.

Active. More than twenty minutes of sustained activity, such as jogging, swimming, competitive tennis, or cross-country skiing, more than three times per week or more than forty-five minutes of recreational tennis, paddle ball, or other activities at least three times per week.

Super Active. At least one and a half hours of vigorous activity (training for competitive athletics, full-court basketball, mountain climbing, weight training, football, wrestling, or other similar activity) four days per week or more than two and a half hours of recreational activity four or more times per week.

Your Daily Caloric Needs

Use Table 2 to determine the number of calories you should consume each day. First, locate your desirable weight along the left-hand column. Making sure you use the correct row for your sex, find the number of calories under the column for your activity level.

This is the calorie level you need to satisfy your energy requirements at the specified activity level. Be sure to replace the sat-fat calories you've removed from your diet with calories from complex carbohydrates (vegetables, whole-grains, fruits) in order to keep your calorie level from dropping. If you want to lose weight, you need to reduce your intake of total fat — not your intake of total calories (see *Choose to Lose*).

The following example will help you understand how to determine your desirable caloric level.

George is 5 feet 9 inches tall. He determines by the wrist test that he is of medium frame. To find how much he should weigh, he locates his height in the left-hand column of Table 1. Looking across the row for 5 feet 9 inches, he finds his weight range under the frame column labeled Medium. His weight range is 146–160. George actually weighs 160 pounds but wants to lose 10 pounds and weigh 150 pounds.

George jogs for thirty minutes five times a week. After reading the descriptions of various activity levels above, he determines that his activity level is Active. He finds his desirable weight (150) in the left-

Table 2: Ideal Caloric Level Based on Goal Weight, Activity Level, and Sex

DESIRABLE WEIGHT	SEX	ACTIVITY LEVEL				
		VERY SEDENTARY	SEDENTARY	MODERATELY ACTIVE	ACTIVE	SUPER ACTIVE
90	M	1170	1260	1350	1440	1530
	F	1053	1134	1215	1296	1377
95	M	1235	1330	1425	1520	1615
	F	1111	1197	1282	1368	1453
100	M	1300	1400	1500	1600	1700
	F	1170	1260	1350	1440	1530
105	M	1365	1470	1575	1680	1785
	F	1228	1323	1417	1512	1606
110	M	1430	1540	1650	1760	1870
	F	1287	1386	1485	1584	1683
115	M	1495	1610	1725	1840	1955
	F	1345	1449	1552	1656	1759
120	M	1560	1680	1800	1920	2040
	F	1404	1512	1620	1728	1836
125	M	1625	1750	1875	2000	2125
	F	1462	1575	1687	1800	1912
130	M	1690	1820	1950	2080	2210
	F	1521	1638	1755	1872	1989
135	M	1755	1890	2025	2160	2295
	F	1579	1701	1822	1944	2065
140	M	1820	1960	2100	2240	2380
	F	1638	1764	1890	2016	2142
145	M	1885	2030	2175	2320	2465
	F	1696	1827	1957	2088	2218
150	M	1950	2100	2250	2400	2550
	F	1755	1890	2025	2160	2295
155	M	2015	2170	2325	2480	2635
	F	1813	1953	2092	2232	2371
160	M	2080	2240	2400	2560	2720
	F	1872	2016	2160	2304	2448
165	M	2145	2310	2475	2640	2805
	F	1930	2079	2227	2376	2524
170	M	2210	2380	2550	2720	2890
	F	1989	2142	2295	2448	2601
175	M	2275	2450	2625	2800	2975
	F	2047	2205	2362	2520	2677
180	M	2340	2520	2700	2880	3060
	F	2106	2268	2430	2592	2754
185	M	2405	2590	2775	2960	3145
	F	2164	2331	2497	2664	2830

DESIRABLE WEIGHT	SEX	ACTIVITY LEVEL				
		VERY SEDENTARY	SEDENTARY	MODERATELY ACTIVE	ACTIVE	SUPER ACTIVE
190	M	2470	2660	2850	3040	3230
	F	2223	2394	2565	2736	2907
195	M	2535	2730	2925	3120	3315
	F	2281	2457	2632	2808	2983
200	M	2600	2800	3000	3200	3400
	F	2340	2520	2700	2880	3060
205	M	2665	2870	3075	3280	3485
	F	2398	2583	2767	2952	3136
210	M	2730	2940	3150	3360	3570
	F	2457	2646	2835	3024	3213
215	M	2795	3010	3225	3440	3655
	F	2515	2709	2905	3096	3289
220	M	2860	3080	3300	3520	3740
	F	2574	2772	2970	3168	3366

hand column of Table 2. Looking across the row for 150 for males (M), he finds his ideal caloric intake level under the Active column. George's ideal daily caloric intake is 2400 calories.

Reduce Saturated Fat to 10 Percent of Total Calories or Less

Now that you have determined *your* calorie level, you can figure out how much saturated fat you should eat each day. Your daily allotment of saturated fat will ultimately depend on the initial level of your blood cholesterol and how much your blood cholesterol drops in response to a lower saturated fat intake.

The first step for everyone, no matter how high your initial blood cholesterol level, is to reduce your saturated fat intake to no more than 10 percent of your total calories. We call this the *Eater's Choice* 10 Percent Plan. (Those with high-risk blood cholesterol levels — see National Institutes of Health recommendations in Chapter 4 — should consider starting directly with the *Eater's Choice* 6 Percent Plan discussed on page 53.)

In practical terms, what does that mean? Here is George again. George should consume 2400 calories a day to maintain his desirable weight. His blood cholesterol level is 250 mg/dL. To lower his blood cholesterol below 200 mg/dL, he must reduce his saturated fat intake to 10 percent or less of his daily calories. Ten percent of 2400 calories is 240 calories of saturated fat. George should eat no more than 240 calories of saturated fat each day.

To help you visualize what 240 calories of saturated fat means in terms of foods, there are:

- 45 calories of saturated fat in 1 cup of whole milk;
- 100 calories of saturated fat in 4 ounces of lean, broiled ground beef;
- 12 calories of saturated fat in 4 ounces of roasted chicken breast without skin;
- 117 calories of saturated fat in a Burger King Double Cheeseburger.

You can use the blank worksheet on page 55 to determine *your* daily Sat-Fat Budget. Use George's worksheet as a guide.

Once you go on the *Eater's Choice* plan, you will want to monitor your blood cholesterol levels periodically to see how you are doing. Remember, it only takes two to three weeks for blood cholesterol levels to respond to changes in eating patterns. At first you should check at more frequent intervals — six weeks, six weeks, three months, six months — until your blood cholesterol stabilizes at its new lower level. Then have it checked every twelve months. Do not get upset if your blood cholesterol level fluctuates slightly — this is normal.

To prevent your blood cholesterol from rising, you must continue to follow the *Eater's Choice* plan, to keep your sat-fat intake at 10 percent or less of your calories. Your blood cholesterol level is affected by what you eat and will jump right back to its previously high level if you return to your old eating habits.

Eater's Choice 6 Percent Plan

If after about three months your blood cholesterol has not fallen below 200 mg/dL, you will need to switch to the *Eater's Choice* 6 Percent Plan. As you might guess, on the 6 Percent Plan you reduce your sat-fat intake to no more than 6 percent of your total calories. In George's case, he would eat no more than 144 (6 percent of 2400) calories of saturated fat a day on the *Eater's Choice* 6 Percent Plan.

Again, once you have brought your blood cholesterol below 200 mg/dL you must continue to follow the *Eater's Choice* 6 Percent Plan.

WORKSHEET TO DETERMINE
YOUR DAILY SAT-FAT BUDGET

Name ____GEORGE_____   Date __1/10/95____

STEP 1: DETERMINE YOUR DESIRABLE WEIGHT

    A. Sex: Male __X____   Female _____

    B. Height: __5__ feet ___9__ inches

    C. Frame (wrist method):

        Small _____   Medium __X__   Large _____

    D. Weight Range (Table 1): _146 – 160_

    E. Desirable Weight: ____150_____

STEP 2: DETERMINE YOUR DAILY CALORIC INTAKE

    A. Activity Level   Very Sedentary _____
        (see text):   Sedentary _____

                         Moderately Active _____

                         Active ___X_____

                         Super Active _____

    B. Daily caloric intake (use Table 2): _2400_____

STEP 3: DETERMINE YOUR DAILY SAT-FAT BUDGET

    DAILY SAT-FAT BUDGET:

    ___10___% of daily caloric intake = _240___

WORKSHEET TO DETERMINE YOUR DAILY SAT-FAT BUDGET

Name _____   Date _____

STEP 1: DETERMINE YOUR DESIRABLE WEIGHT

    A. Sex: Male _____   Female _____

    B. Height: _____ feet _____ inches

    C. Frame (wrist method):

        Small _____   Medium _____   Large _____

    D. Weight Range (Table 1): _____

    E. Desirable Weight: _____

STEP 2: DETERMINE YOUR DAILY CALORIC INTAKE

    A. Activity Level   Very Sedentary _____
        (see text):

                        Sedentary _____

                        Moderately Active _____

                        Active _____

                        Super Active _____

    B. Daily caloric intake (use Table 2): _____

STEP 3: DETERMINE YOUR DAILY SAT-FAT BUDGET

DAILY SAT-FAT BUDGET:

    _____% of daily caloric intake = _____

Monitor your blood cholesterol periodically — six weeks, three months, six months — and then once a year after you are sure your blood cholesterol has stabilized below 200 mg/dL.

For some, moving to a 4 percent plan may be necessary if strict adherence to a 6 percent plan has failed to reduce their blood cholesterol to below 200 mg/dL.

The Appeal of *Eater's Choice*

The main goal of *Eater's Choice* is to help you lower your risk of heart disease. What you may find just as important is that it allows enough personal choice to keep both your psyche and taste buds happy. You will still be able to eat the fatty foods you love, but perhaps less often or in smaller quantities.

The menu plans in Chapter 13 will give you some idea of how well you can eat on an *Eater's Choice* 10 Percent or 6 Percent Plan. The recipes at the end of the book will satisfy your palate without overloading your Sat-Fat Budget. See "Modifying Recipes," pages 133–34 for tips on how to modify high-fat recipes from other cookbooks to create low-fat dishes.

A Balanced Diet

Eater's Choice emphasizes eating less saturated fat to lower your blood cholesterol level, but you must remember that your diet has to be balanced. In your zeal to reduce your intake of fats, you must not forget that you need vitamins, minerals, proteins, fiber, and bulk. (The meal plans in Chapter 13 will give you examples of balanced low-fat meals.)

As you remove saturated fat from your diet, you will have to replace it with something else. Most health experts today recommend replacing the saturated fat calories you eliminate with calories from complex carbohydrates. Complex carbohydrates are found in whole-grain breads, pastas, and vegetables. Enriching your diet with these foods and fruits has the additional advantage of increasing your intake of vitamins, minerals, and fiber.

Insoluble fiber, such as in whole wheat, may help prevent certain cancers, such as colon cancer. Soluble fiber, such as in oat bran products, has been found to lower blood cholesterol levels.

LAST RESORT: DRUGS

If diet does not reduce your blood cholesterol adequately and *you are really following your eating plan to the letter,* you may need to take drugs prescribed by a physician. The preferred drugs are bile acid sequestrants — either cholestyramine (Questran)* or colestipol (Colestid) and nicotinic acid (niacin).

The bile acid sequestrants bind bile acids in the intestine and prevent their reabsorption and return to the liver. The bile acids are excreted in the feces. To compensate for the loss of bile acids, the liver removes large amounts of LDL-cholesterol from the blood. The cholesterol is converted into bile acids, which are then secreted into the intestine, where they help emulsify dietary fats.

Niacin lowers blood cholesterol levels by reducing the formation of VLDL, thereby blocking the formation of LDL. In small amounts (about 100 mg per day), niacin is a vitamin and has no effect on blood cholesterol. In doses large enough to lower blood cholesterol (1000–3000 mg per day), niacin is a potent drug with side effects (such as flushing, an itching rash, gastric upset, and/or blurred vision) and potential toxicities. It is recommended that people taking large doses should be under a physician's supervision and should have their liver function, blood glucose, and blood uric acid monitored periodically. Large amounts of niacin should not be taken by people with the following conditions: peptic ulcers, liver disease, gouty arthritis, or some types of heart rhythm disturbances.

Lovastatin is the first of a new class of potent blood cholesterol–lowering drugs: HMG CoA reductase inhibitors. These drugs work by blocking the synthesis of cholesterol in the liver. To compensate, the liver increases the amount of cholesterol, mainly LDL-cholesterol, that it removes from the blood. At this writing, lovastatin holds much promise but long-term safety has not yet been established.

If this discussion produces a vision of a banana split with four scoops of ice cream covered with chocolate sauce and whipped cream in one hand and a glass of bile acid sequestrant in the other, you will be sorely disappointed. All the drugs have side effects or toxicities and, with the exception of niacin, cost between $800 and $3000 a year, depending on drug and dose. In addition, drug therapy does not make up for eating a high-fat diet. Drugs complement a blood cholesterol–lowering diet. In fact, the more you lower your blood cholesterol by diet, the more effective will be your use of drugs. In a study showing the role of diet on effectiveness of drug therapy, 80 percent of people who ate a low-fat diet in com-

(*continued on next page*)

---

*Questran was the drug used in the Coronary Primary Prevention Trial to lower blood cholesterol levels and incidence of heart attacks.

LAST RESORT: DRUGS (continued)

bination with the cholesterol-lowering drug, lovastatin, lowered their LDL to the recommended level. In contrast, only 50 percent of those taking lovastatin while continuing to eat a high-fat diet were able to lower their LDL-cholesterol to the recommended level. The more you lower your blood cholesterol by diet, the more effective the drug will be. And remember, a low-fat, cholesterol-lowering diet has additional benefits that drugs do not have, such as weight control, reduced risk of some common cancers, regularity, low cost, no unpleasant side effects, and great taste.

ADDED BENEFITS OF *EATER'S CHOICE*

Weight Loss

One of the loveliest benefits of *Eater's Choice* is a natural loss of weight. Many people report losing 10–15 pounds, and some as much as 40. You will be eating less fat and thus fewer calories without necessarily eating less food.

"But," you ask in disbelief, "if I replace saturated fat with complex carbohydrates, won't I turn into a tub? Everyone knows carbohydrates are fattening." If this is what you think, get this myth out of your head.

All fats — saturated, polyunsaturated, and monounsaturated — contain 9 calories per gram. Proteins and carbohydrates, on the other hand, contain only 4 calories per gram. Carbohydrates have less than half the calories per unit weight than fats (4 versus 9) and thus twice the bulk per calorie. Carbohydrates fill you up at half the caloric cost. Carbohydrate calories, even in excess, are not stored as fat tissue. Excess fat calories are stored as fat tissue. Fat makes fat!

It is not the potato that makes you fat, it is what you do to it. A medium baked potato has a trace amount of fat. You glob 3 tablespoons of sour cream (23 fat calories per tablespoon) on top, and the innocent potato now contains 69 fat calories. A piece of bread has 9 fat calories per slice. When you slather it with butter or mar-

Fat makes fat! is the theme of our book, *Choose to Lose. Choose to Lose* specifically focuses on total fat for weight loss. It is true that by reducing saturated fat in their diet, many people lose weight. However, just reducing saturated fat is not always enough. There are foods such as olive oil and margarine that are very low in saturated fat but very high in total fat, and thus fattening. So to lose weight you have to target total fat. Learn what your Fat Budget is and how, by reducing fat in your diet, increasing your intake of complex carbohydrates, and exercising aerobically (walking) every day, you can become lean and stay that way forever.

garine at 100 fat calories per tablespoon, it becomes 109 fat calories or more per slice. It is the huge amount of fat in the American diet that leads to overweight and obesity.

Dr. William Castelli, director of the Framingham Heart Study, aptly concurs:

If you take the lowly potato, it's about 100 calories, let's say. If you chop it up and cook it in fat, you're up to 275 to 300 calories from that original hundred calories. If you slice it up real fine and make potato chips, you're up to 400 calories over that original potato. Now what's the difference? Just fat. What kind of fat? Well, frequently it's totally saturated fat. Why? Well, someone learned that if you cook potato chips in a totally saturated fat, they stay crispier longer. The shelf life, you know, of the potato chip goes on and on and on and on. The shelf life of the person who eats it doesn't. That's our problem.

Expanding Your Palette

A whole new world of foods will be open to you as you replace your saturated fats with complex carbohydrates. Both your food palette and taste palate will be expanded as you explore new recipes that fit into your Sat-Fat Budget. For starters, try Indian Vegetables (page 288) or Indonesian Chicken with Green Beans (page 214) or Calzone (page 313).

Regularity

An added benefit of removing fat from your diet and increasing fiber, particularly whole grains, fruits, and vegetables, is the increased regularity of your excretory system.

Remember:

1. *Eater's Choice* is a simple method for lowering blood cholesterol by limiting the amount of saturated fat you eat while giving you control over your food choices.
2. Step-by-Step Guide to *Eater's Choice:*
   a. Have your total blood cholesterol measured; if it is above 200 mg/dL, have all your lipoproteins measured — total cholesterol, LDL, HDL, and triglycerides.
   b. Set your blood cholesterol goal (not to exceed 200 mg/dL).
   c. Determine how much you should weigh.
   d. Determine how many calories you must eat to maintain that weight. Calorie requirements depend on your sex, frame size, and activity level.
   e. Multiply your total daily calorie allotment by 10 percent (or 6 percent) to determine your maximum daily saturated fat budget; follow eating plan and monitor blood cholesterol levels in three months.
   f. If blood cholesterol is still above 200 mg/dL after three months, begin the 6 Percent (or 4 Percent) eating plan.

MAKING THE RIGHT CHOICES

Now THAT YOU or your physician have figured out how many calories of saturated fat you should eat each day, you are probably eager to put *Eater's Choice* into action.

Obviously, since you are setting limits on the saturated fats you consume, you will have to know the saturated fat contents of foods that you eat. The Food Tables at the end of the book list foods, their caloric value, and the number of calories of fat and saturated fat they contain. After you determine the number of calories of saturated fat in a given portion of food, you can budget it into your daily food intake in one of two ways.

If planning is impractical or not in your nature, you can keep a running total of what you eat for the day. When you reach your daily allotment of saturated fat, that is it — no more saturated fat until tomorrow.

If you are a planner type, you can determine what your meals will be for the day or a week and add up the saturated fat calories in advance. You can make choices before you eat. "Hmmm," you think, "I'll spend ——— sat-fat calories on ——— and ——— sat-fat calories on ———." Planning ahead also makes you a more efficient grocery shopper.

If you plan ahead, you can save up sat-fat calories for a particular day or special occasion. Perhaps you are going out to dinner Saturday night and want to splurge on a big steak and a rich dessert. By not spending your total Sat-Fat Budget each day, you may be able to save enough sat-fat calories to eat a 6-ounce lean and trimmed porterhouse steak (78 sat-fat calories), 2 tablespoons of sour cream (28 sat-fat calories) on your baked potato, and a piece of cheesecake (89 sat-fat calories).

Likewise, even if you have spent your Sat-Fat Budget for the day and your Aunt May insists that you try the strawberry whipped cream cake she has made *just for you*, you may take a piece without dropping dead on the spot. Blood cholesterol levels do not respond to a single day's food intake; they reflect the sum of the fats you have eaten over the past several weeks. To make up for the splurge, eat fewer sat-fat calories than allowed on your budget for the next few days. But try to limit overdrawing your Sat-Fat Budget in emergency situations or your arteries will pay the penalty.

Keeping Track

The only way to *really* know if you are eating within your Sat-Fat Budget is to write everything down. It is not enough just to *think* you are eating a low-sat-fat diet. Suppose you ate a piece of chicken because you know that chicken is a low-fat food. Did you eat a KFC (Kentucky Fried Chicken) thigh at 69 sat-fat calories? Or two at 138? Or was it a batter-fried chicken breast with skin at 44 sat-fat calories? Or perhaps you grilled a breast with no skin at 4 sat-fat calories? It makes a big difference. To lower your cholesterol and keep it low, you have to know *exactly* what you are eating and the only way to know is to keep an honest and accurate food record.

Keeping a food record is THE SKILL that will give you insight into the reason your cholesterol is elevated and the mastery to control it. (See pages 583–591 for details on how to keep a food record.)

Recording the sat-fat calories of the foods you eat gives you power. You learn which foods are making your cholesterol high so you can make changes. You analyze your food record to discover which high-sat-fat foods you can't live without, which ones you can eat less of, and which ones you can eliminate altogether. You know how many sat-fat calories you have eaten so you can make room for splurges. You learn if your diet is balanced; if it is filled with enough fruits, vegetables, whole grains, and low- or nonfat dairy foods. How could you know if you don't write everything down?

You may think adding up sat-fat calories will take all the spontaneity out of eating. However, you probably eat a limited number of foods and a limited number of dishes (whether you cook them or eat them out). Sooner than you think, you will know their sat-fat values as well as you know the telephone numbers of your friends. Within a short time, you will learn which combinations and amounts of your favorite foods will fit into your Sat-Fat Budget. For example, you will learn that if you want to have cheese on a bagel for breakfast, you might choose a turkey sandwich for lunch. If you want ice cream for dessert, you might choose scallops for dinner.

To help you keep track of your sat-fat intake, you may want to use the order form at the end of the book to send away for a handy, pocket-sized Passbook.

Another approach to determining the sat-fat content of the foods you eat is to use a computer nutrient-analysis program. Many such programs are available. The DINE System is a nutritionally comprehensive system with a database of 5500 food items. This user-friendly program will analyze the saturated fat content in the foods you eat and in recipes. It will also provide the amounts of fourteen other nutrients: monounsaturated and polyunsaturated fats, protein, complex carbohydrates, sugar, cholesterol, and key vitamins and minerals, including sodium, potassium, and calcium. The analysis compares your diet with current dietary guidelines. The DINE System is available for Apple and IBM computers. You can get more information by writing to: DINE Systems, Inc., 5 Bluebird Lane, West Amherst, New York 14228.

Monitor Your Sat-Fat Intake Every Six Months. Just as you should have your blood cholesterol level measured periodically to make sure you are maintaining a level below 200 mg/dL, you should monitor your sat-fat calories for one or two days every six months. This will help you know you are still eating within your Sat-Fat Budget.

FOOD TABLES

The Food Tables at the end of the book can help you see how much saturated fat lurks in the foods you eat. This information gives you the power to take control and make your own food choices — choices that allow you to lower your blood cholesterol and enjoy eating at the same time.

The Food Tables are arranged in the following groups: beverages; dairy products and eggs; fast foods; fats and oils; fish and shellfish; frozen, refrigerated, and microwave foods; fruits and fruit juices; grain products; meats; nuts and seeds; poultry; restaurant food;

sauces, gravies, and dips; sausages and luncheon meats; snack foods; soups; sugars and sweets; vegetables and legumes; miscellaneous items. Within each group, items are arranged in alphabetical order.

FOOD TABLES INDEX

To help you locate specific foods in the Food Tables, use the Food Tables Index on page 576.

Data for meats, fish, and poultry are usually given in 1-ounce amounts, to help you compare the fat contents of foods, and sometimes also in a measure commonly used for cooking or eating. For instance, if you eat 7 ounces of chicken, you would multiply the sat-fat content by 7 to determine the amount of saturated fat you actually ate.

Be careful. These Food Tables make meats look like low-fat foods because the fat values are given for 1-ounce amounts. Rarely does anyone eat only 1 ounce of meat.

Measuring

In order to use the Food Tables, you will need to measure the actual amounts of the foods you eat. In addition to measuring spoons and measuring cups, you might find an inexpensive kitchen scale useful.

Use these measuring tools to determine the size of the serving you actually eat and see how many times larger or smaller it is than the listed amount. Then calculate the actual numbers of calories you are consuming. For example, if 1 ounce of cheddar cheese contains 54 calories of saturated fat and you eat ½ ounce, then you are consuming 54 × ½ calories or 27 calories of saturated fat.

How the Food Tables Help You

By focusing on saturated fat rather than foods, the Food Tables allow you to choose, based on your own preferences, combinations of foods that can fit into your daily Sat-Fat Budget.

You may be able to eat less of a certain food rather than eliminate it entirely. Since the cup of ice cream you long for contains 80 sat-fat calories, then ½ cup has only 40 sat-fat calories. Maybe your Sat-Fat Budget can accommodate the smaller helping.

Using the Food Tables, you may be able to find a low sat-fat substitute for a food you normally eat. For example, during the course of a day, you may eat a total of six pats of butter — on toast, sandwiches, and a baked potato. Since each pat of butter contains 23 calories of sat-fat, butter is contributing 23 × 6 or 138 calories of sat-fat to your daily Sat-Fat Budget. In place of butter, substitute margarine at 6 calories of sat-fat per teaspoon (equivalent to a pat). The margarine will contribute only 6 × 6 or 36 calories of sat-fat to your daily Sat-Fat Budget at a savings of 102 sat-fat calories.

Here are some other benefits of using the Food Tables:

1. Hidden sources of saturated fat will jump out at you. "Wow! My nondairy, cholesterol-free coffee whitener has 26 calories of sat-fat per ounce. My daily 3 cups of coffee with 3 ounces of whitener equals 78 calories of sat-fat — that's a third of my Sat-Fat Budget for the whole day, and I haven't even eaten anything!" You can determine if it is really worth eating those fatty foods once you know their sat-fat content.
2. You can check to see if foods that you always considered low-fat are truly low in fat. Take veal, for one: a fiction has developed that veal is less fatty than other beef. Check out the food tables and see how false this assumption is.
3. You can use the Food Tables to check and modify recipes. For example, a pie recipe uses 1 cup of sour cream, or 270 calories of saturated fat. Replace the sour cream with an equivalent amount of low-fat yogurt, and you only add 3 calories of saturated fat to the pie.

KEEPING A FOOD RECORD

Read pages 583–591 and get the inside scoop on keeping a food record — the KEY to lowering your blood cholesterol.

And Coming in the Next Chapter...

Hold on to your seats: the next chapter will tell you all the juicy gossip about the fats in the foods you eat.

Remember:

1. Budget saturated fat into your daily food intake by keeping a running total for each day or planning ahead for the week.
2. The Food Tables list saturated fat contents of common foods. They help you:
   a. keep track of your saturated fat intake;
   b. choose a variety of foods you like with different sat-fat values to fit into your Sat-Fat Budget;
   c. check and modify recipes.

WHERE'S THE FAT?   7

THE FOCUS of *Eater's Choice* is on limiting saturated fat in your diet while still allowing you to make food choices that reflect your food preferences. There is no large source of saturated fat concentrated in just one food. Nearly every food contains some fat, and most of the fat is hidden. Fats added at the table, such as spreads and salad dressings, account for only about one-fourth of the fat intake, while three-quarters of the fat is invisible or hidden in foods such as red meat, dairy products, baked goods, frozen dinners, and fat used in food preparation.

To help you analyze and change your daily meal plan, the list below will focus your attention on the high sat-fat foods you may have been eating — often without realizing they are high sat-fat foods. For example, do you think of beef as full of fat, or do you think of beef as protein? Is milk on your list of high-fat foods? Do you know how much fat is in a glass of whole milk?

The Top 50 Percent. The following food items contributed about 50 percent of the total saturated fat consumed by Americans during the time period 1976–1980. In descending order of importance, they were: hamburgers, cheeseburgers, meat loaf; whole milk and whole-milk beverages; cheeses, excluding cottage cheese; beef steaks and roasts; hot dogs, ham, and luncheon meats; doughnuts, cookies, and cake; eggs.*

The Next 28 Percent. Another 28 percent (for a cumulative total of 78 percent) of the saturated fat intake was contributed by, in descending order: pork, including chops and roasts; butter; white bread,* rolls,* and crackers; ice cream and frozen desserts; marga-

---

*These foods are relatively low in saturated fat, but the large amounts consumed contribute substantial saturated fat calories to the American diet.

rine; 2% milk; mayonnaise and salad dressings; french fries and fried potatoes; salty snacks; bacon; nondairy coffee creamers; sausage.

Do these foods sound familiar? Do they contribute heavily to your saturated fat intake? Check the Food Tables to see how much saturated fat these and other foods actually contain. You might be surprised — even shocked. Your immediate reaction might be that you must eliminate these foods, *now,* if not sooner.

Not a Bare-Bones Eating Plan. Relax. Any food can be fitted into *Eater's Choice*. No food need be completely eliminated. The Food Tables will help you determine *how much* and *how often* you can eat certain foods. Of course, the higher the saturated fat content of a food, the less often or the smaller the amount you will be able to fit into your personalized daily Sat-Fat Budget.

Use Food Tables as You Read This Chapter. As we discuss the fat contents of common foods in this chapter, check back to the Food Tables to compare foods. Soon, you will have learned the sat-fat contents of the foods you commonly eat and will find you no longer need to look up every food in the tables.

MEATS

Since ground beef is number one on the saturated fat hit parade, let us look at the meat category. All the meat, poultry, and fish entries in the food tables are given in 1-ounce portions to help you compare the different meats. You can easily calculate the sat-fat content by multiplying the number of ounces of meat you eat times the saturated fat contained in 1 ounce. For instance, 1 ounce of braised lean flank steak has 16 calories of saturated fat per ounce. If you eat 6 ounces of flank steak, you are consuming 6 × 16 or 96 calories of saturated fat.

Hamburger — Three Times Fattier. You're thinking about dinner. The refrigerator is bare. Should you buy round steak or ground beef? You look at the beef section of the Food Tables. Trimmed, lean, round steak happens to be the leanest cut of red meat. It contains 7 calories of saturated fat per ounce. Check out the broiled lean ground beef: 25 calories of saturated fat for the same portion size. If you eat 6 ounces of either meat, the round steak will contribute

7×6 or 42 sat-fat calories, while the ground beef will contribute 25×6 or 150 sat-fat calories. The round steak has less than one-third the calories of saturated fat found in the broiled lean ground beef. Would this comparison help you decide?

Admittedly, hamburger is a convenience food. It's fast and tasty. However, it is so chock full of saturated fat your arteries shudder when a mere whiff of hamburger floats under your nose. If you need to prepare a delicious meal in a hurry, sauté scallops with garlic and ginger (5 minutes), cover a white fish with lemon yogurt and bake for 5–10 minutes, or cut round steak thin and sauté with onions and green peppers (15 minutes).

For those of you who would rather give up your right arm than give up hamburgers, here are several hints to make your hamburger healthier. Broil rather than pan-fry hamburgers so some of the fat drips away. Immediately after cooking, place hamburgers between paper towels to absorb excess fat. Mix ground beef with bread crumbs to make your hamburger half as fatty.

The Veal Story. According to the newly published U.S. Department of Agriculture Food Tables, many cuts of lean veal are relatively low in saturated fat. When trimmed of fat, braised veal leg has 5 sat-fat calories per ounce. Roasted veal shoulder blade, trimmed of fat, has 7 sat-fat calories per ounce. However, you must still be cautious when choosing veal cuts that have not been trimmed. For example, braised veal breast, untrimmed of fat, contains 156 calories of saturated fat per 6 ounces — that's a pretty big chunk out of a daily Sat-Fat Budget of 200.

RED MEATS — BIG SATURATED FAT DONORS

In general, the higher the grade of meat, the more fat and saturated fat it contains. Take note: regardless of the grade or cut, the fat of all red meats is predominantly saturated (about 50 percent of the fat) and very little polyunsaturated fat (2 percent of the fat). Although some fat is lost through broiling and some fat can be trimmed, much of the fat is marbled throughout the meat and remains in it even after cooking.

Under the Wool, a Lot of Fat. The saturated fat content of lamb is comparable to all but the fattiest cuts of beef. Even the leanest cuts of lamb — lamb leg and lamb loin — are moderately high in saturated fat, containing about 60 calories of saturated fat per 6 ounces. Lamb shoulder and rib chops contain about 84 calories per 6 ounces.

Pork, Both High and Low. Pork has a reputation as a high-fat food. But the amount of fat (sat-fat) in pork dishes depends on the cut and the way you prepare it. For example, some pork dishes are relatively low in saturated fat, such as roasted lean tenderloin (24 sat-fat calories per 6 ounces) or broiled lean center loin (54 sat-fat calories per 6 ounces), while other dishes are high in sat-fat, such as roasted center rib loin with fat (132 sat-fat calories per 6 ounces) and pan-fried loin blade with fat (204 sat-fat calories per 6 ounces).

TAKE NOTE: Trim the fat from pork before cooking and you remove half the sat-fat calories. Save another 3 to 5 calories of sat-fat per ounce of meat by braising, broiling, or roasting instead of pan-frying.

By far the worst pork product in terms of saturated fat content is bacon. Three medium slices of cooked bacon contain 30 calories of saturated fat. A healthier alternative to bacon is Canadian bacon, which has about one-sixth as much saturated fat. Thus, an amount of Canadian bacon equivalent to 3 slices of regular bacon contributes only 5 calories of saturated fat.

What If You Still Want Red Meat?

You can see that all red meat contains too much saturated fat to be healthy for your coronary arteries. But can red meats fit into your *Eater's Choice* budget? The answer is yes — a yes that depends on the cut of meat, the amount, and how it is prepared. And because red meats are so high in saturated fat, you may have to adjust your saturated fat intake from other sources.

For example, if you consume 2000 calories per day, the *Eater's Choice* 10 Percent Plan allows 200 calories of saturated fat, and the *Eater's Choice* 6 Percent Plan allows 120 calories of saturated fat. One 4-ounce lean hamburger provides 100 sat-fat calories, 50 percent of the daily saturated fat allotment on the *Eater's Choice* 10 Percent Plan and 83 percent on the *Eater's Choice* 6 Percent Plan. That leaves 100 (10 Percent Plan) or 20 (6 Percent Plan) sat-fat calories for the rest of the day. Maybe every once in a while you have to have red meat or you will bite a passing stranger. Fine, have the red meat. On the other hand, you have other choices.

Meat Leaves Center Stage

If red meats are to be eaten on the *Eater's Choice* plan, you have two choices: either you limit the rest of your saturated fat intake for that day, or you use meat as a condiment. Eventually you will stop thinking of meat as the centerpiece of the meal — a 12-ounce steak with a vegetable on the side. Instead, you will use a meat such as thinly sliced flank steak to provide taste and texture to, say, a rice-based or a vegetable-based dish or a pasta.

Good Meat: Chicken

Chicken is very low in sat-fat compared to other meats. Six ounces of roasted chicken breast without skin contain 6 calories of saturated fat, versus 42 for round steak and 150 for ground beef.

Chicken breast is the part of the bird lowest in fat and thus your best choice.

CHICKEN PART (WITHOUT SKIN)	SAT-FAT CALORIES PER 6 OZ
breast	6
drumstick	12
wing	12
leg	18
thigh	18
back	24

In addition, chicken breast is one of the most versatile of meats and can be substituted for beef or pork in many recipes. Lemon Chicken (page 215), Chicken Fajitas (page 255), and Sesame Chicken Brochettes (page 225) are but a few of the millions of interesting, delicious, and often quick and easy recipes using chicken breasts without skin.

Skin the Beast. Chicken breast scores high as a heart-healthy food as long as it is prepared properly. Bake a breast without skin for 4 calories of sat-fat. Bake it with the skin on, and your sat-fat calories climb to 19. Batter-dip and fry it with the skin on, and your sat-fat calories soar to 44. TAKE NOTE: skin must be removed *before* cooking or the fat from the skin will be absorbed by the meat.

Better Meat: Turkey

The leanest poultry meat is roasted turkey breast without skin (see box below) which contains only 3 calories of saturated fat per 6 ounces. Dark meat turkey, such as the leg, contains six times as much saturated fat (18 calories), but compared to even the leanest red meats, it is low in saturated fat.

Turkey breast or cutlets ground in a food processor or meat grinder make an excellent low sat-fat ground beef substitute for making burgers, adding to spaghetti sauces and chilis, etc. However, be aware that ground turkey purchased at the grocery store may be loaded with large amounts of turkey fat and skin, and thus may not be a low-fat choice. For example, one commercially ground turkey product contains 36 calories of fat per ounce. Considering that plain white turkey meat contains less than 2½ calories of fat per ounce, the food manufacturer must be adding 33½ calories of fat and skin per ounce to the ground turkey. That's a lot of fat. At about 11 calories of sat-fat per ounce (44 sat-fat calories per 4 ounces), this brand of ground turkey is a better choice than lean ground beef at 25 sat-fat calories per ounce (100 sat-fat calories per 4 ounces). However, it is a choice that should not be eaten with abandon. To make matters worse, the fat content of commercially ground turkey is often not given. To ensure that your ground turkey is low in fat, grind it yourself.

WARNING: Pay attention to turkey labels. Do not buy Butterball turkeys or turkeys that have been shot up with coconut or other hydrogenated oils. Buy plain ol' natural unadulterated turkeys. Cook them breast down and they will still be juicy.

Best Meat: Fish

All animals that live in the water — shellfish, fish, and even marine mammals — contain a special kind of fat called omega-3 polyunsaturated fat. Omega-3 polyunsaturated fats are especially potent in lowering blood triglyceride levels. So, if high blood triglycerides are your problem, eating plenty of fish may be your salvation. Omega-3 polyunsaturated fats also reduce blood clotting. It is the small clots floating through the blood stream that often get caught in clogged arteries, causing heart attacks. The fewer clots that are formed the better.

Not only do fish contain the risk-reducing omega-3 polyunsaturated fats; they also are low in saturated fat. Lean fish such as flounder and sole contain only about 1 calorie of saturated fat per ounce. Even fatty fish such as red salmon have only about 5 calories of saturated fat per ounce — and the fattier the fish the more omega-3 polyunsaturated fat they contain. However, be advised — deep-frying fish or cooking them in cream or butter sauces turns a heart-healthy food into a heart-risky one.

Eat the Fish, Not the Capsule. The best way to get omega-3 polyunsaturated fats is by eating fish. Fish oil capsules are not the answer.

- Fish oil capsules are not regulated by the Food and Drug Administration, and thus may contain either very little or a lot of omega-3 polyunsaturated fat. You have no way of judging the potency of different brands.
- All the fat-soluble contaminants found in fish are concentrated in the fish oil in the capsules.
- Fish oil capsules add unnecessary fat and calories to your diet.
- Fish oil capsules are expensive.

A TIP: tuna packed in water tastes delicious and has 12 fewer calories of saturated fat per 3½-ounce can than tuna packed in oil. The oil used is soybean oil and not fish oil. If you are only able to purchase tuna packed in oil, wash the tuna with water to remove excess oil before eating. This will remove unwanted fat and calories.

Ruining Chicken, Turkey, and Fish

We often hear protests: "I eat only chicken, fish, and turkey, and yet my cholesterol is pushing 280 mg/dL. Am I one of those people whose cholesterol isn't affected by diet?" No! Even heart-healthy foods can be made heart-risky by the way they are prepared.

Nutritious and low in fat, chicken, turkey, and fish are often transformed into cholesterol-raising high-fat foods when they are processed into frozen dinners. This is how it works: pollack is a fish with trace saturated fat — that means a tiny bit more than 0 calories of saturated fat. A food processing company takes the pollack, cuts it into fish sticks, breads it, fries it in partially hydrogenated vegetable oil, and packages it. Now, according to the label the serving size of 4 pollack fish sticks contains 90 calories of fat and 45 calories of saturated fat. The food processing company took an almost totally fat-free, heart-healthy food and increased its fat content by more than 9000 percent.

Fast-food restaurants commit similar crimes when preparing chicken and fish. Foods with negligible saturated fat become sat-fat gold mines when breaded and deep-fried in saturated oils. Remember — just because it's chicken, turkey, or fish does not mean it's heart-healthy.

Low in Fat but Not Much to Eat

Supermarket freezer cases are bulging with new, healthier frozen dinners that are truly low in saturated fat. But like all frozen dinners, they are no substitutes for freshly prepared food. In addition, the factor that makes them so low in saturated fat also creates another problem. Many of these dinners contain only about 1 to 2 ounces of meat. This is not much meat and not much food. People tend either to eat several of these dinners (which doubles or triples the sat-fat calories). Or, to diminish their hunger, they fill up later on other foods that are often high in saturated fat. Low-sat-fat frozen dinners are only a solution to your cholesterol problem if you eat one dinner and enhance it with plenty of vegetables and whole grains.

Cholesterol in Meats

All the meats — fish, poultry, and red meats — contain approximately equal amounts of cholesterol, about 25 mg per ounce or about 150 mg per 6 ounces. But take a look at the differences in calories of saturated fat. (Remember, these amounts are for only 1 ounce of meat.) Thus, decisions about choosing meats are best made on the basis of saturated fat content and not cholesterol content.

Fish and white meat turkey or chicken without skin are so low in saturated fat that large quantities could be fitted into any heart-healthy eating plan if it were not for their cholesterol contents. However, if you are going to stay within the American Heart Association

CHOLESTEROL AND SATURATED FAT VALUES OF MEAT, POULTRY, FISH, AND SHELLFISH

	CHOLESTEROL MG/OZ	SATURATED FAT CALORIES/OZ
Veal breast	36	26
Lamb loin chop, broiled	26	23
Pork chop, broiled	28	21
Sirloin steak, broiled	26	19
Chicken breast, no skin	24	1
Turkey breast, no skin	20	½
Flounder, baked	20	1
Shrimp	43*	1

*Shrimp has slightly more cholesterol than other meats, but is extremely low in saturated fat (1 calorie per ounce) and contains risk-reducing omega-3 polyunsaturated fats. How much shrimp can you eat? As much as you can afford — unless you are a shrimp fisherman or very wealthy.

guideline of 200–300 mg of cholesterol per day (see Chapter 5), you should not exceed 10–12 ounces per day of even the leanest fish or poultry. If your physician or dietitian has recommended a limit of 100 mg of cholesterol per day, then you should not eat more than about 4 ounces of even the leanest fish or poultry. Don't worry — you won't starve eating even this amount.

Sausages and Luncheon Meats

Sausages and luncheon meats are extremely high in saturated fat as well as extremely high in sodium. They are poor choices to fit into your eating budget.

Consider the sausage. One Polish sausage contributes over 200 calories of saturated fat to your Sat-Fat Budget, more than is allowed for the whole day on the *Eater's Choice* 10 Percent Plan for a 2000 calorie per day intake level.

Smoked link sausages are also very high in saturated fat. Although they are small, each 2.4-ounce sausage link contains about 70 calories of saturated fat, which represents approximately 35 percent of the 200 sat-fat calories allowed on the *Eater's Choice* 10 Percent Plan and 58 percent of the 120 sat-fat calories allowed on the *Eater's Choice* 6 Percent Plan. Thus, eating only one sausage link may mean making severe restrictions in your saturated fat intake for the rest of the day. Two links would completely use up your saturated fat allowance on the *Eater's Choice* 6 Percent Plan.

What's a baseball game or cookout without a hot dog nestled in a warm bun and covered with ketchup or mustard and pickle relish? What about two or three? Beware! A two-ounce all-beef frankfurter contains 63 calories of sat-fat. If that hot dog is in addition to your regular meals, you may be in great danger of having overspent your Sat-Fat Budget — unless you planned ahead.

MILK AND MILK PRODUCTS

Milk — A High-Fat Food

Milk is characterized by its fat content. Thus, whole milk is generally about 3.3 percent fat. This means that 3.3 percent of the total weight is contributed by fat. (This system of rating milk was established many years ago to ensure a minimum fat content as a way of protecting consumers from watered-down milk.)

The amount of fat in whole milk — 3.3 percent — seems so trivial, hardly worth counting. False — do not be fooled. Most of the weight of milk is accounted for by water. In terms of calories, fat accounts for 72 of the total 150 calories in a cup of whole milk, or 48 percent of the total calories. A cup of whole milk contains 45 calories of saturated fat.

Thus, whole milk is a high-fat food. On a 2000 calorie per day eating pattern, 4.4 cups of whole milk would provide 200 calories of saturated fat and would thus account for the entire saturated fat

---

Most (about 64 percent) of the fat in milk products is saturated fat regardless of whether it is whole, 2%, or 1% milk. This is true of all milk products, including yogurt, cream, ice cream, and cheese. **Think before you eat.**

allotment on the *Eater's Choice* 10 Percent Plan. A mere 2.7 cups of whole milk would provide 120 calories of saturated fat, accounting for the entire saturated fat allotment on the *Eater's Choice* 6 Percent Plan.

Move Toward Skim Milk

Low-fat milk (2%) tastes pretty similar to whole milk. If you are a whole milk drinker, start by changing to 2% milk. Although 2% milk contains less fat than whole milk, it still contains 27 calories of saturated fat per cup. After a few weeks, try 1% milk. It contains only 14 calories of saturated fat per cup.

However, the best favor you can do your heart is to drink skim milk. "Yuk," you say, "it looks like blue water." We say, "If you don't love it now, you will. It just takes getting used to. Our kids are revolted by whole milk."

And what great benefits. Skim milk is essentially fat-free, containing at most 3 calories of saturated fat per cup. Look at these statistics:

	WHOLE MILK PER CUP	SKIM MILK PER CUP
Total calories	150	86
Sat-fat calories	45	3
Cholesterol, mg	33	4
Calcium, mg	291	302

It may take time, but it is worth working your way toward skim milk.

More Calcium in Skim Milk Than Whole Milk. Milk is an important source of calcium. Calcium is vital for developing and maintaining strong bones and preventing osteoporosis in later life. Skim milk contains more calcium than whole milk: 302 mg of calcium per cup of skim milk versus 291 mg per cup of whole milk. Most skim milk available today has been fortified with vitamins and thus contains just as many vitamins as whole milk. Skim milk is just as nutritious as whole milk *and* is heart-healthy.

Butter

The creamy sweet taste of butter is irreplaceable, but its saturated fat content is so high you must either use it sparingly or find a suitable substitute. The food industry has invested heavily in producing such substitutes. They range from whipped butter, which has about 25 percent less saturated fat than regular butter, to butter-margarine blends, with about 50 percent less saturated fat, margarines, with about 70 percent less saturated fat, and diet margarines, with about 86 percent less saturated fat.

Cream

Coffee drinkers, did you realize that adding 1 tablespoon of light cream to a cup of coffee uses 18 calories of saturated fat of your Sat-Fat Budget? Three cups of coffee with cream provide 54 calories of saturated fat, about one-quarter of the daily allotment of saturated fat under the *Eater's Choice* 10 Percent Plan for 2000 total calories and almost half of the daily allotment under the *Eater's Choice* 6 Percent Plan. And all that for three dinky little tablespoons of cream. Mind-boggling.

Half-and-half contains half as much saturated fat as light cream while 2% milk provides about a tenth the amount of saturated fat as light cream. How about using 1% or skim milk, or drinking your coffee black?

You must be careful when using nondairy coffee whiteners. Some of the dry creamers still contain tropical oils. The serving size is a mere teaspoon and contains less than 9 sat-fat calories. (Do you use 1 teaspoon?) Even most of the "lite" powdered creamers contain coconut oil, palm kernel oil, or palm oil. One lite creamer that contains hydrogenated vegetable oil instead lists no polyunsaturated fat and no saturated fat, only monounsaturated fat. The hydrogenation process has obviously generated a lot of monounsaturated fat in the trans form (see discussion of trans fats on page 81). The frozen creamers generally contain hydrogenated vegetable oils (trans fats) and contain less than 9 sat-fat calories per tablespoon.

Cheese, Wonderful Cheese, Why Are You Almost All Fat?

The sad story about cheese is that whole milk cheeses are no more than delectable little packages of concentrated fat and saturated fat. One small ounce of Cheddar cheese provides 81 fat calories. One ounce of cream cheese contains 96 calories of fat and 56 calories of saturated fat.

You can include cheese in your *Eater's Choice* eating plan, but you will have to sacrifice other sources of sat-fat in your diet. Just plan ahead. Keep your daily sat-fat intake low and you will be able to sneak in a piece of cheese without sinking your heart-healthy diet boat. However, before you devote your entire Sat-Fat Budget to cheese, be aware that most cheeses are extremely high in sodium.

HINT: Satisfy your cheese hunger with minimal sat-fat calories by using a cheese slicer to shave yourself a thin piece of cheese. Remember: many thin slices make one big fat slice.

Lower-Fat Cheeses. A truly low-fat cheese is 1% cottage cheese. One percent cottage cheese contains one-quarter the saturated fat calories of creamed cottage cheese and tastes just as good. Mix cottage cheese with cut-up fruit for a refreshing low-fat lunch. Cover Honey Whole-Wheat Bread (page 362) with sliced bananas and 1% cottage cheese for a filling, scrumptious breakfast. One percent cottage cheese can be used in cooking as a creamy substitute for higher-fat cheeses, as in Creamy Chicken Pie (page 233), Spinach Quiche (page 318), and Calzone (page 313).

The dairy cases in grocery stores now offer a multitude of lower-fat cheeses ranging from 9 to 45 sat-fat calories per ounce. Be careful to read the label. Just because the cheese is advertised as "low-fat," "lower in fat," or "lite" does not mean that it is actually low in saturated fat. For example, part skim milk ricotta and mozzarella are lower in saturated fat than their whole milk counterparts. One-half cup of part skim milk ricotta contains about half the saturated fat calories of whole milk ricotta: 55 versus 93. One ounce of part skim milk mozzarella contains 28 sat-fat calories versus 40 sat-fat calories for whole milk mozzarella. These cheeses may be lower in saturated fat, but they are still high enough so that you need to monitor them carefully.

And don't forget that although one piece of Kraft Reduced-Fat Monterey Jack may contain only 27 sat-fat calories, two pieces contain 54 sat-fat calories, and three pieces contain 81. If you want to eat a limited amount of low-fat cheeses, fine. However, you might find it more satisfying to eat real (high-fat) cheeses, but rarely and in very small quantities. We guarantee you'll really taste them.

Nonfat Cheeses. For those who find giving up cheese next to impossible, the introduction of fat-free cheeses must seem like a miracle. At 0 fat and 0 sat-fat calories, why not make cheese the main staple of your diet? Here's why not: You must use sense in consuming any nonfat food. A little is okay; a lot pushes out more nutritious foods from your diet. Nonfat cheeses contain a lot of sodium —about 310 mg per slice or about one-third your daily allotment. Although they contain little or no fat, nonfat cheeses perpetuate your high-fat taste. While there is nothing harmful about spreading a tablespoon of fat-free cream cheese on your bagel or eating an occasional cheese sandwich for lunch, those who overdo their use of creamy and cheesy-tasting nonfat foods are less likely to lower their cholesterol because they never give up the taste and craving for fatty foods. If you limit the high-fat or high-fat-tasting foods you consume, eventually you won't even desire them. It's true. Studies have shown that it takes about twelve weeks to change to a low-fat, tasty taste *if* you don't keep subjecting yourself to your old high-fat tastes. The most successful followers of *Eater's Choice* use their Sat-Fat Budget to wean themselves from fatty foods and replace them with high-fiber, nutritious foods.

Yogurt

Several different varieties of yogurt, with vastly different saturated fat contents, are available. They include nonfat, low-fat, and regular high-fat yogurt. Some yogurts are loaded with eggs and cream. Read the label of the yogurt you choose to make certain it has a low saturated fat content.

Nonfat yogurt makes a good substitute for sour cream in many recipes (even in a sweet dessert such as Deep-Dish Pear Pie, page 404). Whole milk plain yogurt contains about a sixth as much saturated fat as sour cream, while skim milk plain yogurt contains almost 1/100.

Do Not Skimp on Low-Fat Dairy Foods

Let us say it again: to stay healthy and to keep your bones and teeth strong, you need the calcium that dairy foods provide. Women especially need calcium to prevent osteoporosis. Children need calcium for strong bones and teeth and for growth. Eat dairy products, but eat low-fat dairy products, such as skim milk, 1% cottage cheese (creamy and good), and low-fat or nonfat yogurt.

You can fit cheeses, cream, sour cream, whole milk, and whole milk yogurt into your Sat-Fat Budget as a splurge, but only as an occasional splurge. Cook with low- or nonfat products. Substitute nonfat yogurt or buttermilk for cream or sour cream. We even substitute skim milk for cream (see Potato Soup with Leeks and Broccoli, page 184, or Mushroom Sauce, page 275) with excellent gustatory results.

FATS AND OILS

Two of the most important and widespread changes made by the American public to lower blood cholesterol levels are the substitution of margarine for butter and the substitution of unsaturated vegetable oils for saturated animal fats such as lard or beef tallow.

Margarine

For years, margarine has been accepted as a good substitute for butter. Whereas butter contains 65 calories of saturated fat per tablespoon, margarine contains only 18.

Enter the Villain *Trans*. We still endorse margarine as a substitute for butter, but the less you use margarine and the more you use olive oil, the better. Here is the scientific explanation. Polyunsaturated fats and oils are hydrogenated (a chemical process that adds hydrogen and results in a more saturated fat) to make them more solid at room temperature and to increase their shelf life — the time they can sit on a shelf without becoming rancid. Food manufacturers use hydrogenated and partially hydrogenated vegetable oils in margarines and many other processed foods exactly because of these properties. Just read food labels to see how pervasive hydrogenated soybean, cottonseed, and corn oil are in commercial foods.

During the process of hydrogenation, a new class of chemical is produced called *trans* fats. (Fats that occur in nature are almost completely of the *cis* form. *Cis* and *trans* refer to the three-dimensional arrangement of the fat.)

Trans fats have several properties that please food manufacturers and several that won't please you. Food manufacturers like trans fats because they are even harder at room temperature than their cis counterparts. Also, because trans fats are monounsaturated, they do not contribute to the saturated fat content of the food. The food appears to be heart-healthy because the food label doesn't show a high-saturated-fat content. In fact, the manufacturer can emphasize the amount of monounsaturated fat on the label.

But the down side of trans fats is that even though hydrogenation has made them into monounsaturated fats, they affect your blood cholesterol more like saturated fats. Studies show that trans fats raise LDL ("bad cholesterol") and lower HDL ("good cholesterol").

So, while foods containing trans fats are probably less heart-risky than those containing saturated fats, it is better to limit your intake of foods containing trans fats. Better still, use more natural (versus man-made), monounsaturated fats such as olive oil. (We use olive oil almost exclusively in the *Eater's Choice* recipes, even in breads, cakes, and pie crusts). The best course of all is to limit the total amount of any type of fat (even heart-healthy monos) you eat to reduce your risk of obesity and colon and breast cancers.

The Vegetable Oil Contest

Olive Oil: Number-One Choice. Olive oil contains mainly monounsaturated fat and little saturated or polyunsaturated fat. It is the most heart-healthy of all the fats. Recent research indicates that olive oil lowers LDL-cholesterol without lowering HDL-cholesterol. In addition, by preventing the oxidation of LDL remnants, olive oil helps prevent the first step of the atherosclerotic process. Epidemiological studies show that populations (such as Greeks and Italians) who use olive oil as the predominant source of fat in their diet have very low rates of heart disease. Choose olive oil even for baking. (Like olive oil, peanut oil is predominantly monounsaturated. However, scientific research has shown that peanut oil causes clogging of coronary arteries in some animals. Why take a chance?)

Canola Oil: Newcomer on the Food Scene. Second choice is canola oil, derived from the rapeseed plant. While it has the lowest amount of saturated fat of all the oils and a lot of monounsaturated fat, canola oil has not been people-tested for a long enough time to assure us that it has no long-term adverse health effects. Why take a chance when you can easily and safely use olive oil?

Polys Have Their Problems. Safflower, sunflower, corn, and soybean oils are primarily polyunsaturated, with small amounts of saturated fat. Safflower contains about 10 percent saturated fat; sunflower, 11 percent; corn, 13 percent; and soybean, about 15 percent. However, as we have mentioned, high intakes of polyunsaturated oils lower HDL levels and may raise the risk of cancer. So don't overdose on polyunsaturated fats.

Cottonseed oil is highly saturated for a polyunsaturated fat. It contains 27 percent of its calories as saturated fat. This is only 1 percent less than vegetable shortening (such as Crisco). Cottonseed is a favorite with food producers. Watch out for it when you buy commercial foods.

Hydrogenated vegetable oils have the problem of containing trans fats (see page 81). The fats that don't become monounsaturated (and trans) during hydrogenation become saturated. Even safflower oil, one of the least saturated fats, loses much of its heart-healthy properties when it is hydrogenated.

Coconut Oil: The Pits. Coconut oil is given to lab rats and other animals normally resistant to developing elevated blood cholesterol levels to produce atherosclerotic plaques and heart disease. With 106 sat-fat calories per tablespoon, it is the most heart-risky fat known. If you are smarter than a rat, you will avoid coconut oil at all costs. Following close is palm kernel oil (100 sat-fat calories/tablespoon) and palm oil (60 sat-fat calories/tablespoon). You should avoid all of these tropical oils. We happily report that tropical oils have almost been entirely eliminated from commercial food products. But, just to be safe, *read the list of ingredients on food labels.*

All Oils Have Equal Calories

You will note that all the oils are really mixtures of polyunsaturated, monounsaturated, and saturated fats. (See Figure 11, page 40.) None contains only one type of fat. We refer to an oil as polyunsaturated or monounsaturated or saturated because it contains predominantly that type of fat. Regardless of the type of oil, they all contain the same number of fat calories because they are 100 percent fat. Fat intake should be limited as much as possible, especially by people trying to maintain their desirable weight, because fat makes fat.

Lard, Chicken Fat, and Other Animal Fats

All animal fats contain large amounts of monounsaturated fat, relatively small amounts of polyunsaturated fat, moderate to large amounts of saturated fat, and moderate amounts of cholesterol. Of the animal fats, chicken fat is the least heart-risky and beef tallow is the most heart-risky. *But no animal fats can be recommended for persons trying to lower their blood cholesterol levels.* The heart-healthy alternative is olive oil.

Keep Short on Shortening

Your mom may have used shortening to bake the flakiest pie crust imaginable, but in this case, don't follow in her culinary footsteps. One tablespoon of shortening has from 30 to 47 calories of saturated fat. For the sake of your heart-health, don't use shortening at home or buy it baked into commercial goods.

Mayonnaise

You will be happy to find something you know and love but do not have to avoid completely: mayonnaise. If you budget carefully, you can fit real mayonnaise into your diet at 11 to 14 sat-fat calories per tablespoon. A better choice is reduced-calorie mayonnaise at 9 sat-fat calories per tablespoon.

Before you feel too happy, take heed. All mayonnaises are almost pure fat and so are high in fat calories. Even reduced-calorie mayonnaises with half the total fat calories contain 45 fat calories per tablespoon, which is still a lot of fat. Use mayonnaise in moderation.

Salad Dressings

Many salad dressings are high in saturated fats as well as total and polyunsaturated fats. A tablespoon of blue cheese dressing or French dressing has 14 calories of saturated fat. Russian has 10, followed closely by Italian with 9, and Thousand Island with 8. One problem with using salad dressing is that one never delicately sprinkles only a tablespoon of salad dressing on one's salad. Another problem is that salad dressings are often high in sodium. Do not ruin the health value of your salad by drowning it in highly fattening and fatty salad dressing.

THE FORK METHOD

Use the fork method to retain the taste of salad dressing without consuming all the fat calories. Have your salad dressing served on the side or pour a small amount into a bowl. Dip your fork into the dressing, then spear your salad greens or vegetables. Voilà! — a tasty low-sat-fat forkful.

A more heart-healthy alternative is to use commercial low-fat dressings. Or make your own: in a jar, combine a little olive oil, vinegar, minced garlic, some herbs (oregano, thyme, or basil, for example), a little Dijon mustard, salt, and pepper — and shake.

DESSERTS

Many Americans enjoy having a sweet, rich dessert to top off their dinner and often their lunch, too. Unfortunately, many of our favorite desserts are rich in saturated fat. A cup of ordinary vanilla ice cream contains 80 calories of saturated fat. Compare this with a cup of vanilla ice milk (32 calories of saturated fat), a cup of orange sherbet (21 sat-fat calories), and a cup of low-fat frozen yogurt (12 sat-fat calories). The low-fat frozen yogurt has less than one-sixth as much saturated fat as the ice cream. Even better are the new nonfat frozen yogurts (such as Colombo Lite) that eliminate all sat-fat calories while retaining the creamy texture and delicious taste.

Fortunately frozen yogurt is becoming increasingly more available in ice cream parlors, restaurants, and grocery stores. But be advised. *Yogurt* is not a synonym for *low-fat*. Ask about the fat content and the ingredients. Many yogurt vendors can provide nutritional information. For example, one popular brand contains 2 grams of fat per 4 ounces. The primary fat is butterfat. This works out to 18 calories of total fat and about 12 sat-fat calories. Another brand contains 0.9 grams of butterfat per ounce. If you eat 4 ounces (about half a cup), you will be eating (4 × .9) 3.6 grams of total fat or about 32 fat calories and about 22 sat-fat calories.

But before you dash over to your frozen yogurt shop, keep in mind that Oreo cookie bits, Heath crunch, Reese's Pieces, chocolate chips, shredded coconut — all the toppings you love to eat — don't become less heart-risky just because they sit atop a nonfat frozen yogurt. Choose a fruit topping (or no topping) to adorn your treat.

Also, be wary of frozen yogurt confections you find in the freezer compartments of your grocery store. A TCBY Vanilla Crunch Yog-A-Bar has 63 sat-fat calories. A half cup of Stonyfield Farm chocolate mint chip frozen yogurt has 27 sat-fat calories.

The Fat Impact of Desserts

A single cake-type doughnut contains 36 calories of saturated fat. A slice of Pillsbury Chocolate Caramel Nut Cake (one-sixteenth of a cake contains 170 sat-fat calories) will eat up a major portion of your Sat-Fat Budget. Coconut custard pie contributes about 81 calories of saturated fat per slice, as does an individual Hostess Apple or Cherry Fruit Pie. A Nestlé Reduced-Fat Crunch Bar contains 45 sat-fat calories. Eat a cup of Ben and Jerry's vanilla ice cream at 180 sat-fat calories and you won't have to worry about making sat-fat choices for the rest of the day.

Commercial cookies are the downfall of many sat-fat counters. Like crackers and nuts, cookie consumption is a miraculous occurrence. Somehow, scores of cookies get from the plate or the box into the mouth without the cookie consumer having put them there. Cookie eaters must pay attention. Cookie packages generally list the amount of saturated fat for one cookie. The only person in the world who ate just one cookie is listed in the *Guinness Book of World Records.* Most people begin with one cookie and end with many cookies. Even at less than 1 gram of saturated fat each (which may mean 8 sat-fat calories), cookie sat-fat calories quickly add up. If you are not a cookie monster and have enough self-control, give yourself a treat and fit just one or two cookies into your Sat-Fat Budget. Otherwise, leave the cookie box in the grocery store.

Being on a low sat-fat diet does not mean you must give up delicious desserts. Why not bake your own? Try the desserts beginning on page 380. Nothing could be simpler or more delicious than Cinnamon Sweet Cakes (page 405) at 8 sat-fat calories per square. What about Deep-Dish Pear Pie (page 404) at 8 sat-fat calories per slice, or Tante Nancy's Apple Crumb Cake (page 398) at 14 sat-fat calories for a trip to the sublime?

Just a note of caution: even desserts that are low in saturated fat are generally more fat-filled than other parts of your meal. You are not going to stay thin by eating baked or frozen desserts at every meal. How about fruit?

Read labels for hidden coconut, palm kernel, palm, or hydrogenated vegetable oil in commercial desserts.

The Good Guys

Many Europeans finish their large meal of the day with a piece of fruit. How about a delicious (and heart-healthy) dessert of sliced fruit mixed with low-fat yogurt? You will see the advantages fruits offer when you consider the saturated fat content of most fruits: none.*

Substituting fruits for rich, sweet desserts will allow you much greater freedom in choosing meats, dairy products, and other foods that contain saturated fats. The choices are yours to make . . . as long as you stay within your own Sat-Fat Budget.

SNACKS

High-fat snacks can be the downfall of any healthy eating plan. Because they are habit-forming, you eat a lot of them. What may start out as a few sat-fat calories per bite quickly ends up bankrupting your Sat-Fat Budget. Even if the sat-fat content is just moderately high, the fat content of most snacks is almost always sky-high. And, remember, eating a diet high in fat increases your risk for cancer, heart disease, diabetes, and obesity.

Of course, all snacks are not high-fat. Read on to find snacks you can eat with moderate abandon.

Popcorn

Potentially Ideal Snack. One of the greatest snacks known to mankind since some ancient American Indian threw dried corn kernels into a fire is popcorn. Fat-free, air-popped** popcorn is high in both insoluble fiber (important for effective bowel function and reducing risk of colon cancer) and soluble fiber (helps to lower blood cholesterol and risk of heart disease). It is filling without being fattening, and it satisfies the hand-to-mouth craving without punishing your budget. Popcorn is truly a treat.

---

*The exception is avocado (41–48 sat-fat calories).
**Air-poppers are inexpensive and easy to care for. They require no cleaning after use. Just drop about 1/2 cup of popcorn kernels into the machine, and in 2 to 3 minutes 12 cups of delicious, healthy popcorn will tumble out.

But Easily Ruined. Drench it in butter at 65 sat-fat calories per tablespoon (would 1/4 cup, or 260 sat-fat calories, be more like it?), and popcorn becomes an ultra-high-sat-fat snack.

Go to the movies and buy a box. Movie popcorn is almost always made with coconut oil. Order it buttered and you can eat up your Sat-Fat Budget for a day (the small size), for two days (the medium size), or blow your budget for half a week (the large, 20-cup tub).

SIZE	SAT-FAT CALORIES	
	POPPED IN COCONUT OIL	POPPED IN COCONUT OIL WITH "BUTTER"
Small (about 7 cups)	171	261
Medium (about 16 cups)	387	504
Large (about 20 cups)	495	657

And as for total fat, pop popcorn in your microwave and you are probably eating from about 20 to 30 fat calories per cup or, more realistically, 200 to 300 fat calories per 10 cups.

Buy it already popped from the grocery store, and even air-popped popcorn is filled with fat. Take Bachman air-popped popcorn at 100 fat calories per 1-ounce serving (about 2¾ cups). Look at the label and try to figure out how a fat-free food (air-popped popcorn) gained 100 fat calories per ounce. The answer: fat was poured on *after* the popcorn was air-popped.

For your best buy, both in terms of health and your wallet, stick with the plain air-popped popcorn you pop at home. At first it may taste a bit like cardboard, but keep eating it and soon you'll even crave it.

HINT: Store popcorn kernels in the refrigerator to keep them fresh and pop-worthy.

Chips and Other Addictive Crunchies

Chips are so easy to eat, you swallow one and crave another and another and another. It takes no effort to inhale an 8-ounce bag all by yourself. The sat-fat and fat calories add up. Look at General Mills Bugles. At 72 calories of saturated fat for 1 ounce, Bugles might help you to see the wisdom of eating a carrot. Pringle's Original chips have 23 sat-fat calories per ounce (90 total fat calories!), but who eats 1 ounce of chips? One ounce of Pringle's Right Crisps (to conform with FDA regulations, Pringles no longer calls these chips "Light") at about 18 sat-fat calories per 14 slender little crisps is not much of a bargain, either, fatwise (60 fat calories). If you have enough self-control to eat just a few chips, fit them in. But don't even open the bag if you and your arteries will regret it later.

Crackers

Since the last edition of *Eater's Choice* was published, hydrogenated and partially hydrogenated vegetable oils have replaced tropical oils in most crackers. This change has lowered the saturated fat content on the food label but has raised the trans fat content of the crackers, and trans fats are no friend to your arteries. Crackers have three additional problems. First, they are usually so small, you hardly notice that you have eaten ten (or more) in one sitting. And, of course, the fats add up, as one cracker after another disappears into your mouth. Next, most crackers are high in total fat. And, finally, crackers prefer not to be eaten alone. When you add up the sat-fat calories of the Cheddar cheese or sour cream and onion dip that tops your cracker, you have a mighty high sat-fat snack.

Nuts

Nuts are a popular snack choice. The trouble with nuts is that they are very high in total fat and thus high in fat calories: about 126 to 196 calories per ounce. (Only 35 shelled peanuts, a small handful, weigh an ounce.) Nuts are also addictive. Who ever heard of eating one peanut? A couple of handfuls disappear without notice — but you and everyone else will notice soon enough if you overdose on nuts. Eat nuts sparingly.

If you must eat nuts, the ones with the least amount of saturated fat are walnuts, pecans, almonds, pistachios, and hazelnuts (about 13 to 17 sat-fat calories per ounce of dry-roasted shelled nuts).

The Bad Guys

Cashews, macadamia nuts, brazil nuts, and coconut contain, in increasing order, greater amounts of saturated fat. Coconut is almost purely saturated fat and should be avoided like the plague.

Peanut Butter

Pure, unadulterated peanut butter is a high-protein food, composed mainly of monounsaturated fats and a relatively small amount of saturated fat (12 sat-fat calories per tablespoon). All-natural peanut butters made from peanuts only, no salt added, are often ground and packaged in your local grocery stores. That is the good news. The bad news is that peanut butter is a high-fat food. It derives 72 of its 95 total calories (per tablespoon) from fat. And, in addition, experiments implicate peanut oil in clogging the arteries of some animals. Beware processed peanut butters, which are filled with added salt, sugar, and partially hydrogenated vegetable fats. Eat peanut butter in moderation.

Seeds

Sunflower seeds are often considered healthy. Any food that contains 36 sat-fat calories (and 135 fat calories) per ounce should not be mistaken for health food. Seeds naturally contain a lot of fat, but when stuck into a little bag with added salt and fat, seeds are a particularly poor choice.

Veggies

Tasty, healthy, and filling, but often overlooked as snacks, are cut-up vegetables. Carrots, cauliflower, broccoli, celery, and cucumbers may be eaten raw or with a low-fat yogurt dip.

Yogurt

A carton of yogurt is a refreshing snack. (See page 80.) Choose nonfat, flavored yogurts. They give you gustatory pleasure without adding a single sat-fat calorie to your Sat-Fat Budget. (Ron says eating Colombo Fat-Free Vanilla Yogurt is like eating ice cream.)

Pretzels

A real treat is a large twisted pretzel with 0 fat and 0 sat-fat calories. (Pretzels vary in fat content, so be sure to check the nutrition label.) You might want to scrape off some of the salt before you begin to munch. Do be careful. A few pretzels are a great snack, but stop at a few. Better to fill up on fruit, vegetables, or whole grains, which provide vitamins, minerals, and fiber.

Muffins, Bagels, Etc.

An *Eater's Choice* Oat Bran Muffin (pages 372–74) with coffee, a slice of Honey Whole-Wheat Bread (page 362) with a glass of skim or low-fat milk, or half a bagel with margarine make excellent snacks. Of course, you know any snack should be eaten in moderation — even healthy ones.

FAST FOODS

You lead a busy life. Fast-food restaurants offer the chance to pop in and get a filling and tasty meal at a moderate price. But is it healthy for your heart?

The road to heart-health does not run through a fast-food restaurant. The bulk of fast-food offerings are high-sat-fat and high-fat. For example, a Burger King Double Whopper with Cheese has a whopping 216 sat-fat calories (and 549 total fat calories!), an Arby's Baked Potato Deluxe contains 162 sat-fat calories. A Jack in the Box Chicken Supreme Sandwich has 90 sat-fat calories. Even though some new offerings can easily fit into your Sat-Fat Budget, it is difficult to resist all the other high-sat-fat and high-fat goodies available.

In addition, what happens to family togetherness when dinner time consists of grabbing a bite to eat at a fast-food restaurant? What are you teaching your children?

- It doesn't matter what you eat as long as it's quick.
- High-fat food tastes great and is good for you.

And what aren't your children learning?

- Vegetables, fruits, and whole grains taste great and are essential for a balanced and healthy diet.

Fast-food restaurants must be approached carefully and rarely. But, if you happen to find yourself in a city that has nothing but fast-food restaurants and you haven't eaten in a week, here are some low-fat choices to consider.

The New Fast-Food Rage — Chicken

Responding to the fat-conscious market, fast-food moguls have introduced a food that people associate with low-fat — chicken. Carl's Jr. claims its Charbroiler BBQ Chicken Sandwich has 18 sat-fat calories. Jack in the Box lists its Chicken Fajita Pita as containing 26 sat-fat calories. Other chicken offerings (such as Burger King's Broiler Chicken Sandwich with no mayo at 27 sat-fat calories or Arby's Chicken Breast Fillet Sandwich at 27 sat-fat calories), while not extremely high in saturated fat, are very high in total fat and thus not a buy, healthwise. Arby's Chicken Breast Fillet Sandwich contains 203 total fat calories. That's two-thirds of a 130-pound woman's total daily Fat Budget. Be careful. Check the *Eater's Choice* Food Tables before you go to a fast-food restaurant and order. Just because the dish is chicken does not mean it is low in sat-fat and/or low in total fat.

Low-Fat Fish + Fat = High-Fat Fish

Likewise, f-i-s-h does not always spell low-fat. The Dairy Queen fish fillet sandwich with no cheese may have only 27 sat-fat calories, but it has too many total fat calories (144) to make it a wise choice. Except for Dairy Queen's fish fillet, fish fillet sandwiches range from a low (which is really quite high) of 216 fat calories at Hardee's to a high of 288 total fat calories at Jack in the Box. Consider other options before you order a fish fillet sandwich.

Salad Bars

Many fast-food restaurants offer salad bars. All the dangers of any salad bar exist (see discussion, page 101), but if you stick to fresh fruit and vegetables and a minimal amount of dressing (note: the small ladle in a fast-food restaurant holds 2 tablespoons of dressing, the large one holds 4 tablespoons), you will not break your sat-fat bank. However, you won't be getting much to eat and may be tempted to supplement your salad with high-fat snacks later.

Overdose on Sodium

In addition to containing large amounts of saturated fat, fast foods contain very large amounts of sodium: a Big Mac contains 1010 mg of sodium, a Dairy Queen Super Brazier hot dog with cheese contains 1986 mg of sodium, Arby's club sandwich contains 1610 mg. Your intake of sodium should be between 1100 and 3300 mg for the whole day. (See Chapter 9.) Each of these items contains more than enough sodium to catapult you over the daily minimum without any additional sources of sodium for the day. With sodium from other foods eaten that day, you are likely to exceed even the maximum allotment of sodium. This is especially a problem if you have high blood pressure.

Underdose on Health

Be sure to check the Food Tables at the back of the book before going to a fast-food restaurant. Do not stray from your original choice when temptation rears its ugly head. And remember, although fast-food restaurants are using fewer saturated fats, the total fat and sodium poured into their offerings are enough to add pounds to your body and subtract years from your life.

FROZEN DINNERS

Take a look at the frozen foods section of your grocery store to get a picture of our changing lifestyle. The freezer cases are jam-packed with microwave dinners for people who don't want to take time to cook. Frozen dinners may be quick, but what are you saving time for? You pay for convenience both in money and health. When you buy a beef sirloin tips dinner (Healthy Choice) you are paying about $28 a pound for the beef and about four times more for the dinner than if you made it yourself. To save a few minutes in the kitchen costs you about 90 sat-fat calories when you stick a Budget Gourmet Chicken with Fettuccine in your microwave. If you prepare Asparagus Pasta with chicken (page 325) instead, it will cost you 5 sat-fat calories and perhaps 20 minutes of preparation time. Steam some broccoli or carrots, bake *Eater's Choice* Potato Skins or a sweet potato, and you have a real feast at a cost of $1.50 (if the chicken is not on sale). For very little expenditure of time and money you will have created a dinner you and your arteries can truly enjoy.

THE JOYS OF REAL FOOD

Perhaps you have to go to a fast-food restaurant or grab a frozen dinner every once in a blue moon. But, on the whole, why not eat real food? Every recipe need not be time-consuming. Try the recipes marked Q in this book, for starters. They are quick and easy. Sitting down with your family in relaxed surroundings is more heart-healthy than spending ten seconds at a fast-food joint, stuffing your mouth with a highly saturated piece of rubbery, salty meat surrounded by airy white bread. Your dinner will also be much more delicious and filling than the contents of a little box heated up in your microwave.

This sentiment needs repeating: take time to make real food. One hour a day to prepare dinner is a small amount of time to devote to an activity that will lengthen and improve the quality of your life.

Remember:

1. Red meats such as beef, veal, lamb, and some pork products are extremely high in saturated fat. The higher the grade of meat, the more saturated fat it contains.
2. Turkey and chicken with the skin removed and fish are all low in saturated fat. (Always remove the skin *before* you cook poultry.) Beware of sat-fat added in preparation.
3. Dairy products are excellent sources of calcium but many are high in fat and saturated fat. Whole milk derives almost half its calories from fat. Most cheeses derive about 80 percent of their calories from fat. Choose low-fat dairy products, such as low-fat yogurt, low-fat cottage cheese, and skim milk.
4. Recent evidence indicates that olive oil, rich in monounsaturated fatty acids, may be the most heart-healthy oil. But before you chug-a-lug a glass of olive oil each morning for breakfast, remember that all fats and oils are fattening and increase your risk for certain cancers, diabetes, and obesity. For long-term good health, reduce all the fats in your diet.
5. Coconut oil, which is found in many commercial foods, is one of the most heart-risky foods you can eat. *Avoid it diligently.*
6. Most fast foods are loaded with sat-fat and sodium. Do your coronary arteries a lifelong favor by staying clear of fast-food restaurants.
7. The cost of frozen dinners can be high in terms of dollars, health, and real enjoyment of food. Cooking from scratch can be quick, easy, healthy, and truly delicious and satisfying.

FROM THEORY TO PRACTICE 8

YOU ARE NOW ready to act. You have already figured out your ideal caloric intake and your daily Sat-Fat Budget. Now you must look at your own eating pattern to see how much saturated fat you actually eat and how to reduce it.

Keep a Record. The best way to find out what you actually eat is to write down everything you consume for two or three days. Include a typical week day and a weekend day. *Write down everything.* Be sure to include that glass of orange juice you drank in the afternoon and that handful of peanuts you grabbed before dinner. Measure everything. (See "The Nitty-Gritty of How to Keep a Food Record," page 583.)

Next, use the food tables to find the total calories and sat-fat calories for the foods you ate and add them up.

This very important exercise may surprise you. You may discover that the Danish pastry you usually eat for breakfast squanders 45 sat-fat calories, without giving you any nutritional value. You may find that most of the saturated fat you eat is concentrated in a few foods, which you can easily change. Analyzing your eating pattern will allow you to make the most effective and enduring changes in the way you eat.

Slow, but Enduring. Having discovered the sat-fat pitfalls in your daily food record, you may be eager to take immediate action and completely revamp your eating pattern. However, slow down! If you make too many changes too fast, you are not likely to stick with them. The changes in your eating pattern will do you and your heart good only if they are permanent.

Remember, it takes years to develop the atherosclerotic plaque that blocks the coronary arteries. Taking a few months to modify your lifelong eating patterns should not cause any harm and will result in more lasting changes.

APPROACH I

One approach to making gradual changes is to focus your attention on the worst culprits. Can you eat these less often, in smaller amounts, or even not at all? Go for the worst first. Change one or a few things at a time.

First, write down your menu for yesterday. Say it looks like this:

	CALORIES	
FOOD ITEM	TOTAL	SAT-FAT
Breakfast		
Soft-boiled egg	79	15
3 slices bacon	109	30
1 slice whole-wheat toast	60	1
1 pat butter	36	23
Coffee + 1 tbsp half-and-half	20	10
Lunch		
Burger King Whopper with cheese	706	144
10 french fries	220	33
Pepsi Lite	1	0
Dinner		
6 oz sirloin steak	372	72
1 small baked potato	105	0
1 pat butter	36	23
1 cup ice cream	270	80
Coffee + 1 tbsp half-and-half	20	10
Snack		
1 cup whole milk	150	45
Total	2184	486

Interesting. If your total calorie intake for the day was supposed to be 2000, 486 is way over your sat-fat allotment of 200 calories allowed on the *Eater's Choice* 10 Percent Plan. You need to eliminate 286 calories of saturated fat to get down to your 200 calorie Sat-Fat Budget.

REPLACEMENT FOOD ITEMS	CALORIES		SAVINGS IN SAT-FAT CALORIES
	TOTAL	SAT-FAT	
Breakfast			
1 *Buttermilk Waffle*	138	2	13
1 tbsp maple syrup	61	0	
1 slice Canadian bacon	43	6	24
1 orange	60	0	1
8 oz nonfat cherry yogurt	190	0	23
Coffee + 1 tbsp 2% milk	8	2	8
Lunch			
Turkey sandwich			
3 oz turkey breast	114	3 ⎫	
2 slices whole-wheat bread	120	2 ⎬	134
1 tsp mayonnaise	33	5 ⎭	
10 french fries	220	33	0
Orange juice	110	0	0
Dinner			
1 serving *Lemon Chicken*	174	4	68
¾ cup rice	149	1	(1)
1 medium baked potato	146	0	0
2 tbsp nonfat yogurt	14	0	23
Steamed broccoli w/ lemon	53	1	(1)
Mixed salad	8	0	
1 tbsp Italian dressing	69	9	(9)
1 slice whole-wheat bread	60	1	(1)
1 tsp margarine	30	5	(5)
1 cup ice milk	184	32	48
Coffee + 1 tbsp 2% milk	8	2	8
Snack			
1 oz Cheerios	110	3	(3)
1 cup 2% milk	121	27	18
Total	2223	138	348

What contributes the most saturated fat for the day? The Burger King Whopper with cheese at 144. How about having a tuna or turkey breast sandwich (3 ounces of either, with 1 teaspoon of mayonnaise) at 10 sat-fat calories each? With the turkey breast, the sat-fat total for the day becomes 352. That's beginning to look a lot better.

Can you do without those fatty strips of bacon? Replace the bacon with Canadian bacon and reduce your sat-fat calories from 30 to 6. Why not eat that egg on a day when your cholesterol intake is not so high? How about eating ice milk (32 sat-fat calories) instead of ice cream (80 sat-fat calories)? And instead of butter (23 sat-fat calories) on your potato, try nonfat yogurt (0 sat-fat calories) or eat it plain. Why waste 72 sat-fat calories on steak? Have a luscious *Eater's Choice* entree such as *Lemon Chicken* (4 sat-fat calories) on rice instead. All the changes listed in the modified meal plan on page 97 bring your daily total sat-fat intake to 138 calories. Great! You've brought your sat-fat intake below your budget and it was painless.

A Few "Sacrifices" for the Old Bod'

By evaluating your eating habits and figuring out what foods you can do without or replace with less fatty substitutes, you can bring your saturated fat total down with little pain. The next stage is to make a few sacrifices. (You will find that these so-called sacrifices are not sacrifices at all. You are substituting foods that are just as satisfying or *more* satisfying than those you ate before.)

Try drinking 1% milk instead of 2%. That's a reduction of 13 calories of saturated fat per cup. How about skipping fatty desserts every day but Sunday? Wow. Watch that sat-fat total drop.

Use small amounts of beef as a condiment with rice or pasta. Choose leaner cuts of beef, such as trimmed round. Instead of having beef four times a week, eat it only twice a week. Perhaps not at all.

Replace some or all of your red meat meals with chicken, turkey, or fish. (This book is filled with scrumptious recipes for chicken, turkey, and fish. Try them.) Notice how much impact the substitution of fish or poultry for beef has on your daily saturated fat intake. Also notice how eliminating sat-fat calories from meat frees up calories that you can spend on a wide variety of foods — foods that are tasty, nutritious, and low or moderate in fat content.

REMEMBER: as you reduce your fat intake, increase your complex carbohydrate intake. Eat more whole-grain cereals and breads, rice, and pasta. Eat more fruits and vegetables. You will feel less lethargic after meals, you will be more regular, you will undoubtedly lose weight, and, who knows, you might have a better sex life.

APPROACH 2

An alternative approach to changing your eating habits is to focus on changing one meal at a time. For example, for the first few weeks only make changes in your breakfast menu. Get rid of that bacon and sausage. Eliminate those doughnuts at 40 calories of saturated fat each, not to mention all that sugar. Avoid granola: it is billed as healthy but look how saturated it is. Notice the coconut they add. It is not worth clogging your arteries for a little crunch.

New Breakfast

How about toast and margarine or jelly? Try low-fat Cinnamon French Toast (page 379) or Buttermilk Pancakes (page 377), 1% cottage cheese in half a cantaloupe, strawberries and nonfat yogurt, oatmeal or oat bran with raisins and cinnamon, or a carton of flavored nonfat yogurt.

Oat bran, which became a national fad several years ago and then faded, is a rich source of soluble fiber. All foods that are high in soluble fiber, such as dried beans and peas, have a modest effect on lowering cholesterol.

If you enjoy hot oat bran cereal or oat bran muffins you bake at home (see Chapter 23 for a variety of tasty muffin recipes), eat away. (Warning: some commercial oat bran muffins contain so much saturated or total fat, they make doughnuts look like health food.) However, before you sprinkle oat bran in your orange juice and eat nine oat bran muffins a day, fill up on oat bran pretzels and oat bran beer, be forewarned that eating oat bran will not save you from the cholesterol-raising effects of a diet high in saturated fat. **A low sat-fat diet is the most effective way to maximize your cholesterol-lowering.**

WHERE TO FIND SOLUBLE FIBER*

FOOD	SERVING SIZE	SOLUBLE FIBER (G)
Grains		
Oat bran	⅓ cup dry	2.0
All-Bran	⅓ cup	1.7
Oat bran muffin	1	1.6
Oatmeal	¾ cup, cooked	1.4
Rye bread	2 slices	0.6
Whole-wheat bread	2 slices	0.5
Dried Beans and Peas		
Black-eyed peas	½ cup, cooked	3.7
Kidney beans	½ cup, cooked	2.5
Pinto beans	½ cup, cooked	2.3
Navy beans	½ cup, cooked	2.3
Lentils	½ cup, cooked	1.7
Split peas	½ cup, cooked	1.7
Vegetables		
Peas	½ cup, cooked	2.7
Corn	½ cup, cooked	1.7
Sweet potato	1 baked	1.3
Zucchini	½ cup, cooked	1.3
Cauliflower	½ cup, cooked	1.3
Broccoli	½ cup, cooked	0.9
Fruit		
Prunes	4	1.9
Pears	1	1.1
Apples	1	0.9
Bananas	1	0.8
Oranges	1	0.7

*From: Nutrition Action Healthletter, Center for Science in the Public Interest, December 1985.

NOW FOR LUNCH

After you have established new and lasting changes in your breakfast, you will be ready to make changes in lunch. If you often eat this meal out, you have an additional challenge. You will have less control over the foods available than if you bring your lunch from home. (See Chapter 10 for tips on how to eat out.)

You might want to consider these options: eating out less often and bringing lunch from home more often; choosing low-fat, low saturated fat items from the menu and passing up the high-fat, heart-risky items; choosing restaurants that offer more low-fat, low saturated fat menu choices. The last option may be especially necessary if you are used to eating lunch in a fast-food restaurant.

If you have to eat at a fast-food restaurant, check the Food Tables first for the choices with the lowest amount of saturated fat. If that is impossible, stick to the salad bar, but be wary.

The Salad Bar: Lettuce, Tomatoes, and Fat

Don't assume that just because salads are composed of vegetables, fruits, and sometimes pastas, they are always healthy choices. The amount of saturated fat and total fat in many salad bar offerings — red potatoes in sour cream dressing, mayonnaise salad with a bit of macaroni, cold cuts swimming in oil — overrides their nutritious

---

YOUR MOTHER WAS RIGHT

Many adults have established the pattern of eating no breakfast and no lunch or a very light lunch. For some, the mistaken notion is that this is a good way to lose weight. For others, breakfast and lunch may be the casualties of life in the fast lane. In any case, it is much healthier to eat three well-balanced meals than to starve yourself all day. Stuffing into one meal all the calories and nutrients needed for functioning at peak efficiency makes for very low efficiency peaks.

The chances are that if you eat only one or two meals a day, you will get hungry and eat snacks. Most snacks are notoriously high in fat, saturated fat, sodium, and/or sugar and appallingly low in vitamins, minerals, and fiber.

The best policy is to make your three meals low-fat (see the meal plans in Chapter 13 for a variety of low-fat meal suggestions) and see if you don't feel better and function at an optimum.

benefits. Even plain salad greens and vegetables become high-fat fare when sprinkled with bacon bits, shredded cheese, and sesame seeds, and covered with a ladle or two or three or four (2 to 16 table-spoons) of high-fat and high-sat-fat dressing. Choose fruits and plain vegetables. Choose low-calorie dressings or make your own dressing with oil and vinegar. If you must use regular salad dressings, use the fork method (see page 84).

But consider a salad — even a low-fat salad — a side dish. A truly low-fat salad for lunch is not enough to eat. It may make you feel virtuous, but it can also leave you very hungry. Better to eat a sat-isfying, low-sat-fat lunch than to starve yourself on a bowl of rabbit food and fill up on high-fat snacks later.

Lunch Options

How about a turkey breast sandwich for lunch (not on a crois-sant, which is loaded with butter)? Most delis and sandwich shops carry white meat turkey sandwiches. Even with mayonnaise, a tur-key sandwich contains a mere 10 calories of saturated fat. How about a bowl of chili *non* carne (peas and beans are rich in protein and fiber and low in fat)? How about a big bowl of sliced fresh fruit mixed with low-fat yogurt or low-fat cottage cheese? How about a chef's salad (hold the cheese) with turkey and ham (optional) and low-fat dressing? Your coronary arteries are looking better and better.

How about filling a pita with last night's dinner and eating it for lunch? How about a pita sandwich of Chili Non Carne (page 322) topped with chopped green pepper, onion, tomato, and lettuce? What about a Bar-B-Que Chicken sandwich? Place Bar-B-Que Chicken (page 244) on a slice of bread, heat the sauce and spoon it over the chicken, cover with tomato and onion slices, and top with a second slice of bread. And, would you believe cheeseless pizza? You can order a vegetarian pizza without cheese at almost any pizza parlor for a real taste treat that is low in sat-fat.

One of the advantages of changing from a high-fat to a low-fat lunch will become evident immediately. You will not feel tired and sluggish after a low-fat meal, so you will be at your peak during the afternoon. You may be so energetic your boss will give you a raise. If you are the boss, you might give yourself a raise.

THE DINNER TACKLE

Finally, after you have both breakfast and lunch under control, you are ready to tackle dinner. Try beginning your meal with a low-fat soup, such as Cucumber Soup (page 192) at 2 sat-fat calories per bowl. Not only is it low in saturated fat, it is cooling, delicious, and one of the easiest-to-make soups known to modern man. Soups help fill you up so you are less tempted to gorge on the higher-fat foods in the main course and in dessert. If you make your own soups, you can control the amount of salt and fat you use. Make a large pot of soup and freeze part for future meals.

Why not eat a low-fat chicken or fish dish? Try Apricot Chicken Divine (page 223) or Shanghai Fish (page 278). Try Turkey Scaloppine Limone (page 259) or Kung Pao Chicken with Broccoli (page 234). There are so many delicious recipes for chicken, turkey, and fish it will take you years to try them all. Vegetable dishes should be explored. As an important part of the meal or as the main dish, vegetables offer interesting flavors and textures as well as vitamins, minerals, and fiber. When not drowned in fat, vegetables fill you up without filling you out. Pastas or rice mixed with a small amount of meat or poultry can make a tasty main dish low in sat-fat calories.

"But I must have beef, too," you cry. *Eater's Choice* allows you to fit beef into your Sat-Fat Budget — perhaps not as often as before, perhaps in smaller portions. Perhaps rather than eating a big fat steak four nights a week, you might eat steak one night, rice mixed with small pieces of beef another, vegetarian chili yet another, and fish, chicken, and turkey the rest of the week.

If you eat dinner in restaurants, many of the same considerations that applied to lunch are relevant.

Togetherness in Health

Since dinner is often the one meal that the whole family eats together, the question arises whether the whole family should eat low-fat, low–saturated fat meals. The simple answer is a loud YES. The American Heart Association recommends that all Americans over the age of two years adopt this new low-fat eating pattern. Both the American Heart Association and the National Cancer Institute recommend it to help prevent heart disease and certain cancers. (For more information about children and diet, read Chapter 12.)

Establish Good Eating Habits Early. If you or your spouse have high blood cholesterol levels, there is a good chance that your children will also have high blood cholesterol levels. Heart-healthy meals will benefit *everyone* in the family. The eating habits that will help you control your blood cholesterol will help your children avoid developing atherosclerosis in the first place. As you have probably already realized, it is hard to change long-established, deep-rooted eating habits. It will be much easier for your children to establish healthful eating habits when they are young than to change them halfway through life.

If everybody in the family eats the same way, you are more likely to stick to the new eating pattern. Of course, this means everyone must learn to eat new foods and recipes and gradually modify their eating pattern. It will be worth it. You will be doing your children and spouse a lifelong favor.

A BALANCED DIET; OR, MAN DOTH NOT LIVE ON LESS SATURATED FAT ALONE

Although *Eater's Choice* focuses on saturated fat, you must take care to eat foods from all major food groups: whole grains and cereals; vegetables; fruits; dairy; meats, fish, and poultry. It cannot be overemphasized that good long-term health depends on eating a variety of foods. You need about 40 different nutrients to stay healthy. These nutrients are in the foods you normally eat — as long as you eat many different types of foods.

See Chapter 11 for examples of foods in each food group and what nutrients they contain.

Tips to Keep Your Eating in Balance

Here are some important tips you should keep in mind as you change your eating habits:

1. Replace fats with filling, fiber-rich nutritious foods, such as whole grains, fruits, and vegetables (not sugars, which have no nutritional value beyond calories).
2. Under normal eating conditions, all the carbohydrates you eat are burned. None is stored as fat. It is not the carbohydrates

(such as potatoes or bread) but the fats (such as butter) added to them that cause weight gain.

3. Dried peas and beans (complex carbohydrates) are rich in protein and fiber and low in fat.

4. Choose whole-grain (such as whole-wheat bread) rather than refined-grain products (such as white bread); refining removes vitamins and fiber from the food.

5. Dried peas and beans and whole-oat products, such as oat bran, are high in soluble fiber and have been shown to lower blood cholesterol levels.

6. Be sure to include adequate amounts of calcium in your diet. Choose low-fat milk products, such as skim milk, low-fat yogurt, and low-fat cottage cheese. They are rich in calcium and low in saturated fat.

7. Certain polyunsaturated fats are required for good health and must be obtained from the diet (just like vitamins); you should not eliminate all sources of fat from your diet.

8. Choose cooking methods that do not add fat to otherwise low-fat, low–saturated fat foods. Baking, roasting, grilling, broiling, poaching, and steaming are preferred to frying (especially deep-frying). Try sautéing in a wok to reduce fat absorption.

9. Avoid fad or crash diets. Even though you are concentrating on removing saturated fat from your diet, you must consume an adequate supply of calories to maintain your desirable weight. It is important to realize that if you consume too few calories (fewer than 1500), your basal metabolic rate will slow down to prevent starvation (your body doesn't know you are starving on purpose) and frustrate your weight loss attempts. Also, if you eat fewer than 1500 calories a day you may not get an adequate supply of vitamins, minerals, and fiber. If you have any doubts about the adequacy of your daily dietary intake, consult a physician or registered dietitian.

Plan Ahead

As we mentioned above, you may find it helpful to develop meal plans for a whole week at a time. It will make shopping easier. But in any case, bring home a variety of foods that provide adequate amounts of vitamins, minerals, and fiber and are not overloaded with calories, refined sugars, sodium, and fats.

Heart-Healthy Storage. Today your cupboard is probably filled with all sorts of horrible, high sat-fat foods that make the new you shudder in disgust. Eventually, you will stock your larder (terrible term) with low-fat foods, herbs, spices, whole grains, and your refrigerator with fresh fruits and vegetables. (See Stocking Up, page 178, for suggestions of foods to keep on hand.)

In fact, the contents of your cupboard and refrigerator are good indicators of how seriously you are taking your cholesterol-lowering. When you are able to throw away that box of cheese crackers that you have been hoarding or that small carton of whipping cream that you just might need for a special occasion, you will know that you have really changed your lifestyle and are waltzing down the path of good living and heart-health — the ultimate goal of *Eater's Choice*.

Honesty Is the Best Heart-Healthy Policy

Eater's Choice only works if you follow it faithfully. Do not fool yourself. "Only one little bite . . . just this time" is the theme song for those who have elevated cholesterol levels. You may fool yourself, but you will not fool your blood cholesterol or your arteries.

Check and Recheck Blood Cholesterol Level

You should have your blood cholesterol level checked at frequent intervals to monitor the effectiveness of the changes you have made in your eating habits, especially at the beginning.

To help you and your physician interpret your numbers, you should also keep a three-day food record some time in the two-week period before your cholesterol test. (Read "The Nitty-Gritty of How to Keep a Food Record," page 583.)

By analyzing these records you will see how your sat-fat intake has affected your blood cholesterol level. You might find that your cholesterol dropped to 188 mg/dL because you eliminated fast-food restaurant-hopping. Or that your cholesterol rose by 50 points because you spent the last two weeks splurging and making exceptions. Or that a 10 percent Sat-Fat Budget is too high to bring your cholesterol number below 200 mg/dL, so you lower your Sat-Fat Budget to 6 or 7 percent. Or that you lowered your cholesterol by 30 points and are now ready to make more changes that will ensure another 30-point drop.

Each blood cholesterol check and food record review will give you insight. You might pat yourself on the back and continue to eat within your Sat-Fat Budget. Or you might shake your head in disgust or disappointment and rethink your diet.

The frequency of blood checks will be determined by your physician. After your blood cholesterol has been stabilized below 200 mg/dL, you probably will not need to have your level checked more than once a year.

Remember:

1. Easy does it. Make changes in your eating pattern *slowly* so that they will be *permanent* changes.
2. To make gradual changes:

   Approach 1: Reduce or change the foods in your daily menu that contribute the most saturated fat. If this does not lower your blood cholesterol level to below 200 mg/dL, make more changes.

   Approach 2: Focus on one meal at a time. First eliminate those highly saturated breakfast foods you can do without and replace them with foods low in saturated fat. After you have established new and lasting changes in breakfast, make changes in lunch and then dinner.

3. Be sure to choose foods from all major food groups: whole grains and cereals; vegetables; fruits; dairy; meats (meat, poultry, fish, dried peas and beans, eggs, and nuts). Only a well-balanced diet will provide all the essential minerals, vitamins, fiber, and calories.
4. Dried peas and beans and oat bran have been shown to have a modest effect on lowering blood cholesterol levels.
5. Have your blood cholesterol measured periodically to learn how much your new eating habits have lowered your blood cholesterol level.

9 OTHER RISK FACTORS FOR CORONARY HEART DISEASE

$\mathbf{W}$E HAVE WRITTEN this book out of our zeal to see coronary heart disease go the way of diphtheria and polio, to see it become a medical curiosity of the past. Our emphasis is on one of the most important risk factors for heart disease: blood cholesterol. Of course, there are other risk factors for coronary heart disease.

Heart disease is the leading cause of death in the United States. It kills three times as many people as all forms of cancer combined. Think of the people you know. According to national statistics, on average, half of the people you know will die of coronary heart disease.

Scientists have identified the major factors that increase risk of heart attacks. You have no control over some of these risks. However, you can affect their influence by modifying those risk factors over which you do have control.

RISKS YOU CANNOT CONTROL

Family History

Heart disease tends to run in families and thus has a genetic or inherited component. If one or both of your parents had a heart attack before the age of sixty, your chances of having one are increased by twofold.

Sex

Men have a greater chance of having a heart attack than women. Fifty-year-old men have a fivefold greater risk of having a heart attack by the age of sixty than do fifty-year-old women. Women seem

108

to be protected from heart disease before menopause by their sex hormones. At the onset of menopause, a woman's risk of heart disease begins to rise. Whereas the rate of heart attacks in men begins to rise at about age forty-five, in women comparable rates are not seen until about age sixty. Lest women feel too complacent about their low rates of heart disease in middle age, they should know that heart disease is the leading cause of death for older women.

Age

In America, risk of heart disease increases with age for both men and women. For men thirty-five to sixty-five years old, risk of heart attack increases twofold for each decade of life. For women forty-five to sixty-five years old, risk increases threefold for each decade of life. In both cases, this increase is *not* a natural result of aging. It is a result of lifestyle. In cultures where a low-sat-fat diet is the norm, both men and women live to ripe old ages unaffected by heart disease.

While heart disease strikes beginning in middle age, it is never too early to change your lifestyle to lower your risk. Remember: the underlying disease process (clogging of the coronary arteries) begins in childhood. Don't let the lack of symptoms fool you into complacency. On the other hand, if you are already middle-aged or older, do not lose hope. It is never too late to lower your blood cholesterol and slow down, stop, or even reverse the blockage of your coronary arteries.

DON'T JOIN THE ODDS, BEAT THEM!

Do not use the fact that you have a bad family history, that you are old, or that you are a male as an excuse to die of a heart attack. Bringing down your blood cholesterol level to below 200 mg/dL by eating a diet low in saturated fat gives you the same odds as people without those risks.

RISKS YOU CAN CONTROL

The fact that you cannot change your age, sex, or parents should not discourage you. The uncontrollable risk factors account for only a part of the total risk. The rest is accounted for by three powerful risk factors over which you do have control: cigarette smoking, high blood pressure, and high blood cholesterol.

Smoking

Most people associate cigarette smoking with lung cancer. While it is true that most lung cancer is caused by smoking, cigarettes cause more coronary heart disease than lung cancer. Smoking one pack a day doubles the risk of a heart attack, while smoking more than one pack a day triples the risk. In addition to heart disease, smoking causes serious diseases of the lungs, such as emphysema and chronic obstructive lung disease, resulting in an estimated 50,000 preventable deaths each year.

If you smoke, you should realize that it is never too late to benefit from quitting. Your risk of coronary heart disease begins to decrease immediately upon stopping. If you smoke one pack a day, your risk of heart disease one to five years after stopping is only 20 percent higher than that of a person who never smoked. Ten years after stopping, you are at no higher risk for heart disease than if you had never smoked. If you smoke more than one pack a day, your risk of heart disease is three times higher than that of a person who never smoked. One year after stopping, your risk drops to one and one-half times higher than that of a person who never smoked. By twenty years after quitting, you are at no higher risk for heart disease than if you had never smoked. So take control of your life and give up the weed. Reduce your risk of heart disease, lung disease, and cancer all in one fell swoop by quitting smoking once and for all.

High Blood Pressure

Both high blood pressure (often called hypertension) and high blood cholesterol are silent killers. They are called silent because there are usually no symptoms or telltale signs. You will not know if you have these risk factors unless you have them measured. Yet they are both deadly. High blood pressure can cause strokes, aneurysms (the weakening and bursting of an artery wall, which causes massive internal bleeding and often sudden death), and coronary heart disease.

About 60 million Americans, or 1 out of every 4 adults, have high blood pressure. High blood pressure is a leading cause of the 500,000 strokes, 175,000 stroke deaths, and 550,000 heart attack deaths each year. High blood pressure is most common in blacks, the obese, diabetics, the elderly, and women taking oral contraceptives. The presence of high blood pressure doubles the risk of coronary heart disease and raises the risk of stroke by sevenfold.

The Joint National Committee of the High Blood Pressure Education Program recommends that blood pressures should be lower than 120/80 mm Hg. The lower the blood pressure, the lower are the risks of strokes, aneurysms, and heart disease.

Like high cholesterol, high blood pressure is under *your* control. Regular aerobic exercise and, when necessary, weight reduction* are potent medicine against hypertension. In addition, people whose blood pressure is sodium-sensitive should reduce their intake of sodium to about 1100 mg per day (see your doctor for a recommendation). Everyone else should reduce intake to between 1100 and 3300 mg per day. (For reference, 1 teaspoon of table salt contains 2132 mg of sodium.) In general, Americans consume far too much sodium. Currently, the average American consumes 4000 to 5000 mg of sodium each day. *The Sodium Content of Your Food* (*Home and Garden Bulletin* Number 233, U.S. Department of Agriculture) is a useful publication to help you keep track of your sodium intake. It is available from the Government Printing Office, Washington, D.C. 20402.

Risks Are Additive

The presence of any one of the three controllable risk factors (high blood cholesterol, high blood pressure, smoking) doubles your risk of heart disease (see Figure 1, Chapter 1). The simultaneous presence of two of these risk factors quadruples your risk. The addition of the third risk factor increases the risk yet another twofold, resulting in an eightfold higher risk of heart disease. The elimination of a risk factor has an equal but opposite effect on risk as does its addition. Thus, smokers with high blood pressure and high blood cholesterol who quit smoking and reduce their blood pressure and blood cholesterol to healthy levels can cut their risk of heart attack by up to eightfold!

Choose to Lose: A Food Lover's Guide to Permanent Weight Loss provides a simple, flexible, and effective plan to lose weight and thus reduce hypertension.

OTHER RISK FACTORS

Diabetes Mellitus

Diabetics have a twofold greater rate of coronary heart disease than do normal people. Moreover, diabetics who survive a heart attack have a poor long-term prognosis. Finally, heart disease is more likely to be fatal in diabetics than in people with normal glucose tolerance. The increased risk of coronary heart disease due to diabetes is independent of the other major risk factors, high blood cholesterol and high blood pressure. But diabetics can lower their risk of coronary heart disease by lowering their blood cholesterol and blood pressure. For diabetics as well as nondiabetics, diet is the first line of treatment for lowering blood cholesterol and blood pressure.

The new dietary recommendations for diabetics are similar to those recommended in this book for persons who want to lower their blood cholesterol levels. Thus, diabetics should reduce their intake of saturated fat and cholesterol and increase their intake of complex carbohydrates and fiber. They should limit their intake of simple or refined sugars.

Obesity

Obese people suffer significantly higher rates of illness and death than people of the same age who are not overweight. Obesity is associated with higher rates of angina pectoris, stroke, and sudden death. High blood pressure and diabetes, risk factors for heart disease, are three times more common in obese people. Death rates from heart disease are 50 percent higher for obese people. In general, the risk of death increases about 2 percent for every pound over "desirable" weight (National Institutes of Health Consensus Conference on Obesity).

Obesity also increases the risk of developing arthritis, respiratory disorders, cancer of the uterus, breast, and cervix in women, and cancer of the colon, rectum, and prostate in men.

An effective way to combat obesity is to follow *Eater's Choice*. Although not designed as a weight-loss diet, responses from readers have shown us that the *Eater's Choice* system often results in weight loss (15–20 pounds is typical; more than 40 pounds has been reported). This is easy to understand. Following *Eater's Choice*, the eater learns to make choices that are heart-healthy — and coincidentally low in fat. And scientific research has shown that fat makes fat. The only drawback in following *Eater's Choice* for weight loss is that it is possible to eat a diet low in saturated fat and not lose weight. This is because some foods, such as olive, safflower, sunflower, and corn oils and margarine, may be low in saturated fat and thus heart-healthy, but are extremely high in total fat, and thus fattening. *Choose to Lose* focuses on reducing total fat for weight loss. Fat has more calories (9) per gram of weight than protein (4) or carbohydrates (4). The fat you eat immediately becomes the squishy, soft pads on your body. The *Choose to Lose* method uses a Fat Budget similar to the *Eater's Choice* Sat-Fat Budget. Based on a diet low in fat, daily aerobic exercise (walking), and an increased consumption of complex carbohydrates (fruits, vegetables, and whole grains), *Choose to Lose* allows you to fit in your favorite high-fat foods, eat loads of delicious low-fat foods, and feel better than ever while your body gets leaner and leaner.

Lack of Physical Exercise

Exercise is an important part of a healthy lifestyle and is essential for cardiovascular fitness. While it may not prevent you from having a heart attack, data suggest it will increase your chances of survival. Regular exercise helps control weight and lower blood pressure.

Most experts recommend moderate aerobic exercise for the maximum cardiovascular benefit. Aerobic exercise involves continuous exertion, usually in a repetitive or rhythmic motion. Examples include running or jogging, walking, rowing, swimming, bicycling, aerobic dancing, and jumping rope. When exercise is aerobic and performed with sufficient intensity and duration, it will raise HDL-cholesterol. But before you wear yourself to a frazzle running fifteen miles a day so you can eat lardburgers at every meal, be advised that exercise does not negate the ill effects of a high-fat diet. The best way to lower your LDL-cholesterol and thus your risk of a heart attack is to reduce your intake of saturated fat.

Aerobic exercise also aids in weight control by building and preserving fat-burning muscle mass. The more aerobic exercise you do, the more fat you will burn from your fat stores and the leaner you will become. Regular aerobic exercise also has many other benefits, such as an improved feeling of well-being, more energy, and reduced risks of osteoporosis and certain cancers.

A WORD OF CAUTION: Exercise may increase the risk of sudden death in people with advanced coronary atherosclerosis. If you are forty or older and have a sedentary lifestyle, it is highly advisable to have a physical examination by a physician, including an electrocardiogram (and even an exercise electrocardiogram) before starting an exercise program. It is also helpful to get professional guidance in designing your exercise program, to ensure that the exercises you choose are not harmful or dangerous, that you start off slowly and intensify your efforts at the appropriate rate, that you vary your exercise program to prevent fatigue, boredom, and drop-out, and, finally, that you get the most cardiovascular benefit from the time and effort you invest.

Like other lifestyle changes that you might be making at this time, exercise will only benefit your cardiovascular system and your overall health if you continue to do it faithfully. It cannot be a sometime thing. Excuse the pun, but it is for life.

High Blood Triglycerides

Many medical experts consider triglycerides to be normal up to 250 mg/dL. However, the combination of triglycerides of 150 or higher with a very low HDL level — below 40 mg/dL — puts you at high risk for heart disease. Generally, people with triglyceride levels above 250 mg/dL have a low HDL and are at increased risk of cardiovascular disease. Those with levels above 500 mg/dL are at additional risk of pancreatitis. For most people, lowering their triglyceride levels will raise their HDL levels and thus reduce their risk of heart disease.

Elevated triglyceride levels can be reduced by the following lifestyle changes: weight loss (if overweight), regular aerobic exercise, restriction of alcohol consumption, and reduced intakes of simple sugars (sweets) and saturated fats (as recommended by *Eater's Choice*). Some people may have to use drugs if diet does not normalize their triglyceride levels.

Stress

It is a commonly held belief that stress increases the risk of coronary heart disease. Scientists have not been able to confirm or deny this relationship. They are hampered by the difficulty in measuring and quantifying stress. What is stressful to you may not be stressful to others. Furthermore, people react to the same stress in different ways.

It is unclear whether stress increases heart disease directly. What is true is that people under stress often give up healthy lifestyle behaviors and thus increase their risk for heart disease. They abandon exercise and eat a diet high in saturated fat. An often quoted study examined accountants at tax time to determine if stress elevates cholesterol. The study was flawed. Yes, cholesterol levels did rise at tax time, but the study neglected to record food intake. Were the accountants stuffing down a Big Mac or two enhanced by french fries and nachos because they felt too stressed to take time out for a real meal?

Type A Behavior Pattern

People with Type A behavior patterns are characterized as hard-driving, impatient, and time-conscious. Type B people, on the other hand, are easygoing. Numerous studies have shown Type A behavior pattern to be a risk factor for developing coronary heart disease. But in all fairness, it must be said that other studies have not confirmed this observation, and so the jury is still out on the importance of Type A behavior in the development of heart disease.

Remember:

1. The major risk factors of heart disease you cannot control are family history of heart disease, sex, and age.
2. The major risk factors you *can* control (in addition to high blood cholesterol) are high blood pressure and cigarette smoking.
3. Other risk factors include diabetes mellitus, obesity, lack of physical activity, and high blood triglycerides.

10 THE REAL WORLD

YOUR NEW eating pattern is for life — in two ways. It will improve your chances for a long and healthy life, and you must follow it for the rest of your life. Following *Eater's Choice* is easy, and you will find that eating heart-healthy foods can be more satisfying than eating your old heart-risky ones.

HONESTY IS THE HEALTHIEST POLICY

Remember: you *must* be honest with yourself. Don't make exceptions — even for special occasions — or before you know it you will be off the eating plan. Face it: we all have an almost infinite capacity to fool ourselves about how much and how often we eat certain foods. We constantly underestimate the calories, fat, and sugar we consume. We make a small change in our diet and feel so sorry for ourselves that we reward ourselves with treats that negate our progress. We don't want to make a fuss or feel embarrassed, so we eat foods we should avoid when we dine out. We see special occasions deserving of exceptions in everyday occurrences, such as office parties, weekends, birthdays, going out to eat, even when this is a weekly or more frequent event. The favorite expressions of the cheater-eater are "Just this one time" and "This little bit couldn't possibly matter."

These problems do not have to be yours. Be strong. It's your life. Cheater-eaters only cheat themselves. *Eater's Choice* eaters don't need to cheat. They plan ahead. *Eater's Choice* is a flexible plan that allows you to eat your favorite foods as well as enjoy an occasional splurge. (See Chapter 13.)

Heart-Healthy Tips

- Avoid eating on the run, which may necessitate eating fast foods or junk food from vending machines. The time you save in the present may cost you dearly in the future.
- To save yourself from a massive pig-out attack, eat *before* you attend a party where you know high sat-fat foods will be served.
- Try to avoid grocery shopping when you are hungry. In a fit of hunger you might satisfy your craving with a tub of ice cream.
- When you feel like eating something sweet, give yourself a cool, refreshing treat. Create a Frothy Fruit Shake in your blender (see page 350).
- Instead of snacking on high-fat foods, make Bagel Chips (page 348). They taste great plain or dipped in Faux Guacamole (page 347).
- Make popcorn (air-popped with no butter added) for a snack while watching TV or visiting friends. Popcorn is a low-fat, low-calorie, high-fiber food, and it's cheap.
- Turn off the TV or leave the room when food ads appear. (Do not go to the kitchen!) Many of the ads on TV are devoted to glorifying the fattiest, most heart-risky foods available to mankind. Watching food ads will make you hungry for these artery cloggers.

BE PROUD OF THE NEW YOU

You should not be ashamed that you are watching your fat intake. By letting your friends, colleagues, and family know that you are serious about your new eating pattern, you can solicit their support. Do not let them make you feel guilty because you are eating healthfully and they may not be.

Truly good friends *will* help, by cooking or serving foods low in saturated fat for you, encouraging you to stay on your new eating plan, suggesting restaurants that offer low-fat entrees. You should never feel pressured either by words or by the situation to stray from your eating plan. Say no politely, but firmly. You'll be respected for your self-control. And who knows, perhaps your friends and relatives will begin to see how good you look, how great you feel, and how well you are eating. You might just have a positive influence on their lifestyles.

EATING OUT

Eating out is no longer a rarity, a twice-a-year entertainment or treat. Eating at home has become the rarity. For those of you who haven't been cooking long or at all, don't give up before you try. You may even enjoy it. For those of you who are veteran cooks and want to retire, don't give up now. Your family's health and taste buds, as well as your own, are counting on you.

When you cook your own food, you control the ingredients. When you eat out, even when you think you are beating the high-fat system, fat sneaks in. Butter is stirred into the rice, chicken is baked with the skin, the yogurt dressing is high in fat. And, really, does the food taste that good? You will do yourself a gigantic favor by cooking food from scratch at home. This does not mean bringing carry-out or frozen dinners home. This means cooking all of the scrumptious *Eater's Choice* recipes and really enjoying eating while making your coronaries croon with joy.

Tips for Survival

For the few, rare times that you eat out, here are a few tips that will help you enjoy yourself and eat within your Sat-Fat Budget.

- First, choose your restaurant wisely. Learn which restaurants serve foods low in saturated fat. Avoid restaurants where you have no choices.
- Be prepared to ask lots of questions. Most restaurants that serve chicken and fish can prepare them without butter, cream sauces, or other added fats. Do not be afraid to ask what the ingredients are and how the dish is prepared. Perhaps you can eat the cream sauce: just ask what's in it.

At the Restaurant: Plan of Action, or Taking Control

1. Ask the maître d' for the menu. Review it for low-sat-fat options before you sit down at a table. (To save yourself a trip, call the restaurant and ask questions *beforehand*.) Do you see any low-sat-fat foods you can eat? Can adaptations be made to reduce saturated fat? If you find no dish acceptable or even adaptable to your needs, leave and find another restaurant.
2. If you decide to stay, you will want to study the menu more thoroughly when you sit down.

a. Unless you have saved for a splurge, eliminate the foods that have absolutely no potential for low sat-fat adaptation, such as a New York sirloin, leg of lamb, duck à l'orange (the saturated fat in duck will demolish your Sat-Fat Budget for a week), blanquette of veal, spare ribs, and breaded pork chops.

b. Next, find the dishes that are composed of foods naturally low in saturated fat, such as chicken, fish, or turkey, and try to determine how they are prepared. Was the dish grilled? or poached? or baked? or broiled? fried? deep-fried?

c. If you are not satisfied with the type of preparation, ask if the dish may be prepared in a different way. Can it be grilled with olive oil instead? Or baked with no fat? Can the skin be taken off the breast *before* cooking?

d. Ask about the ingredients. What's in the creamed soup? What's in the white sauce? What was the chicken marinated in?

e. See if adaptations can be made. Can the sauce be served on the side? Can the sauce be made with whole or 2% milk instead of cream? Can the French onion soup be made without cheese?

f. Ask about the vegetables, too. An overdose of butter is a natural addition to most restaurant rice and vegetables. Are the vegetables cooked with butter? Can margarine be used instead? Can they be steamed without fat? Can the rice be made without fat? The baked potato served plain? The sour cream, butter, or margarine served on the side?

g. Ask for fruit for dessert even if it's not on the menu. A bowl of fresh strawberries (without cream) or a fruit plate make a delightful dessert. To satisfy your sweet tooth, ask your dining companion for a tiny bite of his/her high-fat dessert.

3. When your order arrives, if your chicken comes with skin, your fish swimming in butter, or your potato drowning in sour cream, send it back. That's not what you ordered. Don't be shy. After all, they're your arteries, not the waiter's.

If a restaurant is unable or unwilling to satisfy your low-fat needs, you might consider taking your business elsewhere in the future — and letting them know why.

You can clearly see that the secret to eating out is to *ask*. As you and others ask for low-fat options with increasing frequency, restau-

CHINESE RESTAURANTS: THE MYTH

For years we thought Chinese restaurants were a perfect choice for healthy eating — small amounts of meat and lots of vegetables. However, our awareness of total fat and the resulting health risks have changed our opinion. Although the type of fat used is not heart-risky (Chinese restaurants normally use soy oil), the amount of fat is. Chinese chefs often blanch the meat in oil first. Then they sauté it in oil. They may add oil to the finished dish to make it shiny. That's a lot of fat. Not only does fat make you fat, it also puts you at risk for a multitude of diseases.

Look at some of these sat-fat numbers if you want to choke. These estimated* values are for the whole dish. You have to figure out what part of a dish you eat and how the sat-fat adds up.

DISH	ESTIMATED* TOTAL CALORIES	ESTIMATED* SAT-FAT CALORIES
Barbecued Pork (not fried)	1374	355
Barbecued Spareribs	1863	480
Beef with Vegetables	1572	263
Chicken with Vegetables	1224	102
Chicken with Cashews	1765	186
Egg Roll (each)	152	30
Hunan Shrimp	1068	100
Kung Pao Beef	2458	444
Kung Pao Chicken	1806	158
Kung Pao Shrimp	1068	115
Lemon Chicken	1003	103
Moo Shu Beef	1310	258
Moo Shu Pork	1383	292
Orange Beef	1710	342
Pork with Vegetables	1574	338
Sweet and Sour Pork	1845	389
Sweet and Sour Shrimp	1069	130
Szechuan Pork	1694	356

Gorging is normal behavior at a Chinese restaurant. If you can eat sparingly and carefully, you may want to make Chinese restaurants an occasional splurge.

---

*These estimates are derived from analyses of recipes in Chinese cookbooks and interviews with Chinese cooks. But, beware. Values will vary from restaurant to restaurant.

rants will begin to realize that there is a market for such foods and will respond.

Your Choice. Steering clear of high-fat choices at a restaurant is not easy, but it is not impossible — unless you want it to be. If you insist that you were forced to eat the sour cream in the potato and the chicken "came breaded and deep-fried so what could I do?" you are only fooling yourself . . . not your arteries. Don't blame the restaurant. You chose to eat there and you chose what to eat. If you have no self-control at a restaurant and you really want to lower your cholesterol, don't go out to eat. In fact, even if you have self-control, for the sake of your heart, make your restaurant visits a rarity.

Flying? Call Ahead

Frequent airline travelers know how rarely heart-healthy food graces the airline menu. High-fat meats, sauces, cheeses, butter, and desserts abound, and once up in the air, there are no choices to be had. However, a little forethought may provide you with food you can eat without qualms. At least twenty-four hours before your flight, call the airline reservations clerk and order a special meal. Be as specific as you can in making your request. We usually ask for fish or a chicken breast without skin, and fruit for dessert. You might request a fruit plate for lunch. We also explain that we are on a low-fat diet.

THE ART OF READING FOOD LABELS

Before we begin our discussion of food labels, we take this opportunity once again to give a hearty endorsement for cooking from scratch. For the best-tasting, healthiest food, cook it yourself. Don't zap frozen dinners or frozen dishes in your microwave. Take time to cook. It won't require that much more time and you will know exactly what you are eating. Besides, it will taste better.

We realize that many of you feel harassed and pressed for time and may resort occasionally to grabbing a meal from a box. If this is the case, you have to know exactly what you are consuming if you want to keep your arteries from revolting. Even if you use few processed foods you will need to know how to read a label if you want to survive in the modern world.

U.S. Government Tames a Behemoth

In earlier editions of *Eater's Choice* we warned you about hype on packages — "Lite!" "Lean!" "97% fat-free!" "Cholesterol-free!" What did all the bright letters blazing across the packages really mean? We advised you to ignore the hype and focus exclusively on the nutrition label. With your Sat-Fat Budget in mind, you could easily read the nutrition label and determine if a food was a good choice for you. You were set, but most of the public was not.

FDA Takes on the Food Industry. The Food and Drug Administration (FDA) worried about the misleading labeling. It wanted to make food labels useful for everyone. In an attempt to regulate health and diet claims and standardize serving sizes and nutrition information, the FDA and the Department of Agriculture (USDA) developed new, more restrictive regulations and created a new food label to be used on all commercial foods. The deadline for implementation of the new label rules was August 1994.

Food Labels Tell the Truth. In many ways, the new food labels and rules are a great improvement. Now, if a food is sat-fat-laden, you'll read it on the label because all foods have nutrition labels and all labels now have grams of saturated fat listed. Words such as "Light," "Low-fat," and "Cholesterol-free" can be used only if they meet certain criteria. Serving sizes are supposed to be standardized so that you are not comparing the fat in 1 teaspoon of one salad dressing with the fat in 1 tablespoon of another. Labels list calories of fat and grams of fiber, both of which you need to know to stay in good health.

Watch for Pitfalls. The major downside to the new labels is what the FDA terms Daily Value and % Daily Value. We will discuss them later. Another problem is that although criteria for the use of hype is specific, it may not be restrictive enough. For example, the bread crisps on page 125 carry the claim "Low Cholesterol." People read "Low Cholesterol" and think "healthy." Are these crisps healthy? According to the new rules, Pepperidge Farm may claim only "Low Cholesterol" if the crisps contain less than 20 milligrams of cholesterol per serving (they contain only 5 milligrams) and 1 gram or less of saturated fat per serving (they contain 1 gram). However, seven of these minuscule crackers contain 50 calories of fat — a whopping amount of fat for 1 ounce of food — which makes them a very unhealthy choice.

Reading Labels Made Easy

If you are getting uneasy about the new food labels, relax. In the following section we will show you how to become a label-reading expert. To start, select a can or package from your kitchen so you can examine the label.

Ingredient List

Most packaged foods have a list of ingredients printed somewhere on the package (even if it is so tiny you need a magnifying glass to read it). The ingredients are always listed in descending order by weight. For example, the raspberry sherbet I have before me lists these ingredients: "Skim milk, sugar, water, corn syrup, red raspberries, cream, raspberry juice concentrate, carob bean gum, mono- and diglycerides, natural raspberry flavor, guar gum, dextrose, whey citric acid, polysorbate 80, pectin."

This label tells you there is more skim milk than any other ingredient in the carton. Unfortunately, since the actual weights of ingredients are not provided, you have no way of knowing if the skim milk is 49 or 20 percent of the weight of the sherbet. You know there is less sugar than skim milk, and more cream than raspberry juice concentrate, but you don't know the actual amounts of sugar or cream or any other ingredient.

Ingredient lists can be very beneficial even when they are not quantitative because they may list ingredients you want to avoid. If the first ingredient listed on your frozen yogurt label is cream, you may want to choose another brand. If coconut oil is listed second on your popcorn label, you may decide to leave the bag in the store.

Nutrition Facts

The new law makes it mandatory for almost all food products to have a Nutrition Facts box in addition to an ingredient list. Although nutrition labels look complicated, deciphering them is simple.

First, you should know that the information in the Nutrition Facts box is for one serving of the food. The calories, calories from fat, total fat and cholesterol — all the numbers — are for one serving. And the serving size is listed at the top of the box.

Second, always keep your Sat-Fat Budget in mind. The two numbers on the label that should interest you most are the grams of saturated fat per serving and the serving size. You will also need to read the list of ingredients to find sources of saturated fat.

Let's analyze the Weight Watcher's Chicken Fettuccine label on the right. First look at the information that is most important to you.

Saturated Fat 3g: Since saturated fat is listed in gram amounts and there are 9 calories per gram of saturated fat, multiply by 9 to determine sat-fat calories. The chicken fettuccine has 3 grams or 27 sat-fat calories per serving. You should also check the total fat content because if the total fat is high, you may want to choose another product.

Serving Size: 1 meal (233g)

Servings Per Container: 1. It is not enough to know the number of sat-fat calories. You must check the serving size. The manufacturer's idea of a serving and the amount you consume may differ. In this case a serving is 1 meal (233 grams), which is probably what you eat. There is 1 Serving Per Container.

Chicken Fettuccine

Nutrition Facts
Serving Size: 1 meal (233g)
Servings Per Container: 1

Amount Per Serving	
Calories 280	Calories from Fat 80

	% Daily Value*
Total Fat 9g	14%
Saturated Fat 3g	15%
Cholesterol 40mg	13%
Sodium 590mg	25%
Total Carbohydrate 25g	8%
Dietary Fiber 2g	8%
Sugars 5g	
Protein 22g	

Vitamin A 4%	•	Vitamin C 0%
Calcium 20%	•	Iron 10%

*Percent Daily Values are based on a 2,000 calorie diet. Your daily values may be higher or lower depending on your calorie needs:

		Calories:	2,000	2,500
Total Fat	Less than		65g	80g
Saturated Fat	Less than		20g	25g
Cholesterol	Less than		300mg	300mg
Sodium	Less than		2,400mg	2,400mg
Total Carbohydrate			300g	375g
Dietary Fiber			25g	30g

Calories per gram:
Fat 9   Carbohydrates 4   Protein 4

These listings may also be useful:

Calories from Fat 80. The total fat calories in this product are 80 per serving, a lot of fat for not much food. (To put this number into perspective, the *Choose to Lose* Fat Budget* for a 140-pound woman is 328 fat calories.) If your label lists only grams of fat, multiply the grams of fat times 9 to determine the calories of fat.

Cholesterol 40mg. This number is useful not because you should be concerned with cholesterol content, but because knowing the cholesterol content can help you determine the amount of meat in a product. For example, this product lists 40 milligrams of cholesterol. Since 1 ounce of chicken contains about 24 milligrams of cholesterol, this meal contains about 1½ ounces of chicken (the

---

*See Chapter 2, *Choose to Lose*, to determine your own Fat Budget.

Parmesan cheese accounts for some cholesterol). Of course, it is healthier to eat less meat, but you may be annoyed that you paid as much as you did for so little food and that you are still hungry when you finish eating it.

Daily Value: Ticket to Weight Gain

The great news about the new food labels is that they list calories from fat. You know exactly how much fat you are getting. No more losing fat calories by rounding into grams of fat. No more multiplying by 9.

The bad news is the addition of Daily Value and % Daily Value. You will not need to use this information but you might be interested in finding out what it means.

Daily Value. The FDA was worried that Americans had no way to judge food labels to make healthy food selections. After many months of hearings and debate, it came up with a solution — give all Americans a Nutrition Budget, a Daily Value for fat, saturated fat, cholesterol, sodium, total carbohydrate, and dietary fiber. These Daily Values are based on a 2000-calorie diet. They are the same whether you are a man or a woman, 4 feet 10 inches or 6 feet 7 inches tall, or want to weigh 105 pounds or 195.

Daily Value: Sat-Fat. The Daily Value for saturated fat is based on 9 percent of the 2000-daily-calorie intake or 20 grams (180 sat-fat calories). (This is like your Sat-Fat Budget, but your Sat-Fat Budget is personalized because it is based on your sex, height, frame size, desirable weight, and activity level.) How does this compare with your Sat-Fat Budget? Actually, the daily value for sat-fat is not far off from most budgets and may even be low for many (which is good).

Daily Value: Total Fat. The real problem comes with total fat because the Daily Value for total fat (Fat Budget) is tremendous —

Bread Crisps

Low Cholesterol

Nutrition Facts

Serving Size 1 oz. (28g / about 1/6 of package)
Servings Per Container About 6

Amount Per Serving

Calories 140   Calories from Fat 50

	% Daily Value*
Total Fat 6g	**9%**
Saturated Fat 1g	**4%**
Polyunsaturated 1g	
Monounsaturated 2g	
Cholesterol 5mg	**2%**
Sodium 180mg	**8%**
Total Carbohydrate 18g	**6%**
Dietary Fiber Less than 1g	**2%**
Sugars Less than 1g	
Protein 4g	

Vitamin A 0%	•	Vitamin C 0%	
Calcium 0%	•	Iron 4%	
Thiamine 10%	•	Riboflavin 4%	
Niacin 8%			

* Percent Daily Values are based on a 2,000 calorie diet. Your daily values may be higher or lower depending on your calorie needs:

		Calories:	2,000	2,500
Total Fat	Less than		65g	80g
Sat. Fat	Less than		20g	25g
Cholesterol	Less than		300mg	300mg
Sodium	Less than		2,400mg	2,400mg
Total Carbohydrate			300g	375g
Dietary Fiber			25g	30g

Calories per gram:
Fat 9 • Carbohydrate 4 • Protein 4

585 fat calories. It is 30 percent (too high a Fat Budget) of a 2000-calorie diet — one number chosen for every person in the country. (If you follow *Choose to Lose,* you will determine your own personal Fat Budget based on 20 percent of the calories needed to satisfy your basal metabolic rate.) The Daily Value for fat is more than double the Fat Budget of 285 for a 123-pound woman and even more than the Fat Budget of 429 for a 165-pound man. If either of us were to eat 585 fat calories a day, we would soon become morbidly obese (and have to find a new profession!).

Reading the upper portion of the Pepperidge Farm bread crisps label, you see that these crisps contain 50 fat calories per serving. There are 6 servings in the package. You can eyeball the bag and try to estimate what one-sixth of the package might contain. It turns out to be 7 tiny crackers, which is very, very, *very* little for all that fat. Compared to a Fat Budget of 585, 50 doesn't seem so high, but compare it to a budget of 280 and you'll appreciate the cost.

% Daily Value. This is the *really* confusing part. In the past, when a label listed sat-fat as, say, 5 grams, many people had no way of judging whether the food was high or low in saturated fat because they didn't know what 5 grams meant, and if they did, they didn't know how

Bread Crisps

	% Daily Value*
Total Fat 6g	9%
Saturated Fat 1g	4%
Polyunsaturated 1g	
Monounsaturated 2g	
Cholesterol 5mg	2%
Sodium 180mg	8%
Total Carbohydrate 18g	6%
Dietary Fiber Less than 1g	2%

much sat-fat they should be eating. (Of course, *Eater's Choice* readers knew.)

The FDA solution to helping the public put the gram amount into context is to set a Daily Value for a nutrient and then list what percentage of this Daily Value is represented by one serving of the food.

% Daily Value: Saturated Fat. In the bread crisps example, the % Daily Value for saturated fat is given as 4 percent. This means that the 1 gram (9 sat-fat calories) of sat-fat contained in 7 minute bread crisps represents 4 percent of the Daily Value for saturated fat (20 grams or 180 sat-fat calories). What does this mean to most people? If they eat 14 crackers — and who won't? — do they figure they are eating 8 percent of their DV? Most people will say, "Only 4 percent? That's nothing. I'll eat the whole bag (which turns out to be 9 sat-fat calories/serving × 6 servings = 54 sat-fat calories). How does 54 sat-fat calories fit into your Sat-Fat Budget?

% Daily Value: Total Fat. Again, the real trouble comes with % Daily Value for total fat. One serving of these bread crisps contributed 50 fat calories, which translates into 9 percent of the Daily Value for Total Fat. A natural reaction would be to think, "Only 9 percent? That's not much," and then to finish off the whole bag for a total of 300 fat calories.

The Bottom Line. Consumers would have to be abnormally diligent to add up the % Daily Value for each serving of each food that they eat to make sure they eat less than 100 percent of the Daily Value for each nutrient each day. (Even if they bother to add up all those percentages, we think that the Daily Value for fat is too high and allows — even encourages — people to eat too much fat.) Rather, most people will assume that because the % Daily Values of fat and sat-fat for one serving of most foods are often low, they can eat the food with abandon.

Because they are not adjusting for the number of servings eaten and are not adding up the actual fat and sat-fat calories for the foods they eat all day, they could easily consume much more sat-fat and fat than is healthy.

Serving-Size Savvy

Although the new serving sizes are supposed to be standardized, don't assume that because you know the serving size of one product, you can expect all similar products to have the same serving size. Always check the nutrition label.

Chewy Chocolate Chip Cookies

Nutrition Facts	
Serving Size 3 cookies (36 g)	
Servings Per Container About 14	

Amount Per Serving	
Calories 170	Calories from Fat 70

	% Daily Value*
Total Fat 8g	**12%**
Saturated Fat 2.5g	**14%**
Cholesterol Less than 5mg	**1%**
Sodium 125mg	**5%**
Total Carbohydrate 23g	**8%**
Dietary Fiber Less than 1g	**2%**
Sugars 14g	
Protein 1g	

For example, consider the labels for the Chewy and Chunky Chocolate Chip cookies. The two cookies are almost identical. If you were to read the label for one and assume the information was the same for both, you'd be in big trouble. First look at the serving size of the Chewy Chocolate Chip Cookies. The serving size is 3 cookies weighing a total of 36 grams. The sat-fat calories per serving are 2.5 grams or 23 sat-fat calories. That works out to 8 sat-fat calories per cookie.

Before you stick your hand into the

bag of Chunky Chocolate Chip Cookies and pull out 3 cookies, take a glance at the nutrition label. First check out the sat-fat content per serving — 3 grams or 27 fat calories — almost the same as the chewy model. Look again. The serving size for the chunky cookie is 1 cookie, not 3. One cookie has 27 sat-fat calories — not such a great deal. (The total fat is 40 fat calories — a very un-great deal.) If you were to eat 3 of the chunky cookies, you would be eating 3 × 27 sat-fat calories/serving = 81 sat-fat calories!

**Chunky
Chocolate Chip Cookies**

Nutrition Facts

Serving Size 1 Cookie (17g)
Servings Per Container About 28

Amount Per Serving

Calories 80   Calories from Fat 40

	% Daily Value*
Total Fat 4g	**7%**
Saturated Fat 3g	**14%**
Cholesterol 10mg	**3%**
Sodium 60mg	**2%**
Total Carbohydrate 11g	**4%**
Dietary Fiber Less than 1 gram	**2%**
Sugars 7g	
Other Carbohydrate 4g	
Protein 1g	

Hooray for Fiber!

Fast foods, frozen dinners, convenience foods — besides being full of fat and saturated fat, what do they all have in common? They are all low in fiber. The American diet is deficient in fiber. We owe many of our major health problems to this deficiency, along with a high-fat diet and a sedentary lifestyle.

Now that you know, you can change your low-fiber ways. Actually, by following *Eater's Choice* and eating a diet high in vegetables, fruits, and whole-grains (see Chapter 11, "Ensuring a Balanced Diet"), you will be eating a high-fiber diet. It's important. A high-fiber diet reduces your risk of colon cancer. It helps prevent diverticulosis and hemorrhoids as well as constipation. It can even lower blood glucose levels. The American Dietetic Association recommends eating 20 to 35 grams of fiber a day (more than 50 or 60 grams may decrease the amount of vitamins and minerals your body absorbs). The new food labels list the Daily Value for dietary fiber as 25 grams. By listing dietary fiber, the new food labels allow you to choose higher-fiber foods when possible.

A good way to use dietary fiber information is to comparison-shop in the cereal aisle of your grocery store. Look at the amount of dietary fiber in the Kellogg's Special K. Compare it with the dietary fiber in the Kellogg's All-Bran. Both serving sizes are the same — 31 g/1.1 oz (the cup amount is different). Don't choke down a spoonful of a high-fiber cereal as if it were medicine. If it doesn't appeal to your taste buds, you can get lots of fiber in other foods. But if a cereal

Special K Cereal

Nutrition Facts
Serving Size 1 Cup (31g/1.1 oz.)
Servings per Container 6

Amount Per Serving	Cereal	Cereal with ½ Cup Vitamins A & D Skim Milk
Calories	110	150
Fat Calories	0	0
	% Daily Value **	
Total Fat 0g*	0 %	0 %
Saturated Fat 0g	0 %	0 %
Cholesterol 0mg	0 %	0 %
Sodium 250mg	11%	13 %
Potassium 60mg	2 %	7 %
Total Carbohydrate 22g	7 %	9 %
Dietary Fiber 1g	3 %	3 %
Sugars 3g		
Other Carbohydrate 18g		

All-Bran Cereal

Nutrition Facts
Serving Size 1/2 cup (31g/1.1 oz.)
Servings per Container 13

Amount Per Serving	Cereal	Cereal with ½ Cup Vitamins A & D Skim Milk
Calories	80	120
Calories from Fat	10	10
	% Daily Value **	
Total Fat 1.0g*	2 %	2 %
Saturated Fat 0g	0 %	0 %
Cholesterol 0mg	0 %	0 %
Sodium 280mg	12 %	14 %
Potassium 350mg	10 %	16 %
Total Carbohydrate 23g	8 %	10 %
Dietary Fiber 10g	40 %	40 %
Insoluble Fiber 9g		
Sugars 5g		
Other Carbohydrate 8g		
Protein 4g		

tastes good and also contains 10 grams of dietary fiber per serving, why not choose it over another favorite that has only 1 gram?

Fat-Free, Sat-Fat-Free: The New Math

Fat-free mayonnaise, salad dressings, sour cream, cheeses, cookies, crackers, cake, bread, butter, and on and on. The abundance of fat-free foods is mind-boggling. The label says 0 fat, but do fat-free foods really have no fat?

To discover if a food is truly free of fat or saturated fat, look at the list of ingredients. If you find any fat-containing ingredient, such as partially hydrogenated oil, butterfat, cheese, beef, monoglycerides or diglycerides (these words mean fats), you can assume the food has some fat. Food manufacturers are allowed to call a food fat-free if a serving contains less than half a gram or 4.5 fat calories of fat. Likewise, a food can be labeled sat-fat-free if it contains less than 0.5 grams (4.5 calories) of sat-fat per serving. Since you have no idea of the actual amount in a serving, always assume the food has 4.5 fat or sat-fat calories per serving. You may think so few calories seem trivial, but even few calories can add up, especially if the serving size is small.

Take, for example, this nondairy creamer. Saturated fat is listed as 0 grams. The 1 tablespoon serving supplies 0% of the % Daily Value

Nondairy Creamer

Nutrition Facts

Serving Size : 1 tbsp (15mL)
Servings per Container : 32

Amount Per Serving	1tbsp	1/2 cup
Calories	20	160
Calories from fat	15	120
	% Daily Value*	
Total Fat 1.5g**	2%	20%
Saturated Fat 0g	0%	15%
Polyunsaturated Fat 0.5g		
Monounsaturated Fat 0.5g		
Cholesterol 0mg	0%	0%
Sodium 5mg	0%	2%
Total Carbohydrate 1g	0%	3%
Protein 0g		

Not a significant source of dietary fiber, sugars, vitamin A, vitamin C, calcium and iron.

*Percent Daily Values are based on a 2,000 calorie diet.
**Amount in 1 tbsp serving size.

INGREDIENTS: WATER, CORN SYRUP, PARTIALLY HYDROGENATED SOYBEAN OIL. CONTAINS 2% OR LESS OF THE FOLLOWING: SOY PROTEIN, DIPOTASSIUM PHOSPHATE, EMULSIFIERS (MONO AND DIGLYCERIDES, SODIUM STEAROYL LACTYLATE, POLYSORBATE 80), SALT, SODIUM ACID PYROPHOSPHATE, ARTIFICIAL FLAVOR, COLORED WITH BETA CAROTENE.

for saturated fat. All those zeros certainly make it appear sat-fat-free. Just to be safe, look at the list of ingredients: water, corn syrup, partially hydrogenated soybean oil. . . . Partially hydrogenated soybean oil? Partially hydrogenated soybean oil is a highly saturated fat. Now look at the % Daily Value for ½ cup of this creamer. How did 0 percent become 15 percent? The Daily Value for saturated fat is 20 grams. Multiply 20 grams times 15 percent and you get 3 grams or about 27 sat-fat calories. If you were to pour half a cup of this creamer over your cereal, it would cost you 27 sat-fat calories. Not so sat-fat-free after all. Remember, if a label lists any fat-containing ingredients, assume that one serving contains 4.5 fat calories.

Where Did the Fat Go?

When a nutrition label lists polyunsaturated fat and monounsaturated fat as well as saturated fat (manufacturers are required to list only total and saturated fat), the sum of the three fats often doesn't add up to the amount of the total fat. For example, look at the bread crisps label on page 126. The 1 gram of saturated fat plus 1 gram of polyunsaturated fat plus 2 grams of monounsaturated fat equal 4 grams of fat, not 6 grams of total fat as listed. What happened to the 2 grams of fat?

First, all of the numbers are distorted because calories have been rounded into grams. Let's start with the total fat being 50 fat calories — not the rounded 6 fat grams. Perhaps the 1 gram of saturated fat is really 13 sat-fat calories, the 1 gram of poly is really 7 polyunsat-fat calories, and the 2 grams of mono is really 23 monounsat-fat calories. This adds up to 43 total fat calories. There are also tiny amounts of other unlisted fats that might account for the difference.

Second, it is possible that some of the missing 2 grams of fat could be trans fats.

Trans Fats under Cover

Often polyunsaturated oils (such as corn or soy oil) are listed as hydrogenated or partially hydrogenated. This means that the oil has been treated by a chemical process that converts some or all of the polyunsaturated oil into trans fats. Although these trans fats are monounsaturated, their structure is different from natural mono-unsaturated oils. Trans fats act like saturated fat and raise LDL-cholesterol and thus increase your risk of heart disease. (See the discussion of trans fats on page 81.) Under the FDA regulations, a food manufacturer does not need to list trans fats, but if you subtract the poly, mono, and sat-fats from the total, the difference will be an estimate of the amount of trans fats.

None of the Above

Products are often labeled as containing one or more oils; for example, corn, soybean, palm, or coconut oil. As you know, there are large and important differences among these oils. Olive oil is mono-unsaturated and is the most heart-healthy oil. Soybean is predominantly polyunsaturated and may be cancer-risky in large amounts. Palm, coconut, and palm kernel oils are predominantly saturated and thus heart-risky. Hydrogenated oils contain trans fats and act like saturated oils. In cases where a choice of oils is listed, the manufacturer uses whichever is cheapest at the time. If one of the oils listed is saturated and/or hydrogenated, the best course of action is to avoid the food altogether. You will be happy to learn that when listing the amount of saturated fat on a food label, food manufacturers must base their numbers on the saturated fat content of the most saturated fat listed.

Consumer Beware

Know how to read labels and avoid being misled by the following kinds of advertising claims.

1. CLAIM: Cholesterol-free.
   TRUTH: The average consumer translates "cholesterol-free" to mean "heart-healthy." First, since dietary cholesterol

has a minor effect on raising blood cholesterol, unless it is stupendously high (100 milligrams and above),* the cholesterol content of a food is of little interest. What is significant for your heart health is the amount of saturated fat it contains. Second, cholesterol-free just means that a food contains no animal products because cholesterol is found only in animal products. Every plant product no matter how high in saturated fat is cholesterol-free. Coconut, palm, and hydrogenated plant oils, which are the most heart-risky foods around, are cholesterol-free because they come from plants.

According to the FDA regulations, if a product claims it is cholesterol-free, it must contain no more than 2 grams of saturated fat per serving. If the serving is small, such as one cookie, it must contain no more than 2 grams of saturated fat for 50 grams of the food. For most small cookies, this turns out to be 9 sat-fat calories per cookie. But do you eat one cookie? How about 5 or 6 (45 or 54 sat-fat calories)? Or, for some cookie freaks, 10 or 15 (90 or 135 sat-fat calories)?

2. CLAIM: Lite, light

TRUTH: Food producers bank on the fact that we associate the term "light" with low-fat. However, although a product that advertises itself as "light" must contain one-third fewer calories or half as much fat as the "regular" product, it may still not qualify as low-fat in our book. A "lite" brand of potato chips that contains 45 fat calories per ounce rather than 90 is definitely an improvement, but 45 fat calories is still a whopping amount of fat for so little (and so nutritionally-deficient) food.

3. CLAIM: Lean

TRUTH: Consumers associate the word "lean" with low fat. However, to qualify as "lean" a meat must contain fewer than 10 grams of fat (90 fat calories of fat) or 4 grams of sat-fat (36 sat-fat calories) per 100 grams (3½ ounces) of food. You are not going to remain very lean

---

*See "Cholesterol Contents of Selected Foods," page 42.

if you spend 90 fat calories on a mere 3½ ounces of meat. More likely you will be consuming at least 128 fat calories because you will eat at least 5 ounces of "lean" meat.

4. CLAIM: Extra-lean

TRUTH: Under the FDA regulations, a meat can qualify as "extra-lean" if it contains fewer than 45 fat calories for 3½ ounces of food. This amount hardly seems extra-lean when you compare it with turkey, cod, crab, haddock, lobster, pike, pollock, and scallops at only 7 fat calories for 3½ ounces or skinless chicken breast, red snapper, or sole at only 11 fat calories for 3½ ounces.

Food Label Summary

1. Determine the sat-fat calories per serving by multiplying sat-fat grams by 9. Example: Saturated fat 5 grams. . . . 5 grams × 9 = 45 sat-fat calories.

2. Determine how many servings you eat and adjust for that amount. I eat 2 servings so I multiply 2 × 45 sat-fat calories/serving = 90 sat-fat calories.

3. Compare sat-fat calories for what you eat with your Sat-Fat Budget. My Sat-Fat Budget is 170. So 90 is more than half my budget.

MODIFYING RECIPES

You will find many low-sat-fat recipes in this book. We have chosen only recipes that are low in saturated fat so that you can easily fit them into your daily Sat-Fat Budget. To help you keep track of your saturated fat intake, sat-fat calories are listed at the end of each recipe along with total calories. For those of you who are reducing your total fat intake, total fat calories are also listed.

And you can easily make a whole range of old and new favorites perfect for your new low-fat eating plan with a few simple adaptations.

Substituting Ingredients

Sour Cream Herb Bread can be modified easily without sacrificing taste or texture. Substitute 3 tablespoons of margarine for 3 tablespoons of butter, for a saving of 141 calories of saturated fat. Substitute ½ cup of buttermilk for ½ cup of sour cream for a saving of 135 calories of saturated fat. Buttermilk Herb Bread is just as delicious as Sour Cream Herb Bread and, with 276 fewer calories of saturated fat per loaf, it is much healthier.

Sour Cream Herb Bread	Buttermilk Herb Bread
1 tablespoon dry yeast	same
¼ cup very warm water	same
pinch of sugar	same
3 tablespoons **butter**	3 tablespoons **margarine**
3 cups flour	same
3 tablespoons sugar	2 tablespoons sugar
1 teaspoon salt	same
¼ teaspoon marjoram	same
¼ teaspoon oregano	same
¼ teaspoon thyme	same
½ cup **sour cream**	½ cup **buttermilk**
1 egg	same

	TOTAL CALORIES		SAT-FAT CALORIES	
	LOAF	SLICE	LOAF	SLICE
Sour Cream Herb Bread:	2145	126	351	21
Buttermilk Herb Bread:	1874	110	75	4

Silent Substitutions

These substitutions are termed silent because there is often little or no reduction in the quality (taste and texture) of the final product when ingredients rich in saturated fat are replaced by their low-fat counterparts.

When the recipe calls for:	Use instead:
Butter	Margarine
Lard or solid shortening	Liquid vegetable oil (olive oil is preferable) or margarine
Sour cream	Low-fat yogurt or buttermilk
Whole milk	Skim milk
1 tablespoon chocolate	3 tablespoons cocoa + 1 tablespoon margarine
3 egg yolks	1 egg yolk
2 whole eggs	1 egg + 1 egg white

Pork	Chicken, white meat
Chicken livers	Chicken, white meat
Veal cutlets	Turkey cutlets

COOKING TIPS

Here are some tips for cooking that will help you stay within your Sat-Fat Budget:

- Steam vegetables. Purchase an inexpensive metal steamer that can be placed in any size saucepan. Buy fresh vegetables. Place about an inch of water in the saucepan. Spread out your steamer and place your vegetables on top. Cover the saucepan. Steam the vegetables until they are tender. Overcooking destroys taste, texture, and vitamins.
- Sauté vegetables in 1 teaspoon of olive oil and add splashes of water to steam them.
- Sauté vegetables in broth.
- If the recipe calls for sautéing in ¼ cup oil or butter, use 2 tablespoons of olive oil instead. If the reduced amount works, try 1 tablespoon. If a recipe calls for sautéing in 2 tablespoons of fat, use 1 teaspoon of olive oil or less, plus a splash of water, or sauté in fat-free chicken broth.
- Instead of sautéing chicken breasts in a few tablespoons of olive oil, dredge them in a mixture of flour, salt, and pepper, and then bake them in a single layer in a shallow baking pan. Add no fat. When the breasts are fully cooked, either refrigerate or freeze them for later use or cut them up and add them to the sauce you have just prepared.
- Use a cast-iron griddle to cook turkey cutlets (pound and flour first) or chicken breasts. You will need to add little or no fat.
- Always remove skin *before* cooking chicken. The skin increases the saturated fat content by 2½ times. Bake, broil, or roast chicken. Sauté in a small amount of oil, preferably in a wok.
- Bake, broil, or poach fish. Fried vegetables or meats absorb fat that you do not need. Use a wok for sautéing.
- When cooking beef, trim off all visible fat. Broil or bake on a rack to drain the fat. Remove more fat from the cooked meat with paper towels. Avoid pan-frying.
- *Never* deep-fry foods.

Is Cooking the Low-Fat Way Expensive?

NO. NO. NO. Replacing foods high in saturated fat with vegetables, fruits, and whole grains will save you money as well as improve your health. Convenience foods that are highly processed and full of saturated fat are expensive. Beef is more expensive than chicken, turkey, and many fish. A rice dish with small amounts of chicken or even beef is much less expensive than a steak. Sour cream and sweet cream are costly, both in price and health. Get the picture? Popcorn (made with polyunsaturated oil or air-popped) is one of the healthiest and least expensive snack foods available. In contrast, commercial snack foods such as cookies, chips, and candies are highly saturated, heart-risky, and extremely expensive.

A NEW BEGINNING

You are making a dramatic change in your life. You have learned why it is so important for you to eat heart-healthy foods. In time you will find that a menu low in saturated fat and high in complex carbohydrates will be the most satisfying for you.

Making these changes may not be easy at first, but soon you will find that cooking and eating right is a normal part of your life. I can see you now, sitting in front of the fireplace with your great-great-great-grandchildren, sharing a bowl of air-popped popcorn.

Remember:

1. Take time to eat. Eating junk food from vending machines or at fast-food restaurants saves you time in the present but may cost you dearly in the future.
2. When eating out, *ask* what ingredients are in dishes. Choose broiled, baked, or roasted turkey or chicken without skin or fish. Choose dishes without butter or high-fat sauces. Ask for margarine instead of butter. Ask for dressings and toppings to be served on the side so you can regulate the amount you eat. Don't hesitate to send food back if it is not prepared the way you requested.
3. Learn to read labels carefully. Ingredients are listed in descending order according to weight. Pay particular attention to serving sizes when comparing foods or determining their contribution of saturated fat.

4. Consumer beware: All plant products are cholesterol-free. What they may not be is low in saturated fat. Foods advertised as light, lean, or lower-fat may be high in saturated fat. Some food labels list a choice of vegetable oils. If coconut, palm, palm kernel, or hydrogenated vegetable oils are among the choices, avoid the product.

11 ENSURING A BALANCED DIET

IN YOUR FERVOR to lower your sat-fat intake, don't forget to balance your diet with foods that will give you adequate amounts of vitamins, minerals, protein, and fiber. Eating a well-balanced diet should be no problem if you replace your excess sat-fat calories with a lot of fruits, vegetables, whole grains, and low-fat or nonfat dairy. You'll be amazed at how full and satisfied you'll feel.

The Food Guide Pyramid

More specifically, to maintain your health it is essential that you eat foods from each of the following food groups every day.

WHOLE-GRAIN BREADS, CEREALS, RICE, AND PASTA

For good health and weight control, you should consume 6 to 11 servings of whole-grain breads, cereals, rice, and pasta per day. (See Table 3 on page 143 for sizes of servings.)

The following whole-grain products are rich in starch, fiber, protein, thiamine, riboflavin, niacin, folic acid, vitamin E, iron, phosphorus, magnesium, zinc, and other trace minerals. Choose from:

brown rice	oatmeal	whole-wheat bread
buckwheat groats	pumpernickel	and rolls
bulgur	bread	whole-wheat pasta

The following enriched-grain products contain starch and protein, but thiamine, riboflavin, niacin, and iron have been added. Make

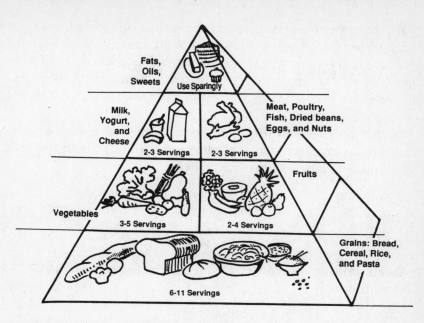

Figure 13: The Food Guide Pyramid *The Food Guide Pyramid proposed by the Department of Agriculture replaces the original four basic food groups wheel. Although both diagrams stress the importance of eating foods from all groups, the pyramid emphasizes the importance of eating more of some foods than others. You should consume whole-grain breads and cereals, rice, and pasta pictured in the base of the pyramid in greatest quantities, followed by vegetables and fruits. Milk products and meat should be eaten in smaller amounts, and fats, oils, and sweets (not even part of the four basic food groups) should be eaten sparingly. In general, Americans have turned this pyramid on its head and have, as a result, been totally out of balance for years.*

sure that saturated fat has not also been added. *Read the labels carefully!* Eat these foods less often. Whole-grain products are far more nutritious.

bagels	French bread	pasta
cereal (ready-to-eat)	noodles	rice

VEGETABLES

Vegetables contribute vital fiber, vitamins, and minerals to your diet. They should be varied and eaten in abundance, at least 3 to 5 servings a day.

The best way to prepare vegetables is to steam them for a short time so they are still crunchy (overcooking causes loss of vitamins and taste). In restaurants, beware of vegetables cooked in butter or drowned in high-fat sauces. To keep them delicious, healthy, and nonfattening, ask that vegetables be steamed with no fat and served with sauces on the side.

Dark green vegetables should be included several times a week. They are an excellent source of vitamins A and C, riboflavin, folic acid, iron, and magnesium. Choose from:

beet greens	endive	spinach
broccoli*	escarole	turnip greens
chard	kale	watercress
chicory	romaine lettuce	

Deep yellow vegetables are an excellent source of vitamin A. Choose from:

carrots	sweet potatoes
pumpkin	winter squash

Other vegetables also contribute varying amounts of vitamins and minerals. Choose from:

artichokes	Chinese cabbage	okra
asparagus	cucumbers	onions
beets	eggplant	radishes
brussels sprouts*	green beans	summer squash
cabbage*	green peppers	tomatoes
cauliflower*	lettuce	turnips*
celery	mushrooms	zucchini

Starchy vegetables are rich in starch, fiber, vitamin B_6, folic acid, iron, magnesium, potassium, and phosphorus. Choose from:

corn	potatoes (white)
green peas	rutabaga*
lima beans	sweet potatoes (rich in vitamin A)

Dried beans and peas are excellent sources of protein, soluble fiber (known to reduce blood cholesterol levels), calcium, magnesium, phosphorus, potassium, iron, and zinc.

---

*These cruciferous vegetables may reduce your risk of colon cancer.

Choose from these dried beans and peas, which should be included as a starchy vegetable several times a week. Dried beans and peas are a healthy substitute for meat, poultry, fish, and eggs. They may be included in both the vegetable and meat food groups in the Food Guide Pyramid.

black beans	lentils	split peas
black-eyed peas	lima beans	other types of dried
chickpeas	navy beans	beans and peas
kidney beans	pinto beans	

FRUITS

Fruits contain vitamins, minerals, and fiber. Eat a variety — at least 2 to 4 servings of fruit daily. Have fruits available around the house instead of nuts, cookies, crackers, or candies. Bananas, oranges, pears, apples, strawberries, peaches, nectarines, cantaloupes . . . all fruits make sweet or crunchy treats. Take a bag of your favorite fruits to work: when hunger or boredom strikes, dip into the bag instead of heading for the vending machine and its high-fat temptations.

Citrus, melon, and berries are rich sources of vitamin C, other vitamins, folic acid, and minerals. Choose from:

blueberries	lemon	tangerine
cantaloupe	orange	watermelon
grapefruit	orange juice	other citrus fruits,
grapefruit juice	raspberries	melons, and
honeydew melon	strawberries	berries
kiwi fruit		

Other fruits are also a rich source of vitamins and minerals. Choose from:

apples	nectarines	prunes
apricots	peaches	raisins
bananas	pears	other fruit
cherries	pineapples	fruit juices
grapes	plums	

MILK, YOGURT, AND CHEESE

Milk products are rich in protein, calcium, riboflavin, vitamin B_{12}, magnesium, vitamin A, thiamine, and, if fortified, vitamin D. Milk products need not be high in saturated fat to contain high amounts of calcium. In fact, skim milk contains slightly more calcium than its high-fat counterparts. Do not skimp on low- or nonfat milk products. Even as an adult, you need all the nutrients they supply. Choose from these foods daily:

nonfat buttermilk   low- or nonfat yogurt
low-fat (1%) cottage cheese   skim milk

Calcium is also found in dark green vegetables.

Women, especially prepubescent girls, need more calcium than men in order to avoid developing the bone-thinning disease osteoporosis.

MEAT, POULTRY, FISH, DRIED BEANS, EGGS, AND NUTS

Meats, poultry, fish, and eggs are good sources of protein, phosphorus, niacin, iron, zinc, and vitamins B_6 and B_{12}. However, Americans eat more meat than is necessary for good health. Limit your meat consumption to no more than 4 to 6 ounces a day.

Choose often from the following:

white meat chicken with no skin
white meat turkey with no skin
fish
shellfish

Choose less often (or not at all) from the following:

beef   lamb   veal
ham   pork   eggs

Eat organ meats such as liver, pancreas, and brain rarely, if at all. They are loaded with cholesterol. Pancreas and brain are also high in fat.

Cooked dried beans or peas, as well as nuts and seeds, may be substituted for meat, poultry, fish, and eggs. However, as these plant foods lack vitamin B_{12}, this vitamin must be supplied by other foods. Nuts and seeds are high in fat and should be eaten in moderation.

Here is a table that will make the recommendations easy to follow.

Table 3: Minimum Basic Nutritional Requirements

FOOD GROUP	RECOMMENDED	DAILY SERVINGS	SERVING SIZE
Fruits and Vegetables	All fruits* and	2–4	½ to 1 cup 1 fruit
	vegetables**	3–5	½ to 1 cup
Dairy		2–3 (adults) 3–4 (children)	
	1% low-fat cottage cheese		½ cup
	Dry-curd cottage cheese		½ cup
	Skim milk		1 cup
	1% low-fat milk		1 cup
	Nonfat yogurt		1 cup
Grain		6–11	
	Whole-grain bread		1 slice
	Bagels		1
	Rice		½ cup
	Bulgur		½ cup
	Whole-grain cereals		1 oz
	Pasta		½ cup
Meat		2	
Poultry	Chicken breast w/o skin**		(2–3 oz)
	Turkey breast w/o skin		
Fish	All fin fish**		(3–4 oz)
	Shellfish**		
	Tuna, water packed		
	Sardines (in fish oil)		
Meat alternatives	Dried beans, peas, lentils		½ cup

*Fresh preferred over canned.
**Not fried.

12 CHOLESTEROL GUIDELINES: FROM TOTS TO TEENS

HEART DISEASE has always been considered a disease of the old. Young people rarely die of heart attacks,* and when they do, it is considered an aberration. Heart disease was thought to be a natural consequence of aging. No more. In recent years, scientific research has shown that heart disease is a disease of lifestyle behaviors and may begin when you are a toddler. The heart attack that took your best buddy last year was not a result of something he did last year or even the year before. It was the accumulation of years of a lifestyle that began when he was just a boy. Do you remember him then — devouring hot dogs, chomping on potato chips?

How do we know heart disease begins when we are young? A variety of studies has shown that the atherosclerotic narrowing of the coronary arteries begins in childhood and is influenced by high blood cholesterol and diet.

EXPERT PANEL PROVIDES GUIDELINES

In 1987 the Adult Treatment Panel of the National Cholesterol Education Program of the National Institutes of Health provided guidelines to physicians and the public about diet and cholesterol in adults. Spurred on by the disturbing evidence that heart disease begins in childhood, a panel of experts was convened to study the problem and make recommendations for children. On April 7, 1991,

---

*About one child in a million has a rare genetic condition called homozygous familial hypercholesterolemia. Because they have no functional LDL receptors, these children have blood cholesterol levels around 700 mg/dL and develop severe atherosclerosis early in life. They suffer heart attacks during childhood, usually dying of heart disease before reaching adulthood.

the National Cholesterol Education Program issued the panel's report on blood cholesterol levels in children and adolescents (ages 2 to 19 years old).

The expert panel cited the following critical evidence to link diet, elevated blood cholesterol, and heart disease in children.

- Autopsies of American children and adolescents who died in accidents revealed fatty streaks in their coronary arteries. Fatty streaks, the earliest visible lesions of the atherosclerotic process, often develop into fibrous plaques, the lesions that narrow the arteries. Fibrous plaques appear in Americans as early as the second decade of life. Autopsies of young (average age: 22 years) American soldiers killed in Korea and Vietnam showed that almost 80 percent had gross evidence of coronary disease.
- High levels of total blood cholesterol and LDL-cholesterol and low levels of HDL-cholesterol have been shown to be directly related to the development of coronary-artery fatty streaks and fibrous plaques.
- As in adults, a diet high in saturated fat causes high blood cholesterol in children. An interesting international study has shown that in countries where the average saturated fat consumption is low, the cholesterol levels of children are also low. In Ghana the average saturated fat intake was 10.5 percent of total calories. The average cholesterol level was 128 mg/dL. The reverse is also true. In those countries where children eat a diet rich in saturated fat, they have higher levels of blood cholesterol. In Finland, where the saturated fat intake was 17.7 percent of total calories, the average cholesterol level was 190 mg/dL. As you might expect, Finland has the highest heart attack rate in the world.
- Children and adolescents in the United States have higher blood cholesterol levels and higher intakes of saturated fat and cholesterol than their counterparts in many other countries. Likewise, U.S. adults have higher blood cholesterol levels and higher rates of coronary heart disease and death than adults in these other countries.

The panel concluded that the fatty streaks and fibrous plaques that develop in the coronary arteries of many American children and adolescents are due largely to a diet high in saturated fat and cholesterol.

Who Is at Risk?

Studies have shown that children and adolescents with high blood cholesterol levels are more likely than the general population to have high levels as adults. Those at highest risk have elevated LDL levels, low HDL levels, a family history of premature heart disease, and the presence of other risk factors.

Are Your Children at Risk? The only way to find out if your children are at risk is to have their cholesterol tested. If you or a member of your family has elevated cholesterol, there is a good chance your children also have high cholesterol levels. Children with elevated blood cholesterol levels, especially those with high LDL levels, often come from families with high rates of coronary heart disease. Elevated blood cholesterol levels cluster in families as a result of both shared heredity and eating patterns.

What Can You Do about It? As we have stressed throughout *Eater's Choice*, a diet low in saturated fat is healthy, regardless of your cholesterol level. This is true for both children and adults alike. You don't have to limit your children to a diet of celery sticks and carrot juice. A low-sat-fat diet can be supremely delicious and satisfying. If you want your children to grow into healthy adults, you will have to put some thought into what you feed them. Before we offer some suggestions, you probably want to know whether to test your children's cholesterol, as well as what are the acceptable cholesterol levels in children.

Who Should Be Tested? In answer to the question, "Should all children have their blood cholesterol measured?" the panel responded "No." They rejected the recommendation of universal screening of children as too expensive. They advise screening only children who are at increased risk of having high blood cholesterol because:

- one parent or both have elevated cholesterol ($\geq$240 mg/dL), **or**
- their parents or grandparents have a history of premature cardiovascular disease.*

---

*A person has premature cardiovascular disease if any of the following criteria is met before the age of 55:
- coronary atherosclerosis documented by coronary arteriography
- balloon angioplasty or coronary artery by-pass surgery
- a documented heart attack, angina pectoris, peripheral vascular disease, cerebrovascular disease, or sudden cardiac death

However, for children or adolescents whose parental or grandparental history is not known, cholesterol screening is advisable, particularly if the children have other risk factors, such as obesity, high blood pressure, or if they smoke. (See pages 593–94 for a flowchart and explanation of recommendations for screening and treatment of children at risk.)

What Do Your Children's Cholesterol Numbers Mean?

The panel defined three categories of risk based on total cholesterol and/or LDL levels:

CHOLESTEROL LEVELS AND RISK FOR CHILDREN

CATEGORY	TOTAL CHOLESTEROL	LDL
Acceptable	<170 mg/dL	<110 mg/dL
Borderline*	170–199 mg/dL	110–129 mg/dL
High*	≥200 mg/dL	≥130 mg/dL

*Classification in the borderline and high categories is based on the average of two measurements and not on a single measurement.

All those with high LDL levels (≥130 mg/dL) should be evaluated for possible causes of elevated blood cholesterol other than a high-sat-fat diet. Some of the other factors commonly present in children and adolescents which raise blood cholesterol levels include:

- obesity
- oral contraceptive use
- isotretinoin (Accutane®)
- anabolic steroid use
- anorexia nervosa

Many of these other causes of high blood cholesterol are potentially reversible.

What Is the Recommended Treatment?

Category: Acceptable. If any of your children fit into the Acceptable category, the panel recommends that they have their cholesterol and/or LDL rechecked in five years and be taught and fed a healthy diet. If they have any of the following risk factors, they should be made aware of the ways to reduce them:

- elevated blood pressure
- low HDL (<35 mg/dL)
- severe obesity (≥30 percent overweight for height)
- diabetes mellitus
- smoking
- physical inactivity

Category: Borderline. If any of your children has cholesterol levels in the Borderline category, they should be eating less than 10 percent of their total calories from saturated fat — the Step 1 Diet (for more on the Step 1 Diet, see Table 4) — with a goal of lowering LDL-cholesterol to <110 mg/dL. They should also be told how to reduce any of the relevant risk factors for coronary heart disease. Children in the Borderline category should be reevaluated in one year.

Category: High Risk. If your child tests in the High category, get ready to gear up for a healthier regime. First, children in the High category should have a clinical evaluation and intensive clinical in-

Table 4: Features of Step 1 and Step 2 Diets

| | RECOMMENDED INTAKE | |
NUTRIENT	STEP 1 DIET	STEP 2 DIET
Total fat	Average of no more than 30% of total calories	Same as Step 1
Saturated fat	Less than 10% of total calories	Less than 7% of total calories
Polyunsaturated fat	Up to 10% of total calories	Same as Step 1
Monounsaturated fat	30% total calories minus (% saturated fat calories + % polyunsaturated fat calories)	Same as Step 1
Cholesterol	Less than 300 mg/day	Less than 200 mg/day
Carbohydrates	About 55% of total calories	Same as Step 1
Protein	About 15–20% of total calories	Same as Step 1
Total calories	To promote normal growth and development and to reach or maintain desirable body weight	Same as Step 1

tervention. They should start with a 10 percent Sat-Fat Budget (see the Step 1 Diet, Table 4) and then move on to a Sat-Fat Budget of less than 7 percent (see the Step 2 Diet, Table 4), with the goal of reducing their LDL-cholesterol to <130 mg/dL at a minimum and ideally to <110 mg/dL.

The expert panel recommends drug therapy for children ten years old and older if the following conditions remain after six months to a year of diet therapy:

- LDL ≥ 190 mg/dL or
- LDL ≥ 160 mg/dL *and* there is a positive family history of premature cardiovascular disease *or* the child or adolescent has two or more other cardiovascular risk factors that persist after energetic attempts to control them.

IMPORTANT!

With few exceptions, you can control your child's cholesterol through diet. Eating delicious food that is low in saturated fat can be a real treat. If you eat healthfully, your child will eat healthfully. Drugs are no panacea. They have side effects, they are expensive, and if diet is not changed, they must be taken forever. Diet also has side effects — weight control; lowering the risk of breast, colon, and prostate cancer; and regularity.

If your child tests High for cholesterol, you should make sure that all members of your family have their blood cholesterol measured.

The Balancing Act of the Pediatric Community

The dietary recommendations reflect the concern of the pediatric medical community that extreme changes in diet might compromise growth and development. The pediatric experts are reluctant to reduce total fat. Because fat has so many calories (9 calories per gram versus only 4 calories per gram for carbohydrates and protein), they fear that reducing total fat will overly reduce total calories, which children need to grow and develop.

Fat Habits Develop Early

On the other hand, children develop food tastes and food habits at a young age. If they eat a high-fat diet at age five, it is likely they will crave a high-fat diet at age thirty-five. And a high-fat diet is not healthy. The high-fat American diet increases the risks of obesity, diabetes, some common cancers, such as colon and breast cancer, and heart disease.

In fact, the total fat intake recommendations of the Step 1 and Step 2 diets may be too high for some children, especially if they are overweight. For such children, a total fat intake of 25 percent of total calories may be closer to the mark. Such a reduction should be made in consultation with your pediatrician, with close monitoring to ensure normal growth and development.

Don't Throw out the Baby with the Fat Calories. Eating too little fat is not an American problem. Our children eat anywhere from 35 to 50 percent of their calories as fat, and when they become adults they suffer the health consequences of such a high-fat diet. The opposite problem, undereating fat, is extremely rare, but occasionally one hears of fanatical parents who reduce their child's fat intake to almost nothing and the child fails to thrive. If you have a tendency toward overzealous behavior, be warned. Too little fat and total calories may cause long-term failure to thrive and seriously impair growth and development.

How Much Fat Do Kids Really Eat? To understand why so many American children are fat and have such high cholesterol levels, take a look at the percentage of fat in the current diets of American children and adolescents as compared to the recommended amounts:

Table 5: Comparison of Current and Recommended Diets of Children and Adolescents

NUTRIENT	CURRENT AVERAGE INTAKE	RECOMMENDED INTAKE STEP 1	STEP 2
Saturated fat	14% of calories	<10%	<7%
Total fat	35–36% of calories	No more than 30%	Same
Cholesterol	193–296 mg/day	<300 mg/day	<200 mg/day

Remember Who's Boss. There is no reason why your children should eat so much fat and saturated fat. An average of 35 percent to 50 percent of calories is a tremendous amount of fat. You are in the fortunate position of being the parent or guardian and keeper of the keys to the kitchen. While your children are young, *you* determine what they eat. They may beg you for a cereal advertised on TV or insist on eating dinner at McDonald's. You are the parent and can just say no!

Good for Everyone

If one of your children has high cholesterol, chances are that you, your spouse, and/or your other children also have high cholesterol. And even if no one else in the family has elevated cholesterol, eating a diet low in saturated fat is healthy and delicious for everyone. Have you heard us say this before?! A diet low in fat and saturated fat is recommended by the American Heart Association for *everyone over 2 years old*.

Everyone in your family deserves the benefits of a low-fat diet. It is never too late for the older members to halt the atherosclerotic process and never too early for the younger members to develop good eating habits, which they can carry with them into old age. Eating healthfully when young will save them the difficulty of un-learning unhealthy eating habits later.

If everyone eats the same healthy diet, you avoid labeling the child who has a cholesterol problem. You do *not* want to single out a child who has high cholesterol by making him feel different and "sick." Why make special dishes just for one when the whole family will enjoy the same mouth-watering low-fat recipes?

IF YOUR CHILD HAS HIGH CHOLESTEROL: A PLAN OF ACTION

First, you have to make sure that *you* are eating a low-fat/high–complex carbohydrate diet. That's a snap now that you have read *Eater's Choice*. With no fanfare, gradually change the way you cook to include more low-sat-fat dishes. Look further on in the book to find almost 300 scrumptious recipes that are low in saturated fat. Try Bar-B-Que Chicken (page 244). It's similar to what your kids are used to. Kung Pao Chicken with Broccoli (page 234) is a dish they may have had in a Chinese restaurant. Try Tortilla Soup (page 208). They'll love the crunchy tortillas at the bottom of the bowl. Serve Divine Buttermilk Pound Cake (page 392) for dessert, and you'll convert the pickiest eater. Soon your family will be openminded about any dish you want to serve.

If your children are not willing to try a new soup or chicken dish, ask them to take just a bite. They'll change their tune after a taste. If they refuse to eat, don't force them, but don't feed them later. They won't starve. Be strong. Don't let food become the basis for a power struggle. Look at it this way. Not eating dinner one night won't kill them, but eating a diet of high-fat snacks may.

In the snack realm, replace chips, cookies, and crackers with fresh fruit, nonfat flavored yogurt, pretzels, homemade air-popped popcorn, cereal (be sure it's low-fat), nonfat frozen yogurt, and raw vegetables like carrot and celery sticks. Your children will soon look forward to a snack of sliced strawberries, half a grapefruit, or a banana. Or whip up a lot of fruit in your blender with ice or nonfat yogurt and create a Frothy Fruit Shake (page 350).

THE SNACK LAW

Never, never, never allow your children to snack — even healthy snacks — too close to dinnertime. You know what time that is. Be firm. If you must, serve dinner earlier or later so you are guaranteed a hungry audience. No matter how wonderful a low-sat-fat meal you prepare, if your children are not hungry, they will not eat it. Then, when they are hungry later, it will be easier to feed them something they won't refuse — high-fat junk. So never, never, never allow your children to snack — even healthy snacks — too close to mealtimes.

A Fly in the Ointment

If your spouse is not willing to cooperate ("I'm a steak and potatoes man. This food is for the birds" or "I can't be bothered changing my style of cooking just for one kid"), explain how vital family cooperation is to the health of your child. High cholesterol in children is a serious, life-threatening problem. Spouses should also read *Eat-*

er's Choice so they can understand the whole problem and see how a low-fat diet will benefit them personally, too.

Bringing Up the Problem

When your children are old enough, if they haven't already confronted you, you will want to tell them that they have high cholesterol. Explain it as a problem that lots and lots of people have. They are not strange or unique. They are lucky because it is a problem that can easily be controlled. Encourage them to read *Eater's Choice*. Treat them like adults. This is *their* problem and they need to make food choices to help them keep their cholesterol low. Being aware of the saturated fat in food will help them make better choices.

Handling the Problem

You might order an Eater's Choice Passbook (see the last page of the book) for them to keep track of their sat-fat calories. Looking up what they eat and recording the sat-fat calories can be extremely insightful. Some children will like the game of it. The adult angle will appeal to some because a Passbook is just like a checkbook. They don't have to keep track of their sat-fat intake forever, but keeping track for even a short period will make a tremendous impact on their future food choices.

IMPORTANT MESSAGE: DOWN WITH FAT — UP WITH COMPLEX CARBOHYDRATES

Eater's Choice emphasizes the reduction of saturated fat to lower blood cholesterol. But reducing fat is not enough. The sat-fat calories that your children eliminate must be replaced by calories of complex carbohydrates — vegetables and whole grains — as well as fruits and low- or nonfat dairy products. Your children need the vitamins, minerals, and fiber that these foods provide. Slip them an orange. Stick a carrot in their lunch. Add banana slices to their cereal. Make sure they are not just cutting out saturated fat. Make sure they are eating lots of vegetables, fruits, whole grains, and low- or nonfat dairy.

A Less Casual Approach

For most children, the changes you make to lower the saturated fat in the family diet will be adequate to lower their cholesterol. However, if your child is in the High category, or his cholesterol doesn't drop low enough with the changes you have made, you might want to try the following approach.

THE SAT-FAT BUDGET

You will notice that *Eater's Choice* has desirable weight tables to help you figure out your Sat-Fat Budget. Such tables do not exist for children. To figure out your child's Sat-Fat Budget:

1. Keep a food record for your child for 3 days. Read "The Nitty-Gritty of How to Keep a Food Record" (page 583) to find out exactly how to do it. (You may want to order a Passbook for keeping the food record. See the order form at the back of the book.) Be exact. Make sure your child's diet is typical of his normal daily food intake.

2. Add up the total calories for each day. Average the totals for the 3 days. Your child consumed an average of _____ total calories a day.

3. To determine the Sat-Fat Budget, take 10 percent of the average total calories consumed a day. Here's how to do it:

$$10\% \times \underline{\hspace{2cm}} = \underline{\hspace{1.5cm}} \text{ sat-fat calories.}$$
$$\text{Total calories}$$

4. Add up the sat-fat calories for each day. Average the 3 totals. Your child consumed an average of _____ sat-fat calories a day.

5. Divide the average sat-fat calories a day by the average total calories consumed.

$$\frac{\text{Average sat-fat calories/day}}{\text{Average total calories/day}} \times 100\% = \underline{\hspace{1.5cm}} \text{ average \%}$$
$$\text{of calories as sat-fat}$$

Your child consumed _____% of calories as saturated fat.

Here is an example to help you determine your child's Sat-Fat Budget. Meet Billy.

1. Billy consumed 1800 total calories on Thursday, 2200 on Friday, and 2000 on Saturday.
2. 1800 + 2200 + 2000 = 6000 total calories.
   6000 total calories ÷ 3 days = 2000 total calories a day.
   Billy consumed an average of 2000 total calories a day.
3. 10% × 2000 = a Sat-Fat Budget of 200 sat-fat calories.
4. Billy ate 400 sat-fat calories on Thursday, 500 on Friday, and 450 on Saturday. 400 + 500 + 450 = 1350 sat-fat calories.
   1350 ÷ 3 days = 450.
   Billy consumed an average of 450 sat-fat calories a day. Remember that his Sat-Fat Budget is 200 sat-fat calories a day.
5. $\dfrac{450 \text{ average sat-fat calories}}{2000 \text{ average total calories}} = 22.5\%$ calories as saturated fat.

Billy consumed an average of 22.5 percent of his total calories as saturated fat and 250 sat-fat calories over his budget. The most important goal is to remove 250 sat-fat calories from Billy's daily diet.

If your child already consumes only 10 percent of total calories from saturated fat and has elevated cholesterol, you might want to reduce his Sat-Fat Budget to 7 percent. But be sure to replace the fat removed with complex carbohydrates so that your child gets enough calories to grow and develop normally. Because complex carbohydrates have twice as much bulk as fat for a given number of calories, your child will be eating much more food. Don't be alarmed. Low-fat food is not fattening. If your child is overweight, consult your pediatrician to see if you should reduce his fat intake.

EATING RIGHT

Knowing your child's Sat-Fat Budget and the sat-fat calories in foods will help you make wise choices in buying and preparing foods. You do not want to make eating into a BIG THING. You want eating healthfully to be a natural part of your child's life.

When your children are young, you have almost complete control over their food choices. Include a variety of fresh fruits and vegetables, breads and cereals (not high-fat) and low- or nonfat dairy in their daily diet. The lure is great, but for the sake of your children's arteries avoid fast-food restaurants. The high-sat-fat temptations are overwhelming. If you must eat out, go to a sub shop instead and order turkey. You might even order a vegetarian pizza without cheese at a pizza parlor.

Cook (and have them help you) *Eater's Choice* or other low-sat-fat recipes, and you will make everyone in the family happy.

It is disturbing to find that your child is at risk for heart disease. But consider how fortunate you are that you can easily prevent this risk. By controlling your child's cholesterol problem, you will be enriching the lives of your children, family, and yourself as well.

TWO WEEKS OF MEALS 13

THE FOLLOWING sample meal plans are provided as an example of how to use your Sat-Fat Budget to plan meals and splurges. Here are two whole weeks of menus with a different breakfast, soup, main course, and dessert for each day to show you the variety of foods you can eat and still stay within your Sat-Fat Budget. All the sample meal plans are based on a total consumption of 2000 calories per day. You can find the recipes for dishes printed in italics in the Cook's Choice section.

The first weekly meal plan provides menus that add up to approximately 200 sat-fat calories a day and thus conform to the *Eater's Choice* 10 Percent Plan. In addition, a 6 Percent Plan (120 sat-fat calories per day) is provided, which illustrates how you can modify your eating in the event the 10 Percent Plan does not lower your blood cholesterol sufficiently. Bold print highlights differences in foods or portion sizes between the 10 Percent and the 6 Percent eating plans.

The second weekly meal plan is based on the 6 Percent Plan. This meal plan illustrates how you can save up sat-fat calories to spend on a splurge later in the week. The saturated fat intake in the meals from Sunday through Friday is lower than allowed on the 6 Percent budget. Despite the fact that you will actually be eating more like a 5 Percent *Eater's Choice* Plan, you will have a most satisfying week. You will even have scrumptious desserts each day.

By eating below your Sat-Fat Budget all week, you will be able to save up calories (in this plan, you will save 205 sat-fat calories) to spend at the end of the week. You can spend these calories any way you wish. Of course, since you ate so well all week, you might choose not to spend these calories at all. Eating less saturated fat than is in your Sat-Fat Budget is always an option — a healthy option.

Armed with your own personal Sat-Fat Budget and using the skills you have learned in this book, you can devise delicious and interesting meal plans based on your own food preferences.

MEAL PLANS — WEEK 1

		10% PLAN			6% PLAN	
FOOD	PORTION	TOTAL CALORIES	SAT-FAT CALORIES	PORTION	TOTAL CALORIES	SAT-FAT CALORIES
SUNDAY — WEEK 1						
Breakfast						
French Toast	2	212	16	2	212	16
Syrup	1 tbsp	61	0	1 tbsp	61	0
Orange juice	**6 fl oz**	83	0	**8 fl oz**	110	0
Coffee	1 cup	0	0	1 cup	0	0
2% milk	1 tbsp	8	2	1 tbsp	8	2
Breakfast subtotal		364	18		391	18
Lunch						
Potato Soup with Leeks and Broccoli	1 cup	113	2	1 cup	113	2
Oriental Chicken Salad	1 serving	140	6	1 serving	140	6
French Bread	**1 piece**	87	2	**2 pieces**	174	4
Coffee	1 cup	0	0	1 cup	0	0
2% milk	1 tbsp	8	2	1 tbsp	8	2
Apple				1 large	125	1
Lunch subtotal		348	12		560	15
Dinner						
Vegetable Soup Provençal	1½ cups	87	0	1½ cups	87	0
Calzone	1 serving	296	4	1 serving	296	4
2% milk	1 cup	121	27	1 cup	121	27
Mixed salad	1 serving	23	0	1 serving	23	0
Italian dressing	1 tbsp	69	9			
Low-cal Italian				1 tbsp	16	2
Ice cream	1 cup	269	80			
Ice milk				½ cup	92	16
Chocolate Cake with Cocoa Frosting	1 slice	273	13	1 slice	273	13
Dinner subtotal		1138	133		908	62
Daily total		1850	163		1859	95

MEAL PLANS — WEEK 1

FOOD	10% PLAN			6% PLAN		
	PORTION	TOTAL CALORIES	SAT-FAT CALORIES	PORTION	TOTAL CALORIES	SAT-FAT CALORIES

MONDAY — WEEK 1

Breakfast

Water bagel	1	200	3	1	200	3
Margarine	2 tsp	60	12			
Edam cheese	1 oz	101	45			
Peanut butter				1 tbsp	95	12
Jam				1 tbsp	55	0
Orange juice	6 oz	83	0	6 oz	83	0
Coffee	1 cup	0	0	1 cup	0	0
2% milk	1 tbsp	8	2	1 tbsp	8	2
Breakfast subtotal		452	62		441	17

Lunch

Turkey sandwich						
White meat turkey w/o skin	3 oz	114	2	3 oz	114	2
Mayonnaise	1 tbsp	99	11			
Low-cal mayonnaise				1 tbsp	35	5
Whole-wheat bread	2 slices	140	8	2 slices	140	8
Tomato	¼ tomato	6	0	¼ tomato	6	0
Potato chips	1 oz	210	32			
Coffee	1 cup	0	0	1 cup	0	0
2% milk	1 tbsp	8	2	1 tbsp	8	2
Pear	1	100	0	1	100	0
Lunch subtotal		677	55		403	17

Dinner

Carrot Soup	1½ cups	104	0	1½ cups	104	2
Chicken Kiev	1 serving	175	6	1 serving	175	6
Rice	½ cup	113	1	½ cup	113	1
Sesame Broccoli	1 serving	50	3	1 serving	50	3
Mixed salad	1 serving	23	0	1 serving	23	0
Thousand Island dressing	1 tbsp	59	8			
Low-cal Thousand Island				2 tbsp	48	4

MEAL PLANS — WEEK 1

	10% PLAN			6% PLAN		
FOOD	PORTION	TOTAL CALORIES	SAT-FAT CALORIES	PORTION	TOTAL CALORIES	SAT-FAT CALORIES
Coffee	1 cup	0	0	1 cup	0	0
2% milk	1 tbsp	8	2	1 tbsp	8	2
Ice milk	1 cup	184	32			
Applesauce Cake				1 slice	250	14
Dinner subtotal		716	52		771	30
Snack						
Mixed nuts				1½ oz	254	27
Daily total		1845	169		1869	91

TUESDAY — WEEK 1

Breakfast

Cheerios	1 oz	110	3	1 oz	110	3
2% milk	1 cup	121	27			
Skim milk				1 cup	86	3
Whole-wheat bread	**2 slices**	140	8	**1 slice**	70	4
Margarine	**2 tsp**	60	12	**1 tsp**	30	6
Jelly	1 tbsp	50	0	1 tbsp	50	0
Coffee	1 cup	0	0	1 cup	0	0
2% milk	1 tbsp	8	2	1 tbsp	8	2
Orange juice	**6 fl oz**	83	0	**8 fl oz**	110	0
Breakfast subtotal		572	52		464	18

Lunch

Arby's Junior roast beef sandwich	1	218	32	1	218	32
French fries	1 serving	220	33			
Apple juice				1 cup	115	0
Coffee	1 cup	0	0	1 cup	0	0
2% milk	1 tbsp	8	2	1 tbsp	8	2
Apple	**1 small**	80	1	**1 large**	125	1
Lunch subtotal		526	68		466	35

Dinner

Zucchini Soup	1 cup	80	0	1 cup	80	0
Scallop Creole	1 serving	177	6	1 serving	177	6

MEAL PLANS — WEEK 1

FOOD	10% PLAN			6% PLAN		
	PORTION	TOTAL CALORIES	SAT-FAT CALORIES	PORTION	TOTAL CALORIES	SAT-FAT CALORIES
White rice	½ cup	113	1	½ cup	113	1
Caraway Carrots	1 serving	35	2	1 serving	35	2
Mixed salad	1 serving	23	0	1 serving	23	0
Russian dressing	1 tbsp	76	10			
Low-cal French dressing				2 tbsp	44	2
Coffee	1 cup	0	0	1 cup	0	0
2% milk	1 tbsp	8	2	1 tbsp	8	2
Tante Nancy's Apple Crumb Cake	1 serving	220	14	1 serving	220	14
Dinner subtotal		732	35		700	27
Snack						
Swiss cheese	1 oz	107	45			
Wheat Thins	4	35	5			
Skim milk	1 cup	86	3			
Ice milk				1 cup	184	32
Daily total		2058	208		1814	112

WEDNESDAY — WEEK 1

Breakfast

FOOD	PORTION	TOTAL CALORIES	SAT-FAT CALORIES	PORTION	TOTAL CALORIES	SAT-FAT CALORIES
Whole-wheat toast	2 slices	140	8	2 slices	140	8
Peanut butter	1 tbsp	95	12	1 tbsp	95	12
Orange juice	**6 fl oz**	83	0	**8 fl oz**	110	0
Coffee	1 cup	0	0	1 cup	0	0
2% milk	1 tbsp	8	2	1 tbsp	8	2
Breakfast subtotal		326	22		353	22

Lunch

Tuna sandwich

FOOD	PORTION	TOTAL CALORIES	SAT-FAT CALORIES	PORTION	TOTAL CALORIES	SAT-FAT CALORIES
White tuna (water packed)	3.25 oz	146	3	3.25 oz	146	3
Whole-wheat bread	2 slices	140	8	2 slices	140	8

MEAL PLANS — WEEK 1

	10% PLAN			6% PLAN		
FOOD	PORTION	TOTAL CALORIES	SAT-FAT CALORIES	PORTION	TOTAL CALORIES	SAT-FAT CALORIES
Mayonnaise	1 tbsp	99	14			
Low-cal mayonnaise				1 tbsp	35	5
Apple	**1 small**	80	1	**1 large**	125	1
Coffee	1 cup	0	0	1 cup	0	0
2% milk	1 tbsp	8	2	1 tbsp	8	2
Lunch subtotal		473	28		454	19
Dinner						
Sirloin steak	**6 oz**	372	72	**4 oz**	248	48
Spinach, cooked	½ cup	20	0	½ cup	20	0
Baked potato w/skin, large	1	220	1	1	220	1
Margarine	**2 tsp**	60	12	**1 tbsp**	90	18
Mixed salad	1 serving	23	0	1 serving	23	0
French dressing, **regular**	2 tbsp	134	28			
low calorie				2 tbsp	44	2
Coffee	1 cup	0	0	1 cup	0	0
2% milk	1 tbsp	8	2	1 tbsp	8	2
Ice milk	½ cup	92	16			
Fruit cocktail				1 cup	185	0
Dinner subtotal		929	131		838	71
Snack						
Grapes				2 cups	194	2
Popcorn	**4 cups**	220	20	**2 cups**	110	10
Daily total		1948	201		1949	124

THURSDAY — WEEK 1

Breakfast

Oat bran cereal	½ cup dry	165	2	½ cup dry	165	2
Raisins	1 tbsp	27	0	1 tbsp	27	0
Margarine	1 tsp	30	6	1 tsp	30	6
Orange juice	**6 fl oz**	83	0	**8 fl oz**	110	0
Coffee	1 cup	0	0	1 cup	0	0
2% milk	1 tbsp	8	2	1 tbsp	8	2
Breakfast subtotal		313	10		340	10

MEAL PLANS — WEEK 1

	10% PLAN			6% PLAN		
FOOD	PORTION	TOTAL CALORIES	SAT-FAT CALORIES	PORTION	TOTAL CALORIES	SAT-FAT CALORIES
Lunch						
Hamburger, lean broiled	**4 oz**	324	100	**3 oz**	243	75
Hamburger roll	1	115	5	1	115	5
Coleslaw	½ cup	42	2	½ cup	42	2
Coffee	1 cup	0	0	1 cup	0	0
2% milk	1 tbsp	8	2	1 tbsp	8	2
Grapes	1 cup	97	0			
Apple				1 large	125	1
Popcorn		___	___	2 cups	110	10
Lunch subtotal		586	109		643	95
Dinner						
Mushroom Soup	1 cup	90	2			
Minestrone				1½ cups	165	2
Turkey Scaloppine Limone	1 serving	246	14			
Turkey Mexique				1 serving	153	5
Steamed Zucchini Matchsticks	1 serving	17	0	1 serving	17	0
Whole-wheat bread	2 slices	140	8			
Rice	½ cup	113	1	½ cup	113	1
Cucumber Salad	1 serving	20	0	1 serving	20	0
Carrot Cake sans Oeufs	1 serving	122	5			
Apricots, canned				1 cup	215	0
2% milk	1 cup	121	27		___	___
Dinner subtotal		869	57		683	8
Snack						
Nonfat fruit yogurt	8 oz	200	0			
Anjou pear				1 pear	120	0
Skim milk		___	___	1 cup	86	3
Daily total		1968	176		1872	116

MEAL PLANS — WEEK 1

		10% PLAN			6% PLAN	
FOOD	PORTION	TOTAL CALORIES	SAT-FAT CALORIES	PORTION	TOTAL CALORIES	SAT-FAT CALORIES
FRIDAY — WEEK 1						
Breakfast						
Whole-wheat toast	**1 slice**	70	4	**2 slices**	140	8
Banana slices	**½ banana**	53	1	1 banana	105	2
1% cottage cheese	**¼ cup**	41	4	**½ cup**	82	7
Cantaloupe	½ melon	95	1	½ melon	95	1
Coffee	1 cup	0	0	1 cup	0	0
2% milk	1 tbsp	8	2	1 tbsp	8	2
Breakfast subtotal		267	12		430	20
Lunch						
Dijon Chicken Rice Salad	1 serving	267	7	1 serving	267	7
Apple Oat Bran Muffin	1 muffin	125	4	1 muffin	125	4
Orange	1 fruit	60	0	1 fruit	60	0
Coffee	1 cup	0	0	1 cup	0	0
2% milk	1 tbsp	8	2	1 tbsp	8	2
Pear				1 large	125	1
Lunch subtotal		460	13		585	14
Dinner						
Cucumber Soup	1 cup	78	0	1 cup	78	0
Rib chops	**2**	480	120	**1**	240	60
Potato Skins	1 serving	66	1	1 serving	66	1
Italian Mixed Vegetables	1 serving	27	1	1 serving	27	1
White wine	3½ fl oz	80	0	3½ fl oz	80	0
Coffee	1 cup	0	0	1 cup	0	0
2% milk	1 tbsp	8	2	1 tbsp	8	2
Cinnamon Sweet Cakes	2	296	16			
Apple				1 large	125	1
Dinner subtotal		1035	141		624	66

MEAL PLANS — WEEK 1

FOOD	10% PLAN			6% PLAN		
	PORTION	TOTAL CALORIES	SAT-FAT CALORIES	PORTION	TOTAL CALORIES	SAT-FAT CALORIES
Snack						
Nonfat yogurt w/fruit	8 oz	200	0			
Grapes				1 cup	97	1
Skim milk				1 cup	86	3
Daily total		1962	166		1822	104
SATURDAY — WEEK 1						
Breakfast						
Buttermilk Waffles	1 square	138	2	1 square	138	2
Syrup	1 tbsp	61	0	1 tbsp	61	0
Grapefruit	1 fruit	95	0	1 fruit	95	0
Coffee	1 cup	0	0	1 cup	0	0
2% milk	1 tbsp	8	2	1 tbsp	8	2
Breakfast subtotal		302	4		302	4
Lunch						
Pawtucket Chili	1½ cups	158	2	1½ cups	158	2
Anjou pear	1 fruit	120	0	1 fruit	120	0
Popcorn	4 cups	220	20	4 cups	220	20
Coffee	1 cup	0	0	1 cup	0	0
2% milk	1 tbsp	8	2	1 tbsp	8	2
Lunch subtotal		506	24		506	24
Dinner						
Pesto on Spaghetti	1 serving	287	14	1 serving	287	14
Pink salmon steak	6 oz	246	12	6 oz	246	12
Cauliflower Sauté	1 serving	47	3	1 serving	47	3
Baked sweet potato	1	115	0	1	115	0
Margarine	1 tsp	30	6	1 tsp	30	6
Mixed salad	1 serving	23	0	1 serving	23	0
Blue cheese dressing	1 tbsp	77	14			
Low-cal Italian dressing				1 tbsp	16	2
Ice cream	½ cup	135	40			
Sherbet				½ cup	135	11

MEAL PLANS — WEEK 1

FOOD	10% PLAN			6% PLAN		
	PORTION	TOTAL CALORIES	SAT-FAT CALORIES	PORTION	TOTAL CALORIES	SAT-FAT CALORIES
Coffee	1 cup	0	0	1 cup	0	0
2% milk	1 tbsp	8	2	1 tbsp	8	2
Dinner subtotal		964	91		903	50
Snack						
Blue cheese	1 oz	100	48			
Wheat Thins	8	70	10			
Oat Bran Muffin		—	—	1	160	6
Daily total		1942	177		1871	84

MEAL PLANS — WEEK 2

FOOD	PORTION	TOTAL CALORIES	SAT-FAT CALORIES
SUNDAY — WEEK 2			
Breakfast			
Buttermilk Pancakes	3	93	3
Syrup	3 tbsp	183	0
Orange sections	1 cup	85	0
Coffee, black	1 cup	0	0
Breakfast subtotal		361	3
Lunch			
Gazpacho I	1 cup	79	1
Scallop Curry	1 serving	187	7
Rice	¾ cup	170	2
Keema Eggplant	1 serving	86	1
Mixed salad	1 serving	23	0
Low-cal Russian dressing	1 tbsp	23	1
Banana Cake	1 slice	263	12
Lunch subtotal		831	24
Dinner			
Corn Chowder	1½ cups	266	8
Tomato Quiche	1 slice	220	21
Spinach with mushroom salad	1 cup	15	0
Dressing (oil, vinegar, Dijon mustard)	2 tbsp	119	16
Coffee, black	1 cup	0	0
Kiwifruit	1	45	0
Dinner subtotal		665	45
Daily total		1857	72
6% Plan sat-fat daily budget		120	
+ Carry-over		0	
Total		120	
− Day's expenditure		− 72	
New carry-over		48	

MEAL PLANS — WEEK 2

FOOD	PORTION	TOTAL CALORIES	SAT-FAT CALORIES
MONDAY — WEEK 2			
Breakfast			
Strawberries	1 cup	45	0
w/nonfat yogurt	½ cup	55	0
Oat Bran Muffins	2	320	12
Orange juice	6 fl oz	83	0
Coffee, black	1 cup	0	0
Breakfast subtotal		503	12
Lunch			
Tuna salad sandwich			
water-packed tuna	3¼ oz	146	3
whole-wheat toast	2 slices	140	8
low-cal salad dressing	1 tbsp	45	9
Orange	1	60	0
Sugar Cookies	2	130	4
Skim milk	8 fl oz	86	3
Lunch subtotal		607	27
Dinner			
Watercress Soup	1 serving	74	0
Indonesian Chicken with Green Beans	1 serving	135	4
Rice	1 cup	226	1
Indian Vegetables	1 serving	72	1
Cucumber Salad	1 serving	20	0
Apple Cake	1 slice	220	13
Dinner subtotal		747	19
Daily total		1857	58
6% Plan sat-fat daily budget		120	
+ Carry-over		48	
Total		168	
− Day's expenditure		− 58	
New carry-over		110	

MEAL PLANS — WEEK 2

FOOD	PORTION	TOTAL CALORIES	SAT-FAT CALORIES
TUESDAY — WEEK 2			
Breakfast			
Cocoa	1 cup		
Cocoa	1 tsp	20	7
Sugar	2 tsp	30	0
Skim milk	8 fl oz	86	3
Low-fat cottage cheese	¼ cup	41	4
Honey Whole-Wheat Bread	1 slice	130	2
Orange juice	6 fl oz	83	0
Banana	1	105	2
Breakfast subtotal		495	18
Lunch			
Ginger Carrot Soup	1 cup	80	1
Peppery Chicken	1 half breast	172	4
Whole-Wheat Bagels	2	230	2
Carrot sticks	1 carrot	30	0
Grapes	1 cup	97	1
Lunch subtotal		609	8
Dinner			
Lentil and Everything Soup	1 cup	85	0
Broiled Monkfish with Orange Sauce	1 serving	194	13
Rice Pilau with Apricots	½ cup	96	1
Cauliflower Sauté	1 serving	47	3
Mixed salad	1 serving	23	0
Dressing made with olive oil, vinegar, herbs	2 tbsp	179	24
Ice milk	¾ cup	138	24
Skim milk	8 fl oz	86	3
Dinner subtotal		848	68
Daily total		1952	94
6% Plan sat-fat daily budget		120	
+ Carry-over		110	
Total		230	
− Day's expenditure		− 94	
New carry-over		136	

MEAL PLANS — WEEK 2

FOOD	PORTION	TOTAL CALORIES	SAT-FAT CALORIES
WEDNESDAY — WEEK 2			
Breakfast			
Oat bran cereal	½ cup dry	165	2
Raisins	1 tbsp	14	0
Margarine	1 tsp	30	6
Orange	1	60	0
Breakfast subtotal		269	8
Lunch			
Fruit Salad with Cottage Cheese	1 serving	280	7
Honey Whole-Wheat Bread	1 slice	130	2
Margarine	1 tsp	30	6
Popcorn (air-popped)	8 cups	240	0
Lunch subtotal		680	15
Dinner			
Avgolemono Soup	1 cup	99	2
Chicken Kiev	1 serving	175	6
Sweet potato, baked	1	115	trace
Sliced tomato	1	23	0
Skim milk	8 fl oz	86	3
Cocoa Brownie	1 square	115	9
Dinner subtotal		613	20
Snack			
Focaccia	2½ pieces	290	5
Daily total		1852	48
6% Plan sat-fat daily budget		120	
+ Carry-over		136	
Total		256	
− Day's expenditure		− 48	
New carry-over		208	

MEAL PLANS — WEEK 2

FOOD	PORTION	TOTAL CALORIES	SAT-FAT CALORIES
THURSDAY — WEEK 2			
Breakfast			
Nonfat yogurt w/fruit	8 fl oz	200	0
Whole-wheat toast	2 pieces	140	8
Jelly	1 tsp	15	0
Coffee, black	1 cup	0	0
Breakfast subtotal		355	8
Lunch			
Curried Tuna Salad w/Pears	1 serving	175	7
Apricot Oat Muffin	2	270	8
Fresh blueberries, cherries, or grapefruit sections	1 cup	80	0
Skim milk	8 fl oz	86	3
Lunch subtotal		611	18
Dinner			
Apple Squash Soup	1 cup	122	0
Turkey Cutlets with Artichokes and Cream Sauce	1 serving	230	15
Rice	¾ cup	170	2
Acorn Squash	1 serving	55	3
Eastern Spinach Salad	1 serving	55	3
Mocha Cake with Mocha Frosting	1 square	174	13
Dinner subtotal		806	36
Daily total		1772	62

6% Plan sat-fat daily budget	120
+ Carry-over	208
Total	328
− Day's expenditure	− 62
New carry-over	266

MEAL PLANS — WEEK 2

FOOD	PORTION	TOTAL CALORIES	SAT-FAT CALORIES
FRIDAY — WEEK 2			
Breakfast			
Cheerios	1 oz	110	3
Skim milk	½ cup	43	1
Banana, sliced	½	53	1
Orange juice	6 fl oz	83	0
Whole-wheat toast	1 piece	70	4
Margarine	1 tsp	30	6
Coffee, black	1 cup	0	0
Breakfast subtotal		389	15
Lunch			
Turkey submarine sandwich			
White meat turkey	3 oz	114	2
Low-cal mayonnaise	1 tbsp	45	9
Submarine roll	1	215	8
Bosc pear	1	100	0
Skim milk	8 fl oz	86	3
Lunch subtotal		560	22
Dinner			
Broccoli Soup	1 cup	99	0
Pizza	2 pieces	232	2
Mixed salad	1 serving	23	0
Low-cal Italian dressing	2 tbsp	32	4
Green Beans Basilico	1 serving	42	2
Deep-Dish Pear Pie	1 slice	236	11
Coffee, black	1 cup	0	0
Dinner subtotal		664	19
Snack			
Popcorn (air-popped)	8 cups	240	0
Daily total		1853	56

6% Plan sat-fat daily budget	120	
+ Carry-over	266	
Total	386	
− Day's expenditure	− 56	
New carry-over	330	

MEAL PLANS — WEEK 2

FOOD	PORTION	TOTAL CALORIES	SAT-FAT CALORIES
SATURDAY — WEEK 2 — Day to Splurge			
Breakfast			
Poached egg	1	79	15
Canadian bacon	2 slices	86	12
Buttermilk Waffles	2 squares	276	4
Orange juice	6 fl oz	83	0
Coffee, black	1 cup	0	0
Breakfast subtotal		524	31
Lunch			
Chili non Carne	1½ cups	176	2
with salad vegetables	¼ cup	15	0
Bran Muffin	1	116	4
Tangerine	1	35	0
Skim milk	8 fl oz	86	3
Lunch subtotal		428	9
Dinner			
Rib roast (lean, trimmed)	6 oz	420	102
Large baked potato	1	220	0
with sour cream	2 tbsp	52	28
Mixed salad	1 serving	23	0
Low-cal Italian dressing	1 tbsp	16	2
Cheesecake	1 slice	280	89
Coffee, black	1 cup	0	0
Dinner subtotal		1011	221
Daily total		1963	261
6% Plan sat-fat daily budget		120	
+ Carry-over		330	
Total		450	
− Day's expenditure		− 261	
New carry-over		189	

TWO

COOK'S CHOICE

INTRODUCTION

COOK'S CHOICE is different and special. In the following pages, you will find only recipes that are *very low* in saturated fat. Not only are these recipes healthy, they make for delicious eating.

We wrote Cook's Choice to show you that low-sat-fat, heart-healthy foods can be just as tasty and satisfying as heart-risky foods. This is especially important for people who need to lower their blood cholesterol. It is also a must for those who want to lower their blood pressure or lose weight, and for diabetics.

But beyond any health considerations, this cookbook is for people who want to eat well. Dishes need not be filled with cream, sour cream, or cheese to taste good. Try Spinach Quiche (page 318), try Key Lime Pie (page 400), try Watercress Soup (page 194) — in fact, try any of the following recipes for a real taste treat.

Be advised: Because the Goor oven is not necessarily calibrated the same as your oven, and your chicken breasts or swordfish steaks may be thicker or thinner than ours, etc., consider the baking time in the recipes as an estimate. If the recipe tells you to bake a dish for 45 minutes, check your oven at 30. Your food may be ready.

A NOTE TO SODIUM WATCHERS

If you are monitoring your sodium intake, you may want to cut down on the amount of salt in some of these recipes.

A NOTE TO FAT WATCHERS

If you are monitoring your fat intake, check the fat calories on each Eater's Choice recipe or refer to the list of fat calories for Eater's Choice recipes on pages 595–606.

Here are some tips for superior taste or nutritional benefits without excess effort or expense:

- In the recipes that call for pepper, use freshly ground black pepper. There really is a difference between the stale, tasteless pepper that comes in a can and the bright taste of pepper that has just been ground. It is definitely worth buying a peppermill (not necessarily expensive) and whole peppercorns (available in the spice section of your local grocery store).
- Grate a whole nutmeg (available in the spice section of your local grocery store) with a hand grater for a fresher, nuttier taste.
- Fresh garlic is available at grocery stores and is far superior to garlic powder or garlic salt. It will stay fresh for weeks in the refrigerator.
- Fresh ginger root is available at many grocery stores and is easily kept for months in the refrigerator in a jar filled with sherry. Slice off the outer covering and use ginger root with superior results in recipes that call for ginger.
- In any recipes that call for canned chicken broth, either strain the broth (we often skim the fat off the surface, then pour the broth through a fine tea strainer) or if the fat is hardened, lift it off the soup with a spoon, or use a gravy skimmer.
- Use *unbleached* white flour. When flour is bleached, it loses many of its important nutritional qualities.
- See "Cooking Tips," page 135.

NOTE: Q indicates recipes that are quick and easy to prepare. But beware: some Q recipes require marinating for several hours or overnight. Read recipes through before beginning!

STOCKING UP

For some of you, reducing your saturated fat will mean a big change in the foods you cook. You may wonder what foods will replace the cream in your refrigerator or the Twinkies in your cupboard. What foods should you have on hand to make cooking the following recipes a snap? Here is a list of foods and spices to keep in your cupboard, your freezer, and your refrigerator.

Foods to keep on your shelves:

almonds, slivered	apricots, dried
anchovies	apricot jelly

artichoke hearts in water
baking powder
baking soda
barley
beans, dried (black, pinto, etc.)
beans, kidney, canned
chicken broth
chickpeas
cocoa, unsweetened
cornstarch
flour, unbleached white
flour, whole-wheat
honey
lentils
molasses
oat bran
oatmeal (not quick)
oil, olive
oil, sunflower or safflower
olives, black and green
onions
pastas (spaghetti, noodles, etc.)

pineapple chunks, canned
peaches, canned
peanuts, unsalted
potatoes
prunes
raisins
salt
sesame paste (tahini)
sherry, dry
sugar, brown
sugar, white
sugar, confectioners'
tomatoes, canned
tomato juice
tomato paste (6 oz)
tomato sauce (8 oz)
vanilla
vermouth
vinegar
walnuts, shelled
yeast (if you plan to make
   bread)

Spices:

basil leaves
caraway seeds
cardamom, ground
cayenne pepper
chili powder, hot (if you like)
chili powder, mild
cinnamon, ground
cinnamon sticks
cloves, ground and whole
coriander
cream of tartar
cumin, ground and seeds
curry powder

dillweed
garam masala*
ginger, ground
mustard seed, black
nutmeg, whole
oregano
paprika
pepper, white
peppercorns, black
rosemary leaves
sesame seeds
tarragon
thyme leaves
turmeric

*Available in Indian groceries and specialty stores

Foods from the Oriental food store:
bamboo shoots, canned
bean sauce
black beans (fermented)
chili paste with garlic
hoisin sauce
mushrooms, dried black
sesame chili oil
sesame oil
soy sauce and double black
  soy sauce
water chestnuts, canned

Foods* to keep in your refrigerator:
buttermilk (for baking)
carrots
celery
garlic cloves
ginger root (store in jar with
  sherry)
lemons
limes
margarine
mayonnaise or salad dressing
mustard, Dijon
yogurt, nonfat plain

Foods to keep in your freezer:
boned and skinned chicken
  breasts
corn, frozen
margarine
peas, frozen
turkey cutlets
whole-wheat bread
whole-wheat pita bread

These all-season foods will enhance your meals — keep some on hand:
broccoli
carrots**
celery**
eggplant
mushrooms (always good in
  salads)
peppers, red or green
potatoes, white or sweet**
snow peas (Chinese peapods)
spinach
squash** (acorn, butternut,
  etc.)
tomatoes
zucchini

Buy fruits in season. Apples, oranges, and pears can usually be purchased year-round. Use for baking, cooking, and snacks.

---

*These foods will stay fresh at least several weeks.
**These vegetables will keep fresh at least a week or more.

SOUPS

Soup! What a wonderful invention! Hot, cold, spicy, sweet, thick, thin, bland, tart — an unlimited source of goodness. Soup is the perfect way to start a meal. It is a delight to the senses and it is filling. In fact, a bowl of soup makes you feel so satisfied that by the time you get to the main course, your ravenous hunger is abated and you may eat less for the rest of the meal.

These are the major advantages of making your own soup:

- It will taste much better than anything you can buy.
- You have an enormous choice of great soups to make.
- You need not worry about whether the soup is too salty or fatty because you control the amount of salt and fat in your soup.
- You make the kind of soup you want when you want it: hot soup to warm you in the winter; cold soup to refresh you in the summer.
- You can make a large amount at one time and freeze it in small containers for use at a later time. Frozen soup is like money in the bank.

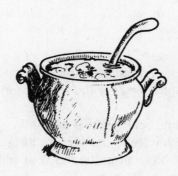

CHICKEN STOCK

Instead of using canned chicken broth, you can make your own chicken stock and freeze it in small amounts. It will be tastier, and it will have no fat or salt. There are many ways to make chicken stock; here is one example.

4 pounds chicken backs, or a
    4–5 pound stewing chicken,
    or 6–8 boneless chicken
    breasts
1 onion, sliced
2 carrots, cut into thirds

1 stalk celery, cut into thirds
1 bay leaf
2 sprigs parsley
¼ teaspoon thyme
1 can (10¾ oz) chicken broth,
    strained

In your largest kettle, combine all ingredients, cover with water, and bring to a boil. Reduce heat, cover, and simmer for 1½ hours.

Remove chicken and vegetables. (You may save both the chicken and the vegetables for another use.)

Refrigerate stock in kettle overnight.

Skim off fat.

Freeze in storage containers.

Q
AVGOLEMONO SOUP
(Greek Lemon Soup)

Avgolemono is a healthy, elegant soup, and it is delicious. Best yet, it is quick and easy to prepare.

½ cup long-grain rice
2 quarts chicken stock, or 3 cans
    (10¾ oz each) chicken broth,
    strained, + 3 cans water
1 teaspoon salt (optional)

1½ cups spaghetti broken into
    1-inch pieces
1 egg
1 egg white
Juice of 1½ lemons

In a soup pot, bring stock to a boil, reduce heat, cover, and simmer with rice until tender (about 20 minutes).

Add salt and spaghetti pieces and simmer for the time specified on the spaghetti package.

Just before serving, beat together egg and egg white.

Slowly add lemon juice to the eggs, beating constantly.

Take 1 cup of the broth from the soup pot and add it to the lemon-egg mixture, beating constantly.

Pour lemon-egg broth back into the soup pot, beating constantly. Bring to a boil and serve immediately.

Makes 9 one-cup servings
Calories per serving: 99 Total; 6 Fat; 2 Sat-fat

☐ MATZO BALL SOUP

Traditional matzo ball soup is made with chicken fat and several eggs. This low-sat-fat version is as light as a feather and is equally tasty.

¼ cup water
2 tablespoons margarine
1 egg
1 egg white
½ cup matzo meal

¼ teaspoon salt (optional)
6 cups chicken stock, or 2 cans (10¾ oz each) chicken broth, strained, + 2½ cans water

Combine water, margarine, egg, and egg white.
Blend in matzo meal and salt and refrigerate for 20 minutes.
Form chilled dough into balls.
Bring chicken stock to a full boil.
Add matzo balls and simmer, covered, for 20 minutes.

Makes 4 one-and-a-half cup servings (2 matzo balls each)
Calories per serving: 167 Total; 26 Fat; 6 Sat-fat

☐ MUSHROOM SOUP

A must! In no more than ten minutes you can make this sophisticated and soothing soup and set it before your family or guests.

½ pound fresh mushrooms, sliced
2 teaspoons olive oil
2 cans (10¾ oz each) chicken broth, strained

Juice of 1 lemon (about ¼ cup)
2 tablespoons dry vermouth
1 tablespoon dry sherry
Dash of Tabasco sauce

In a medium saucepan, sauté mushrooms in olive oil. Add a splash of water and continue to cook until just tender.
Gently mix in strained chicken broth.

Add lemon juice, vermouth, sherry, and Tabasco sauce, and heat until warm.

Makes 5 one-cup servings
Calories per serving: 90 Total; 13 Fat; 2 Sat-fat

POTATO SOUP WITH LEEKS AND BROCCOLI

1 tablespoon olive oil
1½ cups sliced leeks* (white part)
2 tablespoons unbleached white flour
3½ cups hot water
4 cups peeled and sliced potatoes

1 teaspoon salt (optional)
¼ teaspoon freshly ground black pepper
2 cups broccoli flowerets
1½ cups skim milk

In a soup pot, heat olive oil.

Mix in leeks, cover pot, and cook slowly until leeks are soft.

Blend in flour and cook for a few seconds. Remove pot from heat.

Add ½ cup of the hot water and blend thoroughly.

Add the remaining hot water, potatoes, salt, and pepper.

Bring to a boil, reduce heat, and simmer, partially covered, for about 40 minutes or until potatoes are tender.

While the potatoes are cooking, steam the broccoli until it is just tender. Set aside.

Pour the cooked potatoes and their liquid into a blender and purée until they are almost smooth (they should still have some texture).

Return soup to pot, add 1 cup of the skim milk, and blend well.

If the soup is too thick, slowly add more skim milk, ¼ cup at a time. Do not add so much skim milk that the soup becomes too thin. Soup should be *thick*.

Mix in broccoli, correct seasoning, and finish with several twists of your peppermill.

Makes 7 one-cup servings
Calories per serving: 113 Total; 16 Fat; 2 Sat-fat

---

*If you have no leeks, you may use onions, but the special flavor of leeks enhances the soup.

Q
CARROT SOUP

Carrot soup is a great spur-of-the-moment soup because it is simple to make and you probably have the ingredients on hand. It is thick and tasty — wonderful to warm the soul and body on a nippy winter day.

1 medium onion, chopped	1 bay leaf
3 small cloves garlic, minced	Freshly ground black pepper to
1 teaspoon thyme	taste
12 carrots, sliced (about 6 cups)	2 cans (10¾ oz each) chicken
2 potatoes, peeled and sliced	broth, strained
(about 2 cups)	

In a soup pot or large casserole, combine onion, garlic, and thyme.
Mix in carrots, potatoes, bay leaf, and pepper.
Add chicken broth and enough water to cover vegetables.
Bring soup to a boil. Reduce heat, cover, and simmer for 30 minutes.
Remove bay leaf and purée soup in blender.

Makes 11 one-cup servings
Calories per serving: 69 Total; 0 Fat; 0 Sat-fat

Q
CARROT SOUP DES BASQUES

The fennel seeds and cumin combine with the carrots to give this soup a hearty robustness.

¼ teaspoon fennel seeds	1 small onion, minced
2 green onions, sliced	2 cans chicken broth (10¾ oz
4 cups sliced carrots	each), strained
3 cups sliced potatoes	¼ teaspoon marjoram
	½ teaspoon cumin

Crush fennel seeds with the back of a spoon and set aside.
Combine green onions, carrots, potatoes, and onion in a soup pot.
Add chicken broth, plus enough water to cover vegetables.
Add fennel, marjoram, and cumin.

Bring to a boil, reduce heat, and simmer for 30 minutes or until vegetables are soft.

Coarsely purée in a blender.

Makes 7 one-cup servings
Calories per serving: 87 Total; 0 Fat; 0 Sat-fat

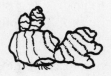

Q GINGER-CARROT SOUP

This soup can be eaten either cold or warm. The lime and ginger give it an interesting flavor.

1 tablespoon minced ginger root
2 cloves garlic, minced
½ cup chopped onion
1 teaspoon olive oil
5 cups sliced carrots

2 cans (10¾ oz each) chicken broth, strained, + 1 can water
¼ cup fresh lime juice (approximately)
Nonfat yogurt, for garnish

In a soup pot or large casserole, sauté ginger, garlic, and onion in olive oil. Add a splash of water and cook vegetables until tender.

Stir in carrots.

Add chicken broth and water and simmer until carrots are tender (about 20 minutes).

Add lime juice and purée soup in blender until smooth.

Chill or serve warm. Top each soup bowl with a large dollop of yogurt.

Makes 7 one-cup servings
Calories per serving: 80 Total; 6 Fat; 1 Sat-fat

Q   # PEANUT BUTTER SOUP

A tasty soup that you can make easily in about 15 minutes.

1 cup chopped celery
½ cup chopped onion
1 teaspoon olive oil
¼ cup natural all-peanut peanut
   butter
1 can (10¾ oz) chicken broth,
   strained, + 1 can water

1 cup tomato juice
½ teaspoon coriander
Freshly ground black pepper to
   taste

In a soup pot or large casserole, sauté celery and onion in olive oil. Add a splash of water and cook until vegetables are tender.
Stir in peanut butter.
Add chicken broth, water, tomato juice, coriander, and pepper.
Bring to a boil, reduce heat, and simmer for 10 minutes.

Makes 5 one-cup servings
Calories per serving: 120 Total; 67 Fat; 11 Sat-fat

APPLE-SQUASH SOUP

Apple-Squash Soup is rich and delicious. Use acorn or butternut squash or even summer squash.

2 cups chopped onion
About 3 pounds squash, peeled,
   seeded, and cubed (about 6
   cups)
2 Granny Smith or other tart
   apples, peeled, cored, and
   cubed
3 cups chicken stock, or 1 can
   (10¾ oz) chicken broth,
   strained, + water to equal 3
   cups

1 teaspoon salt (optional)
5 teaspoons curry powder
1 cup apple cider or apple juice
Freshly ground black pepper to
   taste
1–2 Granny Smith or other tart
   apples, for garnish

In a large pot, combine onion, squash, apples, chicken stock, and salt. Stir in curry powder. Bring to a boil, reduce heat, and simmer for 25 minutes or until squash and apples are tender.

Remove 2 cups of liquid and set aside.

Purée remaining soup in blender and return to soup pot.

Stir cider into puréed soup.

Add liquid that you set aside, a bit at a time, making sure that soup remains thick, but not *too* thick.

If necessary, reheat soup until hot.

Pepper liberally.

Grate or chop apples into tiny pieces *just* before serving and garnish each bowl of soup.

Makes 9 one-cup servings
Calories per serving: 122 Total; 0 Fat; 0 Sat-fat

Q GINGER SQUASH SOUP

½ cup chopped onion

2 tablespoons minced ginger root

6 cups butternut squash, peeled, seeded, and cut into thin slices

2 cans chicken broth (10¾ oz each), strained

1 cup water

½ teaspoon salt (optional)

4 cloves garlic

2–3 tablespoons fresh lime juice

Salt and freshly ground black pepper to taste

In a large soup pot, combine onion, ginger root, and squash.

Add broth, water, salt, and garlic, and bring to a boil.

Reduce heat and simmer, covered, until squash is tender, about 15 minutes.

Purée in blender or food processor.

Return to pot and stir in lime juice, salt, and pepper.

Add more water, a tablespoon at a time, if too thick.

Makes 7 one-cup servings
Calories per serving: 52 Total; 0 Fat; 0 Sat-fat

Q   # TARRAGON SQUASH SOUP

A rich, creamy soup that uses no cream. Puréed bread is the secret ingredient.

2 pounds butternut squash, peeled, seeded, and coarsely chopped
2 cloves garlic, peeled
1 teaspoon salt (optional)
2 cans (10¾ oz each) chicken broth, strained, + ½ cup water

2 slices stale bread, crusts removed
¼ teaspoon freshly ground black pepper
1 teaspoon dried tarragon, or 1 tablespoon fresh tarragon, chopped

In a large pot, combine squash, garlic, salt, chicken broth, and water and bring to a boil. Reduce heat and simmer until squash is tender (about 20–25 minutes).

Tear bread into small pieces and add to squash. Simmer for 3 minutes more.

Purée in blender or food processor.

Just before serving, stir in pepper and tarragon.

Makes 6 one-cup servings
Calories per serving: 122 Total; 3 Fat; 1 Sat-fat

Q   # GREEN TOMATO SOUP

What does one do with all the green tomatoes left on the vine at the end of the summer growing season? Cook tangy, tasty Green Tomato Soup.

1 cup chopped green tomatoes
4 cups sliced green tomatoes
1 cup sliced onion
1 tablespoon olive oil

1 can (10¾ oz) chicken broth, strained, + 1 can water
2 cups shredded fresh spinach

Set aside the 1 cup chopped green tomatoes.

In a medium skillet, briefly sauté sliced green tomatoes and onion in olive oil. Cover and cook at low heat until tender.

Purée tomato-onion mixture in blender or food processor. Pour into casserole or soup pot.

Add chicken broth and water and heat through.

Five minutes before serving, add spinach and reserved chopped tomatoes.

Makes 7 one-cup servings
Calories per serving: 66 Total; 3 Fat; 2 Sat-fat

Q   # SWEET CABBAGE SOUP

4 cups chopped cabbage
3 cups grated carrot
1 large can (28 oz) tomatoes
  with juice
1 teaspoon tarragon

1 teaspoon basil
1 teaspoon salt (optional)
Water
Juice of 1 lemon
¼ cup raisins

In a large pot, combine cabbage, carrots, tomatoes and their juice, tarragon, basil, and salt. Add water to cover.

Bring to a boil. Reduce heat, cover, and simmer until vegetables are tender.

Purée soup lightly in blender so it still has texture.

Add lemon juice and raisins.

Makes 9 one-cup servings
Calories per serving: 56 Total; 1 Fat; 0 Sat-fat

Q   # CAULIFLOWER SOUP

Cauliflower Soup is a treasure. It is simple and quick to make and has a wonderful, delicate taste.

1 large head cauliflower
1 can chicken broth (10¾ oz),
  strained
2 stalks celery, diced
2 green onions, sliced

1 teaspoon olive oil
2 tablespoons unbleached white
  flour
1–2 cups water

Remove and discard cauliflower stem. Steam flowerets until tender. Reserve about ½ to 1½ cups and set aside. (You need about 4–5 cups cauliflower for the soup itself. Make sure you don't reserve too much!)

Purée cauliflower and chicken broth in blender. Set aside.

Sauté celery and green onions in oil until tender.

Reduce heat to medium and stir in flour.

Stir in cauliflower purée. Slowly mix in 1 cup of water, stirring constantly until soup thickens. If soup is too thick, stir in remaining water, ¼ cup at a time. Continue cooking until warmed through.

Cut reserved flowerets into bite-size pieces, add to soup, and serve.

Makes 6 one-cup servings (approximately)
Calories per serving: 47 Total; 7 Fat; 1 Sat-fat

Q **BROCCOLI SOUP**

1 cup chopped onion
½ cup chopped celery
1 cup water
⅓ cup long-grain rice

⅛–¼ teaspoon cayenne pepper
½–1 teaspoon salt (optional)
6 cups broccoli flowerets (about 2 heads)
3 cups skim milk

In a soup pot or large casserole, combine onion, celery, water, rice, cayenne pepper, salt, and broccoli. Bring to a boil and then simmer, covered, for about 20 minutes or until rice is cooked and broccoli is soft.

Place in blender. Add 2 cups of skim milk and blend until smooth. Add remaining milk, a half cup at a time until desired consistency is reached.

Reheat slowly and serve.

Makes 7 one-cup servings
Calories per serving: 99 Total; 0 Fat; 0 Sat-fat

Q

CORN CHOWDER

1 tablespoon margarine
2 tablespoons flour
2 cups skim milk

2 cans creamed corn (16 oz each)
½ teaspoon salt (optional)
½ red pepper or green pepper, chopped

In a large pot, melt margarine.
Remove pot from heat and mix in flour until smooth.
Slowly stir in 1 cup of the skim milk.
Return pot to burner and heat slowly until milk thickens.
Stir creamed corn and salt into milk.
Slowly stir in the remaining 1 cup of skim milk. Heat but do not boil.
Stir in peppers and serve.

Makes 6 one-cup servings
Calories per serving: 177 Total; 23 Fat; 5 Sat-fat

Q

CUCUMBER SOUP

Cucumber soup gets a gold star for excellence. It is as refreshing as a dip in a cool lake on a hot summer day. It is simple, quick, and impressive. Be sure to chill the soup thoroughly.

2 cucumbers
2 cups nonfat yogurt
1 can (10¾ oz) chicken broth, strained

1 clove garlic, crushed
Walnuts, for garnish

Peel cucumbers and cut into bite-size cubes. Salt heavily and set aside.
Spoon yogurt into a medium casserole and stir until smooth.
Stir in chicken broth.
Mix in garlic.
Rinse salt off cucumbers and add them to yogurt mixture. Add salt to taste.

Chill in refrigerator for several hours. Garnish with chopped walnuts.

Makes 5 one-cup servings
Calories per serving: 78 Total; 0 Fat; 0 Sat-fat
Calories per walnut half: 12 Total; 10 Fat; 1 Sat-fat

Q ## ZUCCHINI SOUP

One of the greatest recipes known to mankind. Hot or cold, summer or winter, for family or company, zucchini soup is delicious — and easy. You can even prepare it 20 minutes before you eat. If you want to make more and freeze it, just add a few more zucchini and more broth. This recipe is very flexible. Add more or less of any ingredient, and it will still taste superb.

3 large or 4 medium zucchini (or more or less), sliced
½ cup chopped onion
¼ cup long-grain rice
Chicken stock to cover zucchini, or 2 cans (10¾ oz each) chicken broth, strained, + water to cover zucchini

1 teaspoon salt (optional)
1 teaspoon curry powder (approximately)
1 teaspoon Dijon mustard (approximately)
½–1 cup nonfat yogurt

In a large soup pot, combine zucchini, onion, rice, chicken stock, water, and salt (add more water, if necessary, to cover zucchini).

Simmer for 15 minutes or until zucchini are tender.

Purée in blender, adding curry powder, mustard, and yogurt to taste.

Eat warm or cool.

This soup freezes well. Reheat frozen soup for best results. Eat immediately or cool for later.

Makes 8 (approximately) one-cup servings
Calories per serving: 80 Total; 0 Fat; 0 Sat-fat

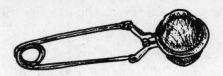

WATERCRESS SOUP

Watercress Soup is thick and creamy in texture but low in fat. It makes a refreshing first course in summer or winter.

1 teaspoon olive oil
1 cup chopped onion
2 bunches watercress, washed and stems removed
2 tablespoons unbleached white flour
5 cups chicken stock, or 2 cans (10¾ oz each) chicken broth, strained, + 2 cans water
1 teaspoon salt (optional)

½ teaspoon freshly ground black pepper
1 teaspoon tarragon
1 teaspoon dillweed
1 quart buttermilk
2 tablespoons fresh lemon juice
1 teaspoon Worcestershire sauce
½ teaspoon curry powder
10 sprigs watercress, for garnish

In a large soup pot, heat olive oil. Add onion and a splash of water and cook until soft.

Stir in watercress.

Cover and cook slowly for 10 minutes or until watercress wilts.

Sprinkle on flour and mix well.

Add chicken stock, salt, and pepper. Cover and simmer for 30 minutes. Add tarragon and dillweed at the last minute.

Cool slightly. Purée in blender or food processor.

Return soup to pot. Add buttermilk, lemon juice, and Worcestershire sauce and stir until smooth.

Add curry powder and heat through.

Cool and refrigerate.

Makes 10 one-cup servings
Calories per serving: 74 Total; 4 Fat; 0 Sat-fat

Q

GAZPACHO I

4 large tomatoes, quartered
1 medium onion, quartered
2 cloves garlic
1 green pepper, coarsely
    chopped
1 cucumber, peeled and coarsely
    chopped

¼ cup white vinegar
1 cup tomato juice
Salt to taste (optional)
Stale bread (1 or 2 slices, or
    bagel)

In a blender, roughly purée tomatoes, onion, garlic, green pepper, cucumber, vinegar, tomato juice, and salt. Chill.

Before serving, make croutons by cutting bread (bagel, whole-wheat bread — whatever you have around) into cubes and toasting until crispy in toaster oven.

Garnish soup with croutons.

Makes 8 one-cup servings

Calories per serving:	Total	Fat	Sat-fat
Without croutons	55	0	0
With croutons	79	1	1

Q

GAZPACHO II

If you hate wasting the juice from canned tomatoes, the following two recipes (Gazpacho II and Tomato-Rice Soup) will appeal to you. Each time you use canned tomatoes, accumulate their juice in a storage container in the freezer for future soups.

8 cups juice from canned
    tomatoes
2 green peppers, coarsely
    chopped
1 medium onion, coarsely
    chopped

2 cloves garlic, minced
1 cucumber, peeled and coarsely
    chopped
¼ cup white vinegar
Salt and freshly ground black
    pepper to taste

Purée all ingredients in blender. Chill.
Add croutons as in Gazpacho I (page 195).

Makes 8 one-cup servings

Calories per serving:	Total	Fat	Sat-fat
Without croutons	53	0	0
With croutons	70	1	1

Q   # TOMATO-RICE SOUP

6 cups juice from canned tomatoes	½ cup long-grain rice
1 tablespoon grated onion	1 cup frozen peas
1 pinch ground cloves	1 cup frozen corn

Combine tomato juice, onion, cloves, and rice and bring to a boil. Reduce heat and simmer for about 25 minutes.

Add peas and corn and cook about 5 minutes more.

Makes 8 one-cup servings
Calories per serving: 93 Total; 0 Fat; 0 Sat-fat

Q   # ORIENTAL NOODLE SOUP

2 cans chicken broth (10¾ oz each), strained, + 2 cans water	¼ teaspoon white pepper
	1 cake tofu,* cubed
	1 green onion, sliced
2 ounces cellophane noodles*	10–15 snow peas
1 tablespoon soy sauce	

Bring broth and water to a boil in a soup pot. Add cellophane noodles.

Simmer about 10 minutes, until noodles are soft.

Add soy sauce and white pepper. Simmer a minute or two.

Add tofu, green onion, and snow peas and serve.

Makes 6 one-cup servings
Calories per serving: 64 Total; 8 Fat; 1 Sat-fat

HOT AND SOUR SOUP

The ingredients in Hot and Sour Soup seem exotic, but they are all available at Oriental food stores. This wonderful soup is worth an extra shopping trip. You may use the ingredients in many other recipes.

NOTE: This soup is spicy hot. Reduce chili oil and white pepper for a milder soup.

10 large dried black mushrooms*
½ cup tree ear fungi*
⅓ cup tiger lily stems (golden needles)*
2 tablespoons cornstarch
3 tablespoons water
¾ cup diced uncooked chicken breast
1 teaspoon olive oil
1 tablespoon soy sauce
1 can (8 oz) bamboo shoots,* sliced

6 cups chicken stock, or 3 cans (10¾ oz each) chicken broth, strained, + 2 cans water
3 tablespoons white vinegar
1 tablespoon double black soy sauce**
2 cakes tofu (fresh bean curd),* cubed
2 teaspoons chili oil*
½–1 teaspoon ground white pepper
2 egg whites, beaten
4 green onions, sliced

Place mushrooms, tree ears, and tiger lily stems in a small bowl and cover with boiling water. In about 15 minutes or when they are soft, drain off the water and chop off stems or any hard parts.

Slice mushrooms and tree ears and pull tiger lily stems into shreds. Set aside.

Combine cornstarch and water into a smooth paste. Set aside.

In a heated wok or skillet, sauté chicken in oil until chicken is cooked through.

Stir in regular soy sauce.

Stir in mushrooms, tree ears, tiger lily stems, and bamboo shoots.

Add chicken stock, vinegar, and double black soy sauce.

Stir cornstarch mixture into soup. Let thicken.

Add tofu and bring soup to a boil.

Stir in the chili oil and white pepper.

---

*Available at Oriental food stores and some supermarkets
**If double black soy sauce is not available, make your own by mixing 2 teaspoons regular soy sauce with 1 teaspoon molasses.

Turn off the heat for 1 minute and then slowly pour the egg whites into the soup, stirring constantly.

Garnish each bowl of soup with chopped green onions.

Makes 10 one-cup servings
Calories per serving: 97 Total; 14 Fat; 4 Sat-fat

Ⓠ MULLIGATAWNY SOUP

Customarily, Mulligatawny Soup is made with cream. Our Mulligatawny Soup dispenses with the cream (at 335 sat-fat calories a cup) or a cream substitute. The spicy flavors and interesting textures make this one of our favorite soups.

½ cup chopped onion
½ cup chopped carrot
½ cup chopped celery
2 teaspoons olive oil
1½ tablespoons flour
2 teaspoons curry powder
5 cups chicken stock, or 2 cans
  (10 oz each) chicken broth,
  strained, + 2 cans water

½ cup diced uncooked chicken
½ cup cooked long-grain rice
¼ teaspoon thyme
1 teaspoon salt (optional)
¼ teaspoon freshly ground
  black pepper
1 apple, peeled and diced

In a soup pot or large casserole, sauté onion, carrot, and celery in oil. Add a splash of water and cook until vegetables are tender.

Stir in flour and curry powder and cook for about 1 minute.

Pour in chicken stock and bring to a boil.

Add chicken. Reduce heat, cover, and simmer for 15 minutes.

Add rice, thyme, salt, and pepper and simmer for 15 minutes more. Add apple and serve.

Makes 6 one-cup servings
Calories per serving: 114 Total; 14 Fat; 2 Sat-fat

☑ MONHEGAN ISLAND FISH CHOWDER

Eating Monhegan Island Fish Chowder will show you that fish chowders need not be made with cream to be delicious. This chowder uses one large can of evaporated skim milk, which has 3 calories of saturated fat. A comparable amount of cream has 335 calories of saturated fat.

3 large potatoes (about 4 cups)
1 cup chopped onion
1 teaspoon olive oil
2 cups water
1 teaspoon salt (optional)
1 teaspoon basil

¼ teaspoon freshly ground
    black pepper
1 pound cod fillets
2 cups frozen corn kernels
1 large can (12 oz) evaporated
    skim milk

Scrub potatoes well and cut into bite-size pieces. *Do not peel.* Steam until just tender. Set aside.

In a large pot, sauté onion in olive oil until tender.

Add potatoes, water, salt, basil, and pepper and bring to a boil. Reduce heat, cover, and simmer for 15 minutes.

Gently place cod fillets on top of potatoes, cover, and simmer until fish flakes easily (about 10 minutes).

Carefully stir in corn and evaporated milk. Heat until corn and milk are hot and serve. Do not allow soup to boil.

Makes 9 one-cup servings
Calories per serving: 156 Total; 13 Fat; 3 Sat-fat

MILD FISH CHOWDER

2 cans (10¾ oz each) chicken
    broth, strained, + 2 cans
    water
3 cups cubed potatoes
2 tablespoons long-grain rice
½ cup sliced carrot
1 teaspoon dillweed
1 cup sliced leeks
2 green onions, sliced

2 teaspoons olive oil
1 tablespoon unbleached white
    flour
1 cup frozen corn
⅓ pound mild white fish (such
    as turbot)
½ can (6½ oz) solid white
    albacore tuna packed in water

In a large pot, combine chicken broth, water, potatoes, rice, carrots, and dillweed.

In a skillet, sauté leeks and green onions in olive oil until soft. Mix in flour until smooth and remove from heat.

Add leek-flour mixture to soup.

Simmer soup until potatoes are fully cooked (about 20 minutes).

Stir in corn, fish, tuna, and tuna liquid. Cook 5 minutes more or until fish is fully cooked.

Makes 7 one-cup servings
Calories per serving: 179 Total; 18 Fat; 1 Sat-fat

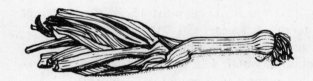

Q MINESTRONE

Almost every Italian restaurant in Italy offers its own minestrone, or vegetable soup. Each one is slightly different and all are wonderful. Take whatever vegetables you have in the refrigerator, add some water or broth, pasta, rice and/or beans, to create your own minestrone.

½ onion, sliced	¼ cup long-grain rice
1 teaspoon olive oil	1 teaspoon basil
2 potatoes, diced	1 teaspoon oregano
4 carrots, sliced	½–1 teaspoon salt (optional)
2 celery stalks, sliced	1 can (15½ oz) kidney beans

In a soup pot or large casserole, sauté onion in olive oil. Add a splash of water and continue to cook until tender.

Mix in potatoes, carrots, and celery. Add water to cover.

Add rice, basil, oregano, salt, and kidney beans.

Bring to a boil. Reduce heat, cover, and simmer until rice is cooked and vegetables are tender (about 25 minutes).

Makes 8 one-cup servings
Calories per serving: 110 Total; 8 Fat; 1 Sat-fat

VEGETABLE SOUP PROVENÇAL

A hearty Mediterranean soup with a distinctive taste. Use whatever vegetables you have on hand. The more the better! The secret ingredient is the pistou. Italy has its pesto and France has its pistou. Both sauces are combinations of basil, garlic, cheese (omitted here because it is so high in sat-fat), and olive oil, added to soups and pasta to enhance and enrich the flavor.

Make a lot of Vegetable Soup Provençal. It freezes well.
CAUTION: Reheat slowly.

1 large onion, chopped
3 cups sliced carrots
2–3 potatoes, diced
2½ quarts water
1 teaspoon salt (optional)
Any vegetables, such as:
   1 zucchini, sliced
   2 cups broccoli flowerets
   1 cup cauliflower flowerets
   2 cups green beans

2 slices stale bread, shredded
½ cup broken pieces of
   spaghetti

Pistou

8 cloves garlic, minced
⅓ cup chopped parsley
1 can (6 oz) tomato paste

3 tablespoons dried basil, or ½
   cup fresh basil

In a large soup pot, combine onion, carrot, and potato.

Add water and salt and heat to boiling. Reduce heat, cover, and simmer for 20 minutes.

Add zucchini, broccoli, cauliflower, green beans, any other vegetables of your choice, bread, and spaghetti and simmer, covered, for 15 minutes more.

Make pistou in food processor, blender, or with a fork by blending garlic, parsley, tomato paste, and basil until smooth.

Stir the pistou into the soup, a little at a time.

Makes 15 one-cup servings
Calories per serving: 58 Total; 1 Fat; 0 Sat-fat

▣ VEGETABLE SOUP WITH SPINACH, POTATOES, RICE, AND CORN

This soup is great! So quick, so easy, and so tasty.

2 cloves garlic, minced
1 teaspoon olive oil
5 ounces fresh spinach, torn into bite-size pieces
1 can chicken broth (10¾ oz), strained, + 2 cans water

½ teaspoon salt, optional
2 small potatoes, peeled and cubed
¼ cup long-grain rice
1 cup frozen corn

In soup pot, sauté garlic in oil until soft.
Stir in spinach and cook for about 1 minute.
Add broth, water, salt, potatoes, and rice, and bring to a boil.
Reduce to a simmer and cook for about 15 minutes or until potatoes are tender and rice is cooked.
Add corn and cook for about 1 minute.

Makes 5 one-cup servings
Calories per serving: 129 Total; 12 Fat; 2 Sat-fat

GREEN PESTO SOUP

3 cups shredded spinach, washed, stems removed
6 green onions, sliced
1 cup shredded leaf lettuce
2 potatoes, peeled and diced (about 2 cups)

8 cups water
1 teaspoon salt (optional)
¼ teaspoon freshly ground black pepper
1 cup broken pieces of thin spaghetti

Pesto

2 cloves garlic
1 tablespoon olive oil
2 tablespoons basil
2 tablespoons chopped parsley

2 cups spinach, washed and
stems removed
½ cup water

In a soup pot, combine spinach, green onions, lettuce, potatoes, water, salt, and pepper.

Cover pot and simmer until potatoes are tender (about 25 minutes).

Add spaghetti and bring soup to a boil. Reduce heat and simmer for 6 minutes.

Meanwhile, make pesto in a blender or food processor by blending garlic, olive oil, basil, parsley, spinach, and water until smooth.

Mix pesto into soup and serve.

Makes 11 one-cup servings
Calories per serving: 53 Total; 11 Fat; 1 Sat-fat

BARLEY-VEGETABLE SOUP

A hearty soup that improves as it ages. Make it in the morning or the night before so it will have time to thicken.

½ cup pearl barley
2 quarts homemade chicken
stock, or 3 cans (10¾ oz
each) chicken broth, strained,
+ 3 cans water
1 small onion, cut into fourths
1 carrot, cut into thirds
1 stalk celery, cut into 1 inch
slices

1 teaspoon thyme
1 bay leaf
Freshly ground black pepper to
taste
3–5 carrots, sliced
2 stalks celery, sliced
½ zucchini, sliced
½ cup onion, chopped
2 cups fresh spinach, chopped

Place barley, chicken stock, onion quarters, carrot thirds, celery slices, thyme, and bay leaf in a large soup pot and bring to a boil. Reduce heat, cover, and simmer for about 1 hour or until barley is tender.

Add sliced carrots, celery, zucchini, and chopped onion and cook until tender.

Add spinach a few minutes before serving.

Makes 9 one-cup servings
Calories per serving: 100 Total; 0 Fat; 0 Sat-fat

Q   ## LENTIL AND EVERYTHING BUT
THE KITCHEN SINK SOUP

Lentils are legumes, which, besides tasting very good, are quite nutritious. They are rich in vitamin C, folic acid, and many minerals. They are a good source of soluble fiber, which has been found to lower blood cholesterol.

1 cup lentils	5 cups water
1 clove garlic, minced	1 cup tomato juice
2 stalks celery, sliced	1 teaspoon salt (optional)
½ cup chopped onion	1 teaspoon thyme
1 teaspoon olive oil	1 tablespoon soy sauce
1 cup grated carrot	⅓ cup brown rice
1½–2 cups coarsely chopped potato	1½ cups frozen corn

Place lentils in a bowl and cover with water.

In a large pot, sauté garlic, celery, and onion in olive oil. Add a splash of water and cook vegetables until tender.

Stir in carrot and potatoes.

Drain water from lentils and add lentils to vegetables.

Add water, tomato juice, salt, thyme, soy sauce, and brown rice. Bring to a boil. Reduce heat, cover, and simmer until lentils and potatoes are tender (about 30 minutes).

Add corn and cook 10 to 20 minutes more.

If soup is too thick, add more water, ¼ cup at a time.

Makes 9 one-cup servings
Calories per serving: 85 Total; 6 Fat; 0 Sat-fat

Q
LENTIL SOUP

½ pound lentils (1⅓ cups)
½ cup chopped onion
1 cup diced carrots
2 stalks celery, diced
1 green pepper, diced
1 teaspoon olive oil
1 teaspoon cumin
1 teaspoon chili powder
¾ teaspoon allspice
1 bay leaf

¼ cup chopped parsley
1 small boiling potato, peeled and diced
1 can chicken broth (10¾ oz), strained
4 cups water
½ teaspoon salt (optional)
Freshly ground black pepper
½ cup nonfat yogurt

Rinse off lentils and cover with water. Set aside.

In a large soup pot, sauté onion, carrots, celery, and green pepper in olive oil. Add a splash of water and cook vegetables until soft. After about 30 seconds, lower the heat to medium.

Mix in cumin, chili powder, allspice, bay leaf, and parsley.

Drain lentils and add to soup. Mix in potato.

Add chicken broth, water, and salt and pepper.

Bring to boil, cover, and reduce to simmer for about 30 minutes or until lentils are tender.

Remove bay leaf. If you wish, purée about ⅞ of the soup. Return purée to pot and mix into remaining soup.

Serve each bowl with a dollop of yogurt.

Makes 8 one-cup servings

Calories per serving:	Total	Fat	Sat-fat
Without yogurt	141	7	1
With yogurt	148	7	1

BEAN SOUPS

Even if you don't like beans, you'll love the following bean recipes: the secret to great bean soup is making a purée of most of the beans instead of leaving them whole. (Of course, you may prefer your beans not puréed at all.) See "Beans," page 293.

CUBAN BLACK BEAN SOUP

Beans are an excellent source of protein, soluble fiber, calcium, magnesium, phosphorus, potassium, iron, and zinc. Experiment with different types of beans to make this hearty, tasty soup. Spoon it over rice and top it with chopped onions.

1 ½ cups dried black beans	1 teaspoon oregano
2 cloves garlic, minced	1 teaspoon salt, optional
1 large onion, chopped	1 ¼ cups cooked rice
1 green pepper, chopped	½ cup chopped onions, for
1 teaspoon olive oil	garnish
1 teaspoon cumin	2 ½ teaspoons vinegar

Cover black beans with cold water and soak overnight, or cover beans with boiling water and let soak for 4 hours.

Drain the beans and place in soup pot. Add water to cover. Simmer until tender (about 1–1 ½ hours).

In a medium skillet, sauté garlic, onions, and green pepper in olive oil until tender. Add a splash of water to help vegetables cook.

Stir in cumin, oregano, and salt. Add 1 tablespoon of water and simmer for one more minute to blend flavors.

Add vegetable mixture to beans. If you wish, purée ⅞ of the soup in blender and return purée to pot.

Place ¼ cup of rice in each soup bowl. Spoon soup over rice. Top with chopped onions and sprinkle with ½ teaspoon of vinegar.

Makes 5 one-cup servings
Calories per serving: 207 Total; 15 Fat; 3 Sat-fat

BEAN SOUP WITH SPINACH, SQUASH, AND TOMATOES

2 cups dried red chili beans (or any other dried bean)
1 can chicken broth (10¾ oz), strained
1 medium onion, minced
3 cloves garlic, minced
1 teaspoon minced ginger root
1 teaspoon olive oil
¾–1 teaspoon cumin
¾–1 teaspoon turmeric
½ teaspoon coriander
¼–½ teaspoon cayenne pepper
½–1 teaspoon salt (optional)
1 medium zucchini, quartered and sliced into ½-inch pieces
5 ounces fresh spinach, torn into bite-size pieces
1 can (16 oz) chopped tomatoes, with juice
1 cup water

Cover beans with boiling water and let soak for 4 hours. Drain. Add water to cover and cook 1 hour or until tender. Drain.

Remove about ⅞ of the beans and purée with chicken broth in blender. Add purée back to the whole beans.

In a large soup pot, sauté onion, garlic, and ginger root in olive oil. Add a splash of water and cook vegetables until soft.

Mix in cumin, turmeric, coriander, cayenne, and salt.

Stir in bean mixture, zucchini, and spinach.

Add tomatoes. If mixture is too thick, slowly add water, a few tablespoons at a time, until desired consistency is reached. Cook 5 minutes.

Makes 10 one-cup servings
Calories per serving: 154 Total; 8 Fat; 0 Sat-fat

GREAT BLACK BEAN SOUP

1½ cups dried black beans
4 carrots, sliced
1 clove garlic, minced
½ cup chopped onion
1 teaspoon olive oil
1 tablespoon cumin
1 teaspoon coriander
¼–½ teaspoon cayenne
2 cans chicken broth (10¾ oz each), strained
½ cup long-grain rice
1 cup water
2 tablespoons nonfat yogurt per serving

Cover beans with boiling water. Let soak for 4 hours. Cook them for 1 hour–1 hour 15 minutes or until tender. Set aside.

Steam carrots until tender. Set aside.

In a large soup pot, sauté garlic and onion in olive oil. Add a splash of water to help vegetables cook.

Stir in cumin, coriander, and cayenne, and cook briefly. Add chicken broth.

Drain beans and add them to the soup. Add all but 1 cup of carrots. Simmer for 5 minutes. Add rice and simmer, partially covered, for 15–20 minutes.

Purée ¾–⅞ of the soup in blender. Return purée to pot. Add remaining carrots.

If soup is too thick, add water a little at a time until soup is a desirable consistency — not too thick and not too watery.

Top with a dollop of yogurt (2 tablespoons) for each serving.

Makes 7 one-cup servings
Calories per serving: 227 Total; 11 Fat; 1 Sat-fat

Q   # TORTILLA SOUP

This instantaneous soup always gets rave reviews.

6 corn tortillas*
1 medium onion, diced
3 cloves garlic, minced
1 teaspoon olive oil
2 tablespoons chili powder
1 teaspoon oregano
1 large can (28 oz) heavy
  concentrated crushed
  tomatoes

1 can (10¾ oz) chicken broth,
  strained, + 1 can water
1 green pepper, diced
1 cup frozen corn
Salt and pepper to taste

About 15 minutes before you serve soup, heat tortillas in a slow oven (325°F), until crisp.

In a soup pot, sauté onion and garlic in oil. Add a splash of water and cook vegetables until soft.

Stir in chili powder and oregano.

Stir in tomatoes, chicken broth, and water.

---

*Corn tortillas can be found in the refrigerator section of most supermarkets. Be sure they contain no lard or other saturated fat.

Bring to a boil and simmer for a few minutes.
Add green pepper and corn.
Add salt and pepper to taste.
For each serving, break a tortilla into small pieces and place at the bottom of a soup bowl. Ladle soup over the tortilla and serve.

Makes 7 one-cup servings
Calories per serving: 144 Total; 10 Fat; 1 Sat-fat

Q   # CANTALOUPE SOUP

Cantaloupe is an excellent source of vitamins A and C and fiber as well as being just plain delicious. Combined with ginger, orange juice, and buttermilk, cantaloupe makes a refreshing and unusual summer soup.

2 cantaloupes, chilled if possible
¼ cup orange juice
1 teaspoon chopped ginger root

3 tablespoons sweet vermouth
½ cup buttermilk

Halve melons, discard seeds, scoop out meat, and place it in blender.
Add orange juice, ginger, vermouth, and buttermilk, and blend.
If cold, serve immediately. Otherwise, chill.

Makes 6 one-cup servings
Calories per serving: 80 Total; 0 Fat; 0 Sat-fat

Q   # CHILLED STRAWBERRY SOUP

Ron says this soup should be in the dessert section. It is sweet and refreshing and easy to make.

2 oranges, peeled and thinly
  sliced
1 cinnamon stick
2 cups water
¼ cup sugar

2 cups sliced strawberries*
Dash of salt
1½ tablespoons cornstarch
1 tablespoon water

*Try peaches, cherries, apricots, or a combination of fruits.

Simmer orange pieces and cinnamon stick in 2 cups of water for 5 minutes.

Remove the cinnamon stick and set aside.

Add sugar, strawberries, and a dash of salt and bring to a boil. Turn heat to low.

Blend cornstarch with 1 tablespoon water and stir into soup until clear.

Chill with cinnamon stick.

Makes 5 one-cup servings
Calories per serving: 90 Total; 0 Fat; 0 Sat-fat

Q   # BLUEBERRY SOUP

This is a wonderful, sweet, refreshing soup that couldn't be easier to make. I have made it with blueberries and with strawberries — each makes an elegant and scrumptious soup. To make more or less soup than the recipe calls for, use the same ingredients, just keep the proportions the same.

3 cups blueberries (or other   ½ cup sugar
   fruit, such as strawberries,   1 cinnamon stick
   raspberries)   1–1½ cups nonfat yogurt
2¼ cups water

Combine fruit, water, sugar, and cinnamon stick in a saucepan.

Bring to a boil and remove from heat. Pour into blender and let cool. (If soup is too hot, it will curdle the yogurt.)

Remove cinnamon stick (but do not discard it) and blend. Add yogurt and blend.

Chill with cinnamon stick. Refrigerate until cold.

Makes 7 one-cup servings
Calories per serving: 96 Total; 0 Fat; 0 Sat-fat

Q   # SOUR CHERRY SOUP

Sour Cherry Soup is a sweet soup. It is ideal for a luncheon or dinner party and *very* simple to make. It has no fat but does have quite a lot of sugar.

2 cans (1 lb each) undrained sour cherries packed in water
¾ cup sugar
1 stick cinnamon

2 tablespoons unbleached white flour
6 tablespoons cold water
2 cups water

Remove about 12 cherries from one can and put aside for garnish. (Or buy another whole can of cherries.)

In a medium saucepan, cook cherries with their juice, sugar, and cinnamon stick for 10 to 15 minutes.

In a small bowl, mix flour and 3 tablespoons of the cold water until smooth. Blend in remaining 3 tablespoons cold water.

Remove cinnamon stick from cooked cherries and set aside.

Pour cherry mixture into blender. Add flour mixture and blend until soup is smooth.

Return soup to saucepan, add 2 cups water, and heat just to boiling.

Return cinnamon stick to soup and chill.

Garnish each bowl of soup with a few cherries before serving.

Makes 6 one-cup servings
Calories per serving: 165 Total; 0 Fat; 0 Sat-fat

15 CHICKEN

CHICKEN IS ONE of the most versatile meats. You can sauté it, bake it, broil it, boil it, roast it, or make it into chicken salad, chicken pot pie, or chicken brochettes. You can cook it with fruit, vegetables, grains, wine, herbs, or spices and it will be different and delicious each time.

Almost all of the following recipes use chicken breasts without skin. Chicken breast without skin is the preferred chicken choice for anyone concerned about saturated fat intake. Both thighs and drumsticks without skin are low in saturated fat (2.6 calories of sat-fat per ounce for a thigh, which amounts to about 6 sat-fat calories per thigh or 12 sat-fat calories for 2 thighs. There are 2 calories of saturated fat per ounce for a drumstick, which amounts to 5 sat-fat calories per drumstick or 10 sat-fat calories for 2). However, chicken breasts without skin are even lower (about 0.8 calories of sat-fat per ounce, which amounts to about 3.5 sat-fat calories per breast) and more versatile. If you do substitute chicken thighs or drumsticks in any of the recipes, make sure you adjust the total sat-fat values to reflect that change.

Chicken breasts may be purchased with bones or already boned. You may have avoided buying *boneless* chicken breasts without skin because of their expense. However, the skin and bones of a chicken breast account for half its weight. You are paying much more for chicken breasts with skin and bones than you think. Look for boned chicken breasts without skin on sale for a real bargain.

If chicken breast tenderloins are available in your supermarket, we recommend them highly. They are wonderfully tender. Substitute about 4 tenderloins for 1 chicken breast. Be sure to pull out the tendon.

COOKING FOR ONE OR TWO

In case you find that one of our recipes makes more servings than you need, just divide all the ingredients proportionately. For example, if the recipe calls for 8 chicken breasts, use 4 or 2, and instead of ½ cup of lime juice, use ¼ cup or 2 tablespoons; instead of 1 teaspoon of ginger, use ½ teaspoon, or ¼ teaspoon, etc. You may also want to make the full or half recipe and eat one half and freeze the rest. If you have a big dinner party, you can double or triple all the ingredients. The recipes are quite flexible, so just relax and adapt them to your needs.

NOTE: It is easier to slice chicken when it is slightly frozen. If you do not mind unusual-looking chicken pieces, the following advice will save you time. Slice slightly frozen (but not rock-hard frozen) boneless chicken breasts without skin lengthwise into 1½-inch-wide chunks. Feed into food processor using the thickest slicer you have. Sauté the chicken in oil and freeze for later use.

If you use canned chicken broth in any of these recipes, either strain the broth (pour it through a fine tea strainer) or, if the fat is hardened, lift it off the surface of the broth with a spoon. You can also use a gravy skimmer to skim off the fat.

SAVING SAT-FAT AND FAT

To save sat-fat and fat calories, flour and bake chicken in a shallow baking pan with no fat instead of sautéing it in oil. When the chicken is fully cooked, either refrigerate or freeze it for later use or substitute it for sautéed chicken in a recipe.

⧉ INDONESIAN CHICKEN WITH GREEN BEANS

A beautiful dish — green beans set against ochre-colored sauce — and very tasty. This is one of our all-time favorites.

6 boned and skinned chicken breasts
½ cup unbleached white flour
¼ teaspoon freshly ground black pepper
½ teaspoon salt (optional)
1 pound green beans, washed and cut into bite-size pieces
10 cloves garlic, minced
1 tablespoon minced ginger root

1 small onion, chopped
1 teaspoon olive oil
Juice of 1 lime (preferred) or lemon
1 tablespoon double black soy sauce*
2 teaspoons brown sugar
2 teaspoons turmeric
1 teaspoon salt (optional)
½ cup water

Preheat oven to 375°F.

Shake chicken in a plastic bag with flour, pepper, and ½ teaspoon salt until chicken is coated.

Place chicken in a single layer in a baking pan and bake until fully cooked, about 20–30 minutes. Set aside. You may bake the chicken the night before and refrigerate it until ready to add to sauce.

Cook green beans in a pot of boiling water for 5–10 minutes until tender but still crisp. Set aside.

Cut chicken into bite-size pieces. Set aside.

Sauté garlic, ginger, and onion in olive oil until soft.

Add lime juice, soy sauce, brown sugar, turmeric, 1 teaspoon salt, and ¼ cup of the water.

Slowly add remaining water, if necessary. Sauce should not be watery.

Add chicken and green beans and stir until completely covered with sauce.

Serve over rice.

8 servings
Calories per serving: 135 Total; 14 Fat; 4 Sat-fat

---

*Double black soy sauce is available at Oriental food stores and some supermarkets. You can make your own by mixing 2 teaspoons soy sauce with 1 teaspoon dark molasses.

Q ## LEMON CHICKEN

A delicate blending of tart and sweet, Lemon Chicken can't help but become one of your most popular family or company dishes.

4 boned and skinned chicken
  breasts
Juice of 2 lemons
½ cup unbleached white flour
¼ teaspoon freshly ground
  black pepper
½ teaspoon salt (optional)

¼ teaspoon paprika
1 tablespoon grated lemon peel
2 tablespoons brown sugar
1 tablespoon lemon juice
1 tablespoon water
1 lemon, sliced thin

Place chicken in a bowl or casserole. Pour lemon juice over breasts and marinate in refrigerator for several hours or overnight, turning chicken periodically.

Preheat oven to 350°F.

Combine flour, pepper, salt, and paprika in plastic bag.

Remove chicken breasts from marinade and coat each with flour by shaking it in the plastic bag.

Place chicken in a baking pan in a single layer.

Either peel the yellow (zest) from a lemon and chop it fine in your food processor (a mini food chopper makes a perfect grater), or grate the zest with a hand grater. Mix 1 tablespoon of the grated peel with the brown sugar.

Sprinkle the lemon zest–sugar mixture evenly over the chicken breasts. Combine 1 tablespoon lemon juice and water and sprinkle evenly over chicken.

Put 1 lemon slice on each chicken breast and bake chicken for 35–40 minutes or until cooked through.

4 servings
Calories per serving: 176 Total; 13 Fat; 4 Sat-fat

LIME-PEANUT-GINGER CHICKEN

Don't be put off by our ho-hum name for this chicken recipe. Although it contains these three ingredients (actually peanut butter), the flavors combine to produce a unique and simply delectable taste.

6 boned and skinned chicken
  breasts
½ cup fresh lime juice
1 clove garlic
1 tablespoon sliced ginger root
1 teaspoon whole black
  peppercorns
1 teaspoon dried basil
1 tablespoon soy sauce
1 tablespoon white vinegar
1 teaspoon honey

1 tablespoon water
1 tablespoon grated lemon peel
2 tablespoons olive oil
1 tablespoon sesame oil
1 tablespoon natural all-peanut
  peanut butter
2–3 cups sliced mushrooms
1 tablespoon cornstarch diluted
  in 2 tablespoons water
¼–½ cup sliced green onions

Cut chicken into bite-size pieces and marinate in lime juice for at least 2 hours in refrigerator.

Make a dressing by chopping garlic, ginger, and peppercorns in food processor or blender until pepper is no longer whole. (It will probably be impossible to break up all peppercorns.)

Blend in basil, soy sauce, vinegar, honey, water, and grated lemon peel.

Pour 1 tablespoon of the olive oil into the processor or blender and process until smooth. Set dressing aside.

Remove chicken from marinade and sauté it in sesame oil and the remaining tablespoon of olive oil until it turns white.

Add dressing and stir until chicken is well coated and sauce is warm.

Mix in peanut butter. Stir in mushrooms. Add cornstarch mixture to thicken sauce.

Sprinkle green onions on top and serve over rice.

8 servings
Calories per serving: 175 Total; 64 Fat; 11 Sat-fat

Q   # CHICKEN KIEV

This recipe is a gem: it uses ingredients you probably have on hand; it takes no time to make; and the resulting dish is so special you can proudly serve it to the most discriminating of guests.

1 clove garlic, finely chopped
½ teaspoon basil
½ teaspoon oregano
¼ teaspoon salt (optional)
1 cup fine bread crumbs made from 1–2 slices of white bread or challah*

4 boned and skinned chicken breasts
1 tablespoon margarine
3 tablespoons dry white wine or vermouth
¼ cup sliced green onions

Preheat oven to 375°F.

Mix garlic, basil, oregano, and salt with bread crumbs and place on a large plate. (You can mince the garlic in a food processor, add bread and process until it becomes crumbs, then add spices and process again.)

Roll each chicken breast in bread crumbs and place it in a shallow baking pan.

Bake near center of oven for 30–45 minutes or until fully cooked.

Melt the margarine. Mix in wine and green onions.

Pour sauce over chicken.

Return chicken to oven for 3–5 minutes or until sauce is hot. Serve over rice.

4 servings
Calories per serving: 175 Total; 38 Fat; 6 Sat-fat

---

*Avoid commercial bread crumbs. They are high in total calories (390 per cup) and high in saturated fat calories (14 per cup). Use your food processor or blender to make your own bread crumbs from a few slices of bread (about 65 total calories and 2 sat-fat calories per slice.

Q INDONESIAN PEANUT CHICKEN

Peanuts are a major ingredient in Indonesian cooking. The spicy peanut sauce that covers this chicken dish is called a satay. The satay may also be used as a dip for vegetables or slices of cold chicken.

4 boned and skinned chicken breasts
½ cup unbleached white flour

½ teaspoon salt (optional)
¼ teaspoon freshly ground black pepper

Satay sauce

1 clove garlic
1 small onion
1 teaspoon ginger root
⅓ cup shelled roasted peanuts, unsalted
2 teaspoons soy sauce
2 teaspoons turmeric

1½ teaspoons lime (preferred) or lemon juice
1–2 hot chili peppers
¾ cup water
1 large onion, sliced
1 teaspoon olive oil

Preheat oven to 375°F.

Shake chicken in a plastic bag with flour, salt, and pepper until coated.

Place chicken in a single layer in a shallow baking pan and bake until fully cooked, 20–30 minutes. Set aside and make satay. You may bake the chicken the night before and refrigerate it until ready to use.

Blend garlic, onion, ginger, peanuts, soy sauce, turmeric, lime or lemon juice, chili peppers, and water in blender or food processor until smooth.

Place sauce in top of double boiler and heat water to boiling. Cover pot and cook sauce for 10–20 minutes or until thick.

Sauté onion rings in olive oil until soft.

Cut chicken into bite-size pieces and warm in a large skillet.

Pour satay sauce over chicken and stir until chicken is well coated. If sauce is too thick, add a small amount of water, 1 tablespoon at a time.

Stir in onion rings and serve over rice.

5 servings
Calories per serving: 148 Total; 61 Fat; 10 Sat-fat

◻ TANDOORI CHICKEN

1 clove garlic, minced
½ tablespoon sliced ginger root
2 tablespoons chopped onion
½ teaspoon Dijon mustard
⅛ teaspoon cardamom
⅛ teaspoon coriander
¼ teaspoon salt (optional)

¼ teaspoon freshly ground
  black pepper
1½ tablespoons fresh lemon
  juice
¾ cup nonfat yogurt
4 skinned chicken breasts

Combine all ingredients except chicken (may be done in food processor, mincing garlic and ginger first) and pour over chicken breasts.

Marinate in refrigerator for at least 24 hours.

Place chicken with marinade in a shallow baking pan.

Bake at 375°F for 30–45 minutes or until chicken is fully cooked.

4 servings
Calories per serving: 152 Total; 13 Fat; 4 Sat-fat

◻ CHICKEN WITH APPLES AND ONIONS

6 skinned chicken breasts
1 cup sliced onion
1 teaspoon olive oil
2 cups sliced tart apples

1 tablespoon margarine
1½ cups apple juice
2 tablespoons honey
½–1 teaspoon salt (optional)

Preheat oven to 350°F.

Place chicken breasts in a shallow baking pan.

In a skillet, sauté onions in olive oil. Add a splash of water and cook vegetables until tender. Add apples and sauté for 1 more minute.

Pour onions and apples over chicken.

Melt margarine in a small saucepan. Combine apple juice, honey, salt, and margarine and pour over chicken and vegetables.

Bake for 30–45 minutes or until chicken is cooked through.

6 servings
Calories per serving: 238 Total; 35 Fat; 9 Sat-fat

▣ CHICKEN SMOTHERED IN VEGETABLES

4 boned and skinned chicken
   breasts
¼ cup unbleached white flour
½ teaspoon salt (optional)
¼ teaspoon freshly ground
   black pepper
1 teaspoon olive oil

1 clove garlic, minced
¾ cup sliced onion
1 green pepper, sliced
1 cup sliced mushrooms
1 teaspoon oregano
10 cherry tomatoes or 3 whole
   tomatoes, sliced

Preheat oven to 375°F.

Cut each chicken breast into four pieces.

Coat chicken by shaking in a plastic bag with flour, salt, and pepper.

Place chicken in baking pan and grind additional pepper over it.

In a large skillet, sauté garlic and onion in oil until soft.

Stir in green pepper, mushrooms, and oregano, add a splash of water, and cook for 1 minute.

Add tomatoes.

Pour vegetables over chicken and bake for 30–45 minutes or until chicken is fully cooked.

4 servings
Calories per serving: 194 Total; 23 Fat; 5 Sat-fat

▣ PEPPERY CHICKEN

A very peppery chicken that tastes good grilled or roasted in the oven.

4 skinned chicken breasts
2 tablespoons soy sauce
2 tablespoons honey
½ teaspoon thyme
½ teaspoon paprika
¼ teaspoon cayenne pepper

1 tablespoon white vinegar
½ teaspoon allspice
1 teaspoon freshly ground black
   pepper
1 cup sliced mushrooms

Place chicken in a shallow casserole.

Combine soy sauce, honey, thyme, paprika, cayenne pepper, vinegar, allspice, and pepper and pour over chicken. Marinate in refrigerator for about 1 hour.

Preheat oven to 375°F.

Bake chicken for 30–45 minutes or until cooked through.

Surround chicken with sliced mushrooms, spoon the sauce over them, and bake 1 minute more.

For grilling: remove breasts from marinade and grill until cooked through, basting periodically with marinade.

Add mushrooms to the marinade and simmer for 1 minute. Spoon over grilled chicken breasts.

4 servings
Calories per serving: 172 Total; 13 Fat; 4 Sat-fat

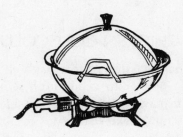

Q ## MA-PO BEAN CURD

This dish may be used as an entree although it barely has any meat (chicken) in it. It is extremely tasty.

1 tablespoon olive oil
1 tablespoon minced ginger root
2 boned and skinned chicken breasts, ground (can be ground in food processor)
3 cakes (each about 3 × 3 × 1¼ inches) tofu (fresh bean curd),* cubed
½ cup water
1½–3 tablespoons soy sauce

½ teaspoon sugar
1–3 teaspoons chili paste with garlic*
1 tablespoon fermented black beans*
1 tablespoon cornstarch mixed with 2 tablespoons water
½ tablespoon sesame oil*
2 tablespoons sliced green onion

*Available at Oriental food stores and some supermarkets

Heat a wok or large skillet to hot. Add olive oil and sauté ginger until fragrant (about 10 seconds).

Add chicken and stir until it turns white.

Stir in tofu, water, 1½ tablespoons of the soy sauce, and sugar.

Reduce heat, cover, and simmer for 5–10 minutes.

Uncover and stir in chili paste with garlic and fermented black beans.

Raise heat and stir in cornstarch mixture and sesame oil until sauce thickens. Taste. Add remaining soy sauce, a teaspoon at a time, if needed for flavor.

Stir in green onion and serve over rice.

6 servings
Calories per serving: 126 Total; 37 Fat; 7 Sat-fat

CHICKEN COUSCOUS

Couscous is the national dish of the Maghreb region of Morocco, Algeria, and Tunisia. The grain, made from semolina, is eaten as a cereal, as a main dish with meat and vegetables, and as a dessert with fruit and nuts. Our Chicken Couscous combines interesting textures and exotic tastes to create a complete meal in one dish.

3 boned and skinned chicken breasts, cut into bite-size pieces
½ cup sliced carrot
¼ cup sliced celery
1 small turnip, quartered
½ cup dry white wine or vermouth
½ teaspoon thyme
¼ teaspoon rosemary
¼ teaspoon salt (optional)

¼ teaspoon paprika
1 tablespoon slivered almonds
1 cup sliced onion
2 teaspoons olive oil
½ teaspoon coriander
2 tablespoons raisins
¾ cup chopped tomatoes
½ teaspoon cinnamon
1 cup quick-cooking couscous
1 teaspoon margarine

In a large casserole, combine chicken, carrot, celery, turnip, wine, thyme, rosemary, salt, and paprika, with water to cover.

Bring to a boil, reduce heat, and simmer, covered, until chicken is cooked (about 10–20 minutes).

Meanwhile, in a medium skillet, toast almonds over low heat until golden. Remove almonds and set aside.

In same skillet, cook onion in olive oil over low heat, covered, until soft, stirring often.

Mix in coriander and raisins and cook slowly for 5 minutes more. Set aside.

When chicken is finished cooking, pour out all but about ½ cup of the liquid.

Add tomatoes and cinnamon to the chicken mixture and mix well. Cook, covered, for 5 minutes more.

Make couscous according to package directions. It takes about 5 minutes. (Add 1 teaspoon margarine instead of any amount of butter they suggest.)

Reheat onion-raisin mixture and sprinkle almonds over it.

Place couscous on a large platter. Cover with onions. Top with chicken and vegetables. Spoon on remaining sauce from casserole.

5 servings
Calories per serving: 283 Total; 24 Fat; 9 Sat-fat

Ⓠ APRICOT CHICKEN DIVINE

One-quarter cup of nonfat yogurt (0 sat-fat calories) replaces ¼ cup of sour cream (68 sat-fat calories) to create this divine chicken.

4 skinned chicken breasts
¼ cup unbleached white flour
½ teaspoon salt (optional)
¼ cup apricot preserves
½ tablespoon Dijon mustard
¼ cup nonfat yogurt
1 tablespoon slivered almonds

Preheat oven to 375°F.

Shake chicken in a plastic bag filled with flour and salt until chicken is coated.

Place chicken in a single layer in a shallow baking pan and bake for 25 minutes.

Combine apricot preserves, mustard, and yogurt.

Spread apricot mixture on chicken and bake for 10–15 minutes more or until done.

Just before serving, brown almonds lightly in toaster oven.

Sprinkle almonds over chicken and serve over rice.

4 servings
Calories per serving: 215 Total; 23 Fat; 5 Sat-fat

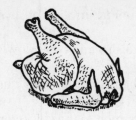

Q̄ GRILLED APRICOT-GINGER CHICKEN

¾ cup dried apricots
Juice of ½ lemon
1 clove garlic, minced
½ teaspoon minced ginger root
¼–½ teaspoon cardamom

⅛–¼ teaspoon cayenne pepper
¼–½ teaspoon salt (optional)
2 teaspoons olive oil
5 skinned chicken breasts

Place apricots in a small saucepan and add water to cover. Add lemon juice, bring to a boil, reduce heat, and simmer until tender.

In a blender or food processor, purée apricots and liquid with garlic, ginger, cardamom, cayenne pepper, salt, and olive oil. Add more water if too thick. Score the chicken breasts several times on each side. Cover with the apricot mixture and marinate in refrigerator for several hours or overnight.

Remove chicken from marinade and reserve marinade.

Preheat oven to broil or prepare grill.

Broil or grill chicken until cooked through.

Heat marinade and spoon over chicken.

Serve over rice.

5 servings
Calories per serving: 191 Total; 29 Fat; 6 Sat-fat

SESAME CHICKEN BROCHETTES

6 boned and skinned chicken
breasts
¼ cup soy sauce
½ cup dry white wine or
vermouth

1 clove garlic, minced
1 tablespoon sesame seeds,
lightly toasted

Cut chicken breasts into 1-inch cubes and place in a bowl or casserole.

Combine soy sauce, wine, and garlic and pour over chicken. Marinate in refrigerator for at least 30 minutes.

Preheat oven to broil or prepare grill.

Remove chicken from marinade and reserve marinade.

Skewer chicken and broil or grill until cooked through, basting occasionally with marinade.

Sprinkle sesame seeds over chicken and serve over rice.

Heat marinade and spoon over chicken and rice.

6 servings
Calories per serving: 160 Total; 20 Fat; 5 Sat-fat

CHICKEN WITH RICE,
TOMATOES, AND ARTICHOKES

4 boned and skinned chicken
breasts
2 cloves garlic, minced
½ cup chopped onion
1 teaspoon olive oil
1 large can (28 oz) tomatoes,
chopped
2 cups water

½ teaspoon thyme
½ teaspoon oregano
1 teaspoon salt (optional)
¼ teaspoon freshly ground
black pepper
1 bay leaf
2 cups uncooked long-grain rice
1 jar (11½ oz) artichoke hearts,
packed in water

Cut chicken into bite-size pieces and set aside.

In a large casserole, sauté garlic and onion in olive oil. Add a splash of water and cook vegetables until soft.

Stir in tomatoes and their liquid, water, thyme, oregano, salt, pepper, and bay leaf and bring to a boil.

Add chicken and rice, cover casserole, and reduce heat to low.

Cook for 25 minutes or until rice is tender, most liquid is absorbed, and chicken is cooked through.

Stir in artichokes and serve.

8 servings
Calories per serving: 274 Total; 12 Fat; 3 Sat-fat

BAGHDAD CHICKEN

¾ cup chopped onion
2 teaspoons garam masala*
1 teaspoon olive oil
⅓ cup uncooked long-grain rice
⅔ cup water
3 tablespoons raisins
3 tablespoons chopped peanuts

¼ cup nonfat yogurt
8 boned and skinned chicken
  breasts
Salt and freshly ground black
  pepper to taste
4 cups cooked long-grain rice
  (optional)

Preheat oven to 375°F.

Sauté onion in garam masala and olive oil. Add a splash of water and cook vegetables until soft. Stir in rice.

Add water, cover saucepan, and cook over low heat until liquid is absorbed (about 20 minutes).

Remove from heat. Stir in raisins, peanuts, and yogurt. Let cool.

Flatten chicken breasts between two sheets of wax paper. Salt and pepper chicken.

Put a portion of the rice mixture in the center of each breast.

Bring together the sides of the breast to enclose the rice.

Place the breast seam-side down in a shallow casserole.

Bake until chicken is cooked through (about 30–45 minutes).

Combine any rice mixture you have remaining with plain rice and serve on the side.

8 servings
Calories per serving: 200 Total; 38 Fat; 7 Sat-fat

---

*Available at specialty food stores. Or make your own by combining ½ teaspoon ground cloves, ¾ teaspoon ground cardamom, and ¾ teaspoon cinnamon.

Q

CHINESE CHICKEN

¼ cup + 2 tablespoons soy
  sauce (approximately)
¼ cup dry sherry
1 clove garlic
3 or 4 shakes ground ginger or 1
  thin slice ginger root
½ cup + 1 tablespoon sugar
  (approximately)

5–6 star anise*
2 cups water (approximately)
10 boned and skinned chicken
  breasts**
2 tablespoons soy sauce
1 tablespoon sugar

Place ¼ cup soy sauce, sherry, garlic, ginger, ½ cup sugar, star anise, and 1 cup of the water in an electric frying pan (or large frying pan). Add chicken in one layer and cook over medium heat for 20 minutes. Sauce will be thick.

Turn chicken. Add remaining 1 cup water, 2 tablespoons soy sauce, and 1 tablespoon sugar.

Taste. If too salty, add more sugar. If too sweet, add more soy sauce.

Cook for 10–30 minutes more or until chicken is cooked through. Keep adding water when sauce gets too thick. Periodically turn chicken. Keep tasting sauce and add soy sauce or sugar if necessary.

Chicken should be a deep brown.

10 servings

Calories per serving:	Total	Fat	Sat-fat
1 breast	183	13	3
1 drumstick	130	19	5
1 thigh	134	24	5

PHYLLO-WRAPPED CHICKEN WITH RICE, ARTICHOKES, AND CREAM SAUCE

What a wonderful combination of tastes and textures! This very elegant chicken can be made a day ahead and refrigerated. (We recommend that you do make this chicken dish ahead because it involves many steps. To cook it along with all the other dishes that comprise a dinner will make you a nervous wreck and frazzled host.)

Phyllo dough that has been stored in the freezer has to be thawed in the refrigerator for 8 hours or overnight and then set out at room temperature for 2–4 hours before using. Take this into account when planning to cook this dish.

Chicken

10 boned and skinned chicken breasts
1 cup dry white wine or vermouth

1 teaspoon salt (optional)
1 1/2 teaspoons thyme
1/2 teaspoon rosemary
1 bay leaf

Rice

1 tablespoon margarine
2 cloves garlic, minced
1/2 cup chopped onion

1/2 pound sliced mushrooms
3/4 cup long-grain rice

Cream Sauce

2 tablespoons margarine
1/4 cup unbleached white flour

1/2 cup skim milk

Assembly

1 package (9 oz) frozen artichoke hearts, thawed, or 1 jar (11 1/2 oz) artichoke hearts, packed in water and drained

3 tablespoons margarine
16 sheets phyllo dough,* thawed (usually comes in 16-oz package)

---

*Available at Greek or Mideast food stores or in the freezer section of many supermarkets.

The Chicken and Broth

In a large pot, combine chicken, wine, salt, thyme, rosemary, bay leaf, and water to cover. Bring to a boil. Reduce heat, cover, and simmer for 25 minutes or until chicken is cooked through.

Remove chicken and cut into bite-size pieces. Set aside.

Boil chicken broth gently, uncovered, until it is reduced to about 3½ cups.

Set aside and make the rice.

The Rice

In a large saucepan, melt margarine.

Add garlic, onion, and mushrooms and cook until tender.

Stir in rice.

Add 1½ cups of the reduced chicken broth. Simmer, covered, until liquid is absorbed (about 20 minutes).

While rice is cooking, make the cream sauce.

The Cream Sauce

Melt margarine over low heat.

Stir in the flour and cook until bubbly.

Remove from heat and slowly stir in remaining 2 cups of broth.

Gradually add skim milk. Return to low heat and stir until thick.

Back to the Rice and Chicken

When the rice is cooked, stir in the artichoke hearts and 1 cup of the cream sauce. Set aside.

Stir remaining cream sauce into chicken pieces. Set aside.

Putting It All Together

Preheat oven to 350°F.

Grease a 13 × 9-inch baking pan with margarine.

Melt the 3 tablespoons margarine.

Unfold phyllo leaves. Cover with plastic or damp towel.

Place 1 phyllo sheet into bottom of pan. Brush lightly with melted margarine.

Repeat procedure with 6 more sheets of phyllo.

Spread half of the rice mixture over phyllo dough.

Spread chicken over rice mixture.

Spread remaining rice mixture over chicken.

Cover with 6 sheets of phyllo, brushing with margarine between each sheet.

Tuck in edges of last sheet and brush the top with margarine.

Cut lightly through 3 or 4 layers of phyllo dough to indicate pieces to be cut later.

Bake chicken for 30–45 minutes or until golden brown and bubbly. Or refrigerate it for up to 24 hours and bake later for 60 minutes.

12 servings
Calories per serving: 270 Total; 56 Fat; 12 Sat-fat

CUBAN CHICKEN

2 potatoes, peeled and cubed
6 boned and skinned chicken
    breasts, cut into thirds
$\frac{1}{2}$ cup unbleached white flour
$\frac{1}{3}$ cup water
1 large can (28 oz) tomatoes
    with juice
1 large green pepper, chopped

$\frac{3}{4}$ cup chopped onion
2 cloves garlic, minced
$\frac{3}{4}$ teaspoon oregano
$\frac{3}{4}$ teaspoon cumin
$\frac{1}{2}$ teaspoon salt (optional)
$\frac{1}{4}$ cup raisins
$\frac{1}{2}$ cup stuffed green olives

Preheat oven to 425°F.

Place potatoes in a saucepan, cover with water, and boil for 10 minutes.

Shake chicken breasts, one at a time, in a plastic bag filled with flour until breast is completely coated.

Arrange floured chicken in a shallow baking pan in one layer. Add water. Place potatoes evenly over chicken.

Reduce heat to 375°F and bake chicken for 20 minutes.

Meanwhile, chop tomatoes either in food processor or by hand and place them with juice in a large bowl.

Add green pepper, onion, garlic, oregano, cumin, salt, raisins, and olives.

Spread tomato mixture over chicken and bake for 10–20 minutes more or until chicken is fully cooked.

Serve over rice.

6 servings
Calories per serving: 252 Total; 35 Fat; 7 Sat-fat

LEMON-MUSTARD CHICKEN

4 skinned chicken breasts
2 teaspoons margarine
1½ tablespoons Dijon mustard

2 tablespoons fresh lemon juice
½ teaspoon tarragon
¼ teaspoon salt (optional)

Preheat oven to 375°F.
Place chicken in a shallow baking pan.
In a small saucepan, melt margarine. Stir in mustard, lemon juice, tarragon, and salt. Pour over chicken.
Bake chicken for 30–45 minutes or until cooked through.
Spoon sauce from pan over chicken.

4 servings
Calories per serving: 147 Total; 33 Fat; 6 Sat-fat

COQ AU VIN

2 whole frying chickens
¾ cup unbleached white flour
¼ teaspoon freshly ground
  black pepper
¼ cup cognac or brandy
2 cups full-bodied red wine (*not*
  Hearty Burgundy)
1 can (10¾ oz) chicken broth,
  strained
2 cloves garlic, minced

1 teaspoon salt (optional)
1 bay leaf
½ teaspoon thyme
12 small white onions, peeled
½–1 pound mushrooms
1 teaspoon olive oil
2 tablespoons margarine
3 tablespoons unbleached white
  flour

Preheat oven to 375°F.
Cut chickens into parts and remove skin. If you cannot remove the skin from a part (such as the wings) do not use that part.
Shake chicken in a plastic bag with flour and pepper until coated. Place chicken in one layer in a shallow pan and bake until fully cooked, 20–30 minutes. Transfer to a large casserole.
Pour cognac over chicken and ignite it. Shake pan while cognac is burning.
When flame subsides, add wine, chicken broth, garlic, salt, bay leaf, thyme, and onions and simmer, covered, until chicken is tender (about 25 minutes).

Remove chicken from casserole and cover to keep warm.

Boil liquid in casserole until it is reduced to about 3 cups (about 10 minutes). Remove from heat.

Sauté mushrooms in olive oil. Add a splash of water and cook mushrooms for about 1 minute and set aside.

Make a paste of the remaining 2 tablespoons margarine and the flour.

Mix the paste into the reduced liquid in the casserole. Reheat slowly until liquid is thickened.

Return chicken and mushrooms to casserole and heat through.

Serve over noodles (shells, rotini, etc.).

10 servings

Calories per serving:	Total	Fat	Sat-fat
1 chicken breast	195	35	9
1 drumstick	140	41	10
1 thigh	148	46	11

Q PINEAPPLE CHICKEN

1 cup unbleached white flour
1 teaspoon salt (optional)
1 teaspoon paprika
¼ teaspoon freshly ground
  black pepper
8 skinned chicken breasts

1 can (20 oz) pineapple chunks
  in heavy syrup
½ cup sliced green pepper
2 green onions, sliced
1 tablespoon brown sugar
¼ cup dry sherry

Preheat oven to 425°F.

Combine flour, salt, paprika, and pepper in a plastic bag.

Piece by piece, coat chicken by shaking it in the bag with the seasoned flour.

Arrange floured chicken in a shallow baking pan in one layer. Bake at 425°F for 20 minutes. Turn chicken.

Combine pineapple, green pepper, green onions, brown sugar, and sherry and pour over chicken.

Lower heat to 375°F and bake until chicken is golden brown and sauce is thick (about 15–30 minutes).

8 servings
Calories per serving: 210 Total; 13 Fat; 4 Sat-fat

CREAMY CHICKEN PIE

Creamy Chicken Pie is a rich and creamy splurge.

Fully baked nonsweet pie crust
(page 398)
1 tablespoon margarine
½ cup chopped onion
3 cups sliced mushrooms
3 tablespoons unbleached white
flour
1 cup low-fat (1%) cottage
cheese

2 cups diced cooked chicken or
turkey breast
⅓ cup chopped parsley
¼ teaspoon freshly ground
black pepper
¼ teaspoon rosemary

Preheat oven to 375°F.
In a large skillet, melt margarine over medium-high heat.
Cook onion and mushrooms until most liquid has evaporated.
Stir in flour. Remove skillet from heat.
Stir in cottage cheese, chicken, parsley, pepper, and rosemary.
Spoon chicken mixture into pie shell.
Bake for 15 minutes or until crust is golden brown.

7 servings
Calories per serving: 156 Total; 60 Fat; 11 Sat-fat

KUNG PAO CHICKEN
WITH BROCCOLI

You can easily make Chinese cooking low-fat and low-sat-fat by limiting the amount of oil you use or by flouring and baking the chicken first and adding it to the sauce. Vegetables or rice are mixed with small amounts of poultry or other meats to create tantalizing combinations of textures and tastes.

6 boned and skinned chicken breasts
½ cup unbleached white flour
½ teaspoon salt (optional)
2 tablespoons cornstarch
2 tablespoons + 1 cup water
2 tablespoons + 2 teaspoons bean sauce*
1 tablespoon + 1 teaspoon hoisin sauce*
1–2 teaspoons chili paste with garlic*

¾ teaspoon sugar
1 tablespoon + 1 teaspoon dry sherry
1 tablespoon + 1 teaspoon white vinegar
2 cloves garlic, peeled and flattened
1 head broccoli, stem trimmed, cut into flowerets
¼ cup unsalted roasted peanuts, shelled
2–4 dried hot red peppers

Preheat oven to 375°F.

Shake chicken in a plastic bag with flour and salt until coated. Place chicken in a single layer in a baking pan and bake until fully cooked, about 20–30 minutes. When chicken is cool enough to handle, cut it into bite-size pieces. Set aside.

Combine cornstarch with 2 tablespoons water. Stir in remaining cup of water. Set aside.

Combine bean sauce, hoisin sauce, chili paste with garlic, sugar, sherry, vinegar, and garlic and set aside.

Steam broccoli in wok or saucepan until tender. Set aside.

Heat chicken in wok or large skillet. Add sauce. Stir until chicken is well coated. Add cornstarch mixture.

When sauce thickens, stir in peanuts and red peppers. Add broccoli and mix until well coated with sauce.

Serve over rice.

10 servings
Calories per serving: 168 Total; 24 Fat; 5 Sat-fat

---

*Available at Oriental food stores and some supermarkets

Q

CHICKEN MARRAKESH

4 boned and skinned chicken
   breasts
3 tablespoons fresh lemon juice
1 tablespoon grated lemon peel
1 clove garlic, minced
2–3 teaspoons thyme

½ teaspoon salt (optional)
½ teaspoon freshly ground
   black pepper
1 lemon, thinly sliced

Place chicken in a bowl or casserole.

Mix together lemon juice, lemon peel, garlic, thyme, salt, and pepper and pour over chicken. Marinate chicken in refrigerator for at least 3 hours.

Preheat oven to 350°F.

Remove chicken from marinade and place in shallow baking dish.

Pour marinade over chicken and bake chicken for 30–45 minutes or until cooked through.

Garnish with lemon slices.

4 servings
Calories per serving: 132 Total; 13 Fat; 4 Sat-fat

CHICKEN PAPRIKASH

Paprikash dishes typically use sour cream. Nonfat yogurt has been substituted here without affecting the taste. Half a cup of nonfat yogurt contains 0 sat-fat calories. Half a cup of sour cream contains about 135 sat-fat calories.

½ cup unbleached white flour
½–1 teaspoon salt (optional)
¼ teaspoon freshly ground
   black pepper
6 boned and skinned chicken
   breasts
3 tablespoons water
1½ tablespoons cornstarch
½ cup chopped onion
2–3 cups sliced mushrooms

2 teaspoons olive oil
1½ teaspoons paprika
½ teaspoon dillweed
½ teaspoon salt
¼ teaspoon freshly ground
   black pepper
1 cup chicken broth, strained
½ cup nonfat yogurt
½–1 cup water

Preheat oven to 375°F.

Place flour, ½–1 teaspoon salt, and ¼ teaspoon pepper in a plastic bag. Piece by piece, coat chicken by shaking it in the bag with the seasoned flour.

Arrange floured chicken in one layer in a shallow baking pan and bake for 30–40 minutes or until chicken is cooked through.

In a small bowl, add water to cornstarch and mix until smooth. Set aside.

Meanwhile, in a large skillet, sauté onion and mushrooms in oil. Add a splash of water and cook vegetables until tender.

Stir in paprika, dillweed, ½ teaspoon salt, ¼ teaspoon pepper, and chicken broth.

Add cornstarch mixture and bring to a boil, stirring constantly. Lower heat to medium.

Cut chicken into bite-size pieces and add to sauce. Stir until chicken is heated.

Remove from heat and stir in yogurt. Add water, ¼ cup at a time, if sauce is too thick.

Serve over rice or noodles.

8 servings
Calories per serving: 152 Total; 23 Fat; 5 Sat-fat

Ⓠ CHICKEN WITH APRICOTS, SWEET POTATOES, AND PRUNES

This dish is colorful to look at and a pleasure to eat. What's more, it is quick and easy and can be prepared ahead of time.

6 boned and skinned chicken breasts
¾ cup dried prunes
½ cup dried apricots
1 tablespoon olive oil
3 tablespoons white vinegar

½ cup dry vermouth
2 cloves garlic, minced
1½ tablespoons brown sugar
1 tablespoon oregano
2 cups sweet potatoes, peeled and cut into ½-inch cubes

Place chicken breasts in a medium-large bowl or casserole.

Combine prunes, apricots, olive oil, vinegar, vermouth, garlic, brown sugar, and oregano and pour over chicken. Cover and marinate in refrigerator for several hours or overnight.

When you are ready to bake the chicken, place sweet potato cubes in saucepan with water to cover. Bring to a boil and boil gently for 3 minutes. Drain and set aside.

Remove chicken from marinade. Arrange in shallow baking pan.

Spread marinade over chicken, cover with sweet potatoes, and bake for 30–45 minutes until chicken is fully cooked.

6 servings
Calories per serving: 301 Total; 34 Fat; 7 Sat-fat

SINGAPORE CHICKEN

Singapore Chicken includes salad greens, but it is more like a main dish than a salad. You can eat it warm or chilled. It tastes even better the second day.

4 boned and skinned chicken breasts
½ teaspoon minced garlic
½ teaspoon minced ginger root
1 tablespoon soy sauce
1 tablespoon hoisin sauce*
½ tablespoon white vinegar
½ teaspoon five-spice powder**
½ teaspoon Dijon mustard
1 teaspoon sugar
¼ cup white vinegar

1 teaspoon soy sauce
1 tablespoon olive oil
½ Chinese celery cabbage, or ½ head lettuce, chopped (about 3 cups)
2 green onions, thinly sliced
1½ tablespoons slivered almonds, toasted
½ tablespoon sesame seeds, toasted

Place chicken breasts in a bowl or small casserole.

Combine garlic, ginger, 1 tablespoon soy sauce, hoisin sauce, ½ tablespoon vinegar, and five-spice powder and pour over chicken. Cover bowl and marinate chicken in refrigerator overnight.

Preheat oven to 350°F.

---

*Available at Oriental food stores and some supermarkets
**Five-spice powder is available at Oriental food stores, or you can make your own by pulverizing the following in a blender: 30 peppercorns, 2 whole star anise (optional), 1 teaspoon fennel seeds, 2 one-inch pieces cinnamon stick, ¼ teaspoon cloves. Store excess in covered jar.

Bake chicken in marinade for 30–45 minutes or until cooked through.

Meanwhile, prepare dressing by combining mustard, sugar, ¼ cup vinegar, 1 teaspoon soy sauce, and olive oil in a jar and shaking well.

Slice chicken into narrow strips and combine with celery cabbage and green onions.

Pour dressing over all and mix until well coated.

Top with almonds and sesame seeds.

Serve or refrigerate overnight.

5 servings
Calories per serving: 164 Total; 50 Fat; 10 Sat-fat

TORTILLAS CON POLLO

Chicken, yogurt, and rice make this tortilla unusual, low-fat, and, of course, delicious.

Tomato Sauce

1 clove garlic, minced
⅓ cup chopped onion
1 teaspoon olive oil
1 large can (28 oz) tomatoes,
    drained and chopped

¼ cup chopped green pepper
½ teaspoon cumin seed
½ teaspoon oregano

Filling

3 cups cooked long-grain rice
1½ cups diced cooked chicken
½–1 teaspoon chili powder

½ teaspoon ground cumin
½ cup nonfat yogurt

8 tortillas*

At least 30 minutes before serving, prepare the tomato sauce: Cook garlic and onion in olive oil until soft. Add tomatoes, green pepper, cumin seed, and oregano and cook until thick (about 30 minutes).

---

*Read the label. Packaged tortillas should contain only corn (perhaps some lime) and should *not* contain any of the following: shortening, fat, salt, or preservatives.

Preheat oven to 350°F. Grease a shallow baking dish with margarine.

Combine rice, chicken, chili powder, cumin, and yogurt.

Place ½ cup rice mixture in center of each tortilla and roll.

Place seam-side down in baking dish.

When all eight tortillas have been placed in baking dish, cover with tomato sauce and bake for 25 minutes.

8 servings
Calories per serving: 207 Total; 16 Fat; 1 Sat-fat

[Q]   # CHICKEN CURRY

6 boned and skinned chicken breasts
½ cup unbleached white flour
½ teaspoon salt (optional)
¼ teaspoon freshly ground black pepper
2 cloves garlic, minced
¾ cup chopped onion

½ cup chopped green pepper
2 teaspoons olive oil
1–2 teaspoons curry powder
½ teaspoon thyme
½ teaspoon salt (optional)
2 cups cherry tomato halves (or whole tomatoes or drained canned tomatoes, chopped)

Preheat oven to 375°F.

Shake chicken in a plastic bag with flour, salt, and pepper until coated.

Place chicken in a single layer in a baking pan and bake until chicken is fully cooked, 20–30 minutes. When chicken is cool enough to handle, cut it into bite-size pieces. Set aside.

Sauté garlic, onion, and green pepper in olive oil. Add a splash of water to help vegetables cook.

Blend in curry powder, thyme, and salt.

Add chicken and stir until well coated with sauce. Stir in tomatoes.

6 servings
Calories per serving: 164 Total; 20 Fat; 5 Sat-fat

Q

KEEMA MATAR

Traditionally, Keema Matar is made with ground lamb or beef. It tastes equally good with ground chicken, and instead of spending 111 sat-fat calories on ground lean beef, you spend a mere 13.

5 boned and skinned chicken breasts

2 tablespoons olive oil

1 tablespoon minced garlic (about 4–5 cloves)

2–3 tablespoons curry powder

1 cinnamon stick

½ teaspoon salt (optional)

1 cup frozen peas

Grind chicken breasts in a food processor or a meat grinder. If you are using a food processor, first cut the cold (but not frozen) chicken breasts into 1-inch cubes. Place the cubes in the work bowl. Press the Pulse/Off button until chicken is ground (not puréed!). In a large skillet, sauté ground chicken in olive oil, stirring constantly, until it is cooked through.

Mix in garlic, curry powder, cinnamon stick, and salt.

Add peas and stir until heated through.

Serve over Indian Rice (page 333).

4 servings
Calories per serving: 249 Total; 76 Fat; 13 Sat-fat

MONGOLIAN HOT POT

Making this dish is a group activity that allows each person to be his own cook. It works like a fondue. Everyone skewers a piece of meat or vegetable and dips it into simmering broth in a large Oriental "hot pot" or in an electric frying pan or wok. When the meat is finished cooking, the enriched broth becomes an after-dinner soup.

6 boned and skinned chicken breasts

Marinade

2 cloves garlic, minced

1 teaspoon olive oil

1 tablespoon white vinegar

2 tablespoons honey

¼ cup soy sauce

1 teaspoon sherry

Sauce

½ cup soy sauce
½ cup dry sherry
5 tablespoons honey

2 tablespoons minced ginger
  root
2 cloves garlic, minced

The Rest

4 ounces cellophane noodles*
½ pound snow peas
1 zucchini, cut into ¼-inch
  slices

½ head celery cabbage, coarsely
  chopped
1 pound bay scallops

Broth

10 cups chicken stock, or 2 cans
  (10¾ oz each) chicken broth,
  strained, + 6 cans water

3 green onions, sliced
1½ teaspoons sliced ginger root
2 cloves garlic, minced

4 cups hot cooked rice

Slice chicken breasts into slender, bite-size pieces. Marinate in garlic, olive oil, vinegar, honey, soy sauce, and sherry in refrigerator for several hours or overnight.

Mix all sauce ingredients together and set aside.

Pour boiling water over cellophane noodles and let stand for 5–10 minutes or until soft. Drain and set aside.

Remove chicken from marinade and arrange artistically on a plate.

Arrange another plate with snow peas, zucchini slices, and celery cabbage. Set aside.

Arrange bay scallops on another plate.

Pour chicken broth and water in a hot pot, chafing dish, or electric wok or frying pan set in the center of the table. Heat to a slow boil.

Mix in green onions, ginger, and garlic.

Give each person a bowl of rice, a plate, and a small custard dish for the sauce. Pass around the trays of chicken, scallops, and vegetables so people may take what they wish. Each person should also have a fondue fork, skewer, or sharp implement to dip chicken, scallops, and vegetables in broth until cooked.

---

*Available at Oriental food stores and some supermarkets

When food is all devoured or everyone is almost full, add noodles and celery cabbage to the broth and cook for 2–3 minutes.
Serve resulting soup in bowls.

8 servings

Calories per serving:	Total	Fat	Sat-fat
2 tablespoons sauce	69	0	0
Meat and vegetables	155	25	4
Broth	184	0	0
Total	408	25	4

Q

SATE AJAM
(BROILED CHICKEN ON SKEWERS)

4 boned and skinned chicken breasts
12 medium mushrooms
1 teaspoon olive oil
2 tablespoons fresh lime juice
⅛ teaspoon freshly ground black pepper
1 teaspoon cumin
1 teaspoon minced garlic

Cut chicken into 1-inch pieces and cut stems off mushrooms.

Alternate pieces of chicken with mushrooms on skewers. (Push skewers through the *tops* of the mushrooms so the mushrooms will not split.)

Place skewered chicken in a shallow casserole.

Combine olive oil, lime juice, pepper, cumin, and garlic and pour over chicken.

Turn skewers to coat chicken and mushrooms with oil mixture.

Refrigerate for at least 30 minutes.

Preheat broiler.

Place skewers on broiler pan and broil 6 inches from heat for about 10 minutes or until cooked through. Turn and baste several times.

Serve over rice and spoon warm marinade over chicken pieces.

4 servings
Calories per serving: 151 Total; 23 Fat; 5 Sat-fat

Q

CAJUN CHICKEN

8 boned and skinned chicken
  breasts

½ cup unbleached white flour
½ teaspoon salt, optional

Seasoning Mix (Use more or less of the peppers for a hotter or milder taste.)

¾ teaspoon oregano
½ teaspoon thyme
½ teaspoon basil
½ teaspoon salt

½ teaspoon paprika
¼ teaspoon freshly ground
  black pepper
½ teaspoon cayenne pepper
¼ teaspoon white pepper

3 cloves garlic, minced
¾ cup chopped onion
2 stalks celery, diced
1 green pepper, chopped
1 tomato, coarsely chopped

1 tablespoon olive oil
1 can (10¾ oz) chicken broth,
  strained
1 small can (8 oz) tomato sauce
1 potato, peeled and diced
2 bay leaves

Preheat oven to 350°F.

Shake chicken in a plastic bag filled with flour and salt until chicken is coated.

Place chicken in a single layer in a shallow baking pan and bake for 25–30 minutes until cooked through.

While chicken is baking, combine oregano, thyme, basil, salt, paprika, and peppers, and set aside.

In a large frying pan, sauté garlic, onion, celery, green pepper, and tomato in oil. Add a splash of water and cook vegetables until soft.

Mix in seasoning mixture and let simmer for about a minute.

Mix in broth and tomato sauce. Bring to a boil, then simmer for 5 minutes.

Lower heat and add chicken breasts, potato, and bay leaves. Cook until potatoes are soft and chicken is done.

NOTE: If you find the finished dish too "hot" for your taste, dilute with an additional can of tomato sauce.

8 servings
Calories per serving: 196 Total; 28 Fat; 2 Sat-fat

Q

BAR-B-QUE CHICKEN

Bar-B-Que Chicken is a popular main dish with food lovers of all ages. It also makes a great sandwich. Place the barbecued chicken on a slice of bread, top with sauce, a slice of tomato, a few slices of onion, and another slice of bread.

2 tablespoons Dijon mustard
¼ cup vinegar
¼ cup molasses
½ cup ketchup
½ teaspoon Worcestershire
  sauce

2 cloves garlic, minced
Dash of Tabasco sauce
8 skinned chicken breasts or
  thighs*

In a large bowl, mix together Dijon mustard, vinegar, molasses, ketchup, Worcestershire sauce, garlic, and Tabasco for marinade.

Pour about half of the marinade over the chicken and refrigerate the rest to use later.

Marinate chicken for an hour (or less, if you haven't planned ahead).

Remove chicken and reserve marinade.

Barbecue, broil, or use a cast-iron pancake griddle to grill chicken for 10 minutes or until fully cooked.

Turn and coat chicken with marinade and continue cooking until done.

Combine reserved marinade with the marinade you refrigerated. Heat to boiling and simmer for 2 minutes. Spoon over chicken before serving.

8 servings

Calories per serving:	Total	Fat	Sat-fat
1 breast	173	13	4
1 thigh	126	24	6

*For a barbecue, you may want greater quantities of chicken. Just double, triple, quadruple, etc., the recipe.

Q GINGER CHICKEN WITH GREEN ONIONS

5 boned and skinned chicken
  breasts
1 teaspoon ground ginger
2 tablespoons cornstarch
1¼ cups water
3 tablespoons soy sauce
2 tablespoons olive oil

2 cloves garlic, minced
2 teaspoons minced ginger root
2 dried red peppers, crushed, or
  1 teaspoon dried red pepper
  flakes
1½ cups green onions cut into
  1-inch pieces

Cut chicken into bite-size pieces, sprinkle with ground ginger, and set aside for 15 minutes.

Make a smooth paste of the cornstarch and 2 tablespoons of the water. Stir in 2 more tablespoons of water and soy sauce. Set aside.

Sauté chicken in oil until cooked through.

Stir in garlic, ginger root, and red pepper flakes.

Mix in soy sauce mixture and heat until the sauce thickens.

If sauce is too thick, add remaining water, ¼ cup at a time, until desired consistency is achieved.

Stir in green onions and serve over rice.

6 servings
Calories per serving: 172 Total; 51 Fat; 9 Sat-fat

Q ORANGE-SOY CHICKEN

4 boned and skinned chicken
  breasts
2 tablespoons soy sauce
1½ tablespoons cornstarch
½ tablespoon hoisin sauce*
3 tablespoons dry sherry
1 cup water
1 clove garlic, minced

1 teaspoon minced ginger root
2 tablespoons orange peel slivers
½ teaspoon olive oil
1 teaspoon marmalade
½–1 teaspoon red pepper flakes
1 orange, peeled and cut into
  bite-size pieces
10–20 snow peas

Place chicken between two pieces of wax paper and pound with a meat mallet to flatten. Then steam in a vegetable steamer or on a steamer tray in a wok until cooked through. Pull or slice chicken into thin strips about 2–3 inches long.

*Available at Oriental food stores and some supermarkets

Mix soy sauce into cornstarch, a tablespoon at a time, creating a smooth paste.

Mix in hoisin sauce, sherry, and water, and set aside.

Sauté garlic, ginger, and orange peel slivers in oil until soft.

Stir in cooked chicken pieces.

Stir in cornstarch mixture and cook until it thickens. Add more water if too dry.

Mix in marmalade, red pepper, orange pieces, and snow peas, and serve over rice.

6 servings
Calories per serving: 119 Total; 12 Fat; 4 Sat-fat

Q   # CHICKEN VERDE

16 spears asparagus	6 anchovies
4 boned and skinned chicken breasts	1 tablespoon olive oil
	2 tablespoons fresh lemon juice
1 clove garlic, minced	1 teaspoon water
1 teaspoon basil	

Preheat oven to 375°F.

Snap off bottoms of asparagus.

Pound breasts between two sheets of wax paper with a meat mallet, until flat. This is important, as they must be thin to cook quickly.

Combine garlic, basil, anchovies, olive oil, and lemon juice into a sauce in blender or food processor, or mash and mix by hand.

In a small rectangular glass casserole, place four asparagus spears closely together and wrap a chicken breast around them. Repeat this process for the rest of the breasts.

Spread sauce over chicken.

Sprinkle teaspoon of water over exposed asparagus.

Cover casserole tightly with aluminum foil.

Bake for 20–30 minutes, or until chicken is cooked through.

DO NOT OVERCOOK. If you cook asparagus too long, it becomes soggy and the sauce becomes watery.

4 servings
Calories per serving: 187 Total; 42 Fat; 8 Sat-fat

VEGETABLES, CHICKEN, AND CELLOPHANE NOODLES

2 ounces cellophane noodles*
2 boned and skinned chicken breasts
8 mushrooms (approximately)
2 carrots
1 zucchini
4 green onions

4 leaves Chinese cabbage*
3 cloves garlic, minced
1 tablespoon olive oil
1 tablespoon sesame oil*
3 tablespoons soy sauce
½ teaspoon sugar
½ teaspoon salt, optional

Cover cellophane noodles with warm water and set aside.

Steam chicken breasts in a vegetable steamer. When cooked through (about 10 minutes), cut them into bite-size pieces and set aside.

Cut mushrooms into thin slices. Cut carrot and zucchini into julienne strips. Cut green onions into 1-inch pieces. Set aside.

Remove the green leaf from the cabbage. Cut into bite-size pieces. Julienne the white part of the leaf. Set aside.

Drain water from cellophane noodles.

Sauté garlic in both oils.

Add vegetables and stir-fry until tender but crisp.

Stir in chicken.

Stir in soy sauce, sugar, salt, and cellophane noodles. Mix to distribute sauce evenly. Serve over rice.

6 servings
Calories per serving: 111 Total; 44 Fat; 7 Sat-fat

Q CHICKEN NUGGETS CHEZ GOOR

The chicken nuggets that you get at fast-food chains are deep-fried in highly saturated oils. Instead of devouring 46 calories of saturated fat per serving, try Chicken Nuggets Chez Goor, marinated in olive oil and garlic and baked in the oven. A mere 5 sat-fat calories per serving.

*Available at Oriental food stores and some supermarkets

4 boned and skinned chicken breasts
1 tablespoon olive oil
2 cloves garlic, minced
¼ teaspoon freshly ground black pepper
1 cup finely ground bread crumbs, made from 2–3 slices French or other bread
¼ teaspoon cayenne pepper
2½ teaspoons honey
2 tablespoons Dijon mustard

Preheat oven to 375°F.

Cut each chicken breast into 8 pieces.

Mix oil, garlic, and pepper with chicken pieces and marinate about 30 minutes.

Combine bread crumbs and cayenne and place on plate.

Roll chicken pieces in bread crumbs and place on large cookie sheet in a single layer.

Bake for about 15 minutes until browned and cooked through. For extra browning, broil for a few more minutes.

Combine honey and mustard. Dip nuggets into honey-mustard sauce.

4 servings

Calories per serving:	Total	Fat	Sat-fat
	191	43	5
With honey-mustard sauce	211	43	5

SHEPHERD'S CHICKEN CHILI PIE

1½–2 pounds potatoes, peeled and cut into chunks
4 boned and skinned chicken breasts
1 can (16 oz) whole tomatoes, with juice
1 large onion, sliced
3 cloves garlic, minced
1 teaspoon olive oil
1½ tablespoons chili powder
½ teaspoon oregano
1 teaspoon cumin
2 tablespoons water
1 tablespoon tomato paste
1 teaspoon margarine
Salt and freshly ground black pepper to taste
1 tablespoon skim milk

Place potatoes in a saucepan with water to cover, bring to a boil, and simmer for about 10–15 minutes, until tender.

Steam chicken pieces in a vegetable steamer or on a steamer tray in a wok until cooked through, about 10 minutes.

Drain tomatoes. Reserve liquid.

Preheat oven to 350°F.

In a large skillet, sauté onion and garlic in olive oil until soft.

Mix in chili powder, oregano, and cumin.

Add water, tomato paste, and tomatoes. Cook until sauce is thick. If sauce becomes *too* thick, add a few tablespoons of the reserved tomato juice.

Mix chicken cubes into sauce.

Drain potatoes and whip them. Add margarine, salt, and pepper. Add skim milk and mix until potatoes are smooth. Add more milk if necessary.

Place chicken mixture in a shallow casserole. Spread potatoes on top. Bake for about 30 minutes.

6 servings
Calories per serving: 204 Total; 15 Fat; 4 Sat-fat

Ⓠ BLACKENED CHICKEN

Ron is in seventh heaven when he bites into a chunk of chicken and the chicken bites back. The spicier it is, the better he likes it. He likes Blackened Chicken a lot.

Spice Mix

1 teaspoon thyme
1 teaspoon basil
½ teaspoon onion powder
¼ teaspoon salt (optional)
½ teaspoon cayenne pepper

½ teaspoon paprika
½ teaspoon white pepper
¼ teaspoon freshly ground
  black pepper

5 skinned chicken breasts

Combine seasonings on a small plate. Roll each breast in seasonings, coating it on both sides and set it aside on a large plate. For a milder chicken, use less seasoning on each breast.

Either grill on a cast-iron pancake griddle or barbecue, broil, or bake chicken until cooked through. Don't overcook.

NOTE: If you are using a cast-iron griddle, don't let it get too hot or it will char the chicken. You may need to turn on your exhaust fan to clear the hot spices from the air.

5 servings
Calories per serving: 130 Total; 13 Fat; 4 Sat-fat

▣ CHICKEN WITH DRIED FRUIT AND LEMON

4 boned and skinned chicken breasts
¼ cup chopped onion
1 tablespoon brown sugar
½ teaspoon ground ginger
¼–½ teaspoon salt (optional)
10 pitted prunes

2 tablespoons raisins
1 lemon, thinly sliced
¼ cup canned beef broth
¼ cup water
1 tablespoon soy sauce
1 tablespoon cornstarch

If you have a clay cooker, soak it in water for 15 minutes. Preheat oven to 450°F.

Place chicken in clay cooker or shallow baking pan.

Distribute onion evenly over chicken.

Combine sugar, ginger, and salt and spread half of the mixture over chicken.

Distribute prunes and raisins evenly over chicken.

Cover with lemon slices.

Sprinkle remaining sugar mixture over lemon.

Combine beef broth, water, and soy sauce and pour over chicken.

Cover clay cooker with top or cover baking pan tightly with aluminum foil.

Cook for 30–45 minutes or until chicken is cooked through.

Remove chicken to plate and cover with foil to keep warm.

Pour remaining liquid and fruit into small saucepan.

Mix cornstarch with about 2 tablespoons of liquid until smooth and add to saucepan. Heat until sauce thickens.

Serve chicken with fruited sauce.

4 servings
Calories per serving: 226 Total; 13 Fat; 4 Sat-fat

Q
SZECHUAN CHICKEN
WITH SWEET RED PEPPER AND PINEAPPLE

The Chinese typically cook chicken by cutting it into small pieces and sautéing it in oil. To save fat calories, the chicken in this sweet-spicy and delectable dish is baked first with no fat, then cut into bite-size pieces and thrown into the sauce.

NOTE: For a different taste, try this recipe with a sliced green pepper and no pineapple.

⅓ cup unbleached white flour
Salt to taste (optional)
¼ teaspoon freshly ground
   black pepper
5 boned and skinned chicken
   breasts
2 tablespoons soy sauce
2 tablespoons dry sherry
1–2 teaspoons chili paste with
   garlic*
1½ tablespoons tomato paste

¼ teaspoon sugar
2 tablespoons cornstarch
1 cup water + 2 tablespoons
1–2 teaspoons chopped ginger
   root
2 green onions, sliced
1 teaspoon olive oil
1 sweet red pepper, sliced
1½ cups pineapple chunks
¼ cup water

Preheat oven to 375°F.

Place flour, salt, and pepper in a plastic bag. Piece by piece, coat chicken by shaking it in the bag with the seasoned flour.

Arrange floured chicken in one layer in a shallow baking pan and bake for 20–40 minutes or until chicken is cooked through.

Meanwhile, combine soy sauce, sherry, chili paste, tomato paste, and sugar. Set aside.

Combine cornstarch with 2 tablespoons water. Then stir in remaining cup of water. Set aside.

When chicken is cooked through, cut into bite-size pieces and set aside.

In a large skillet or wok, sauté ginger and green onions in olive oil for a few seconds.

Remove skillet from heat and mix in soy sauce mixture. Stir in cornstarch-water mixture and return skillet to high heat.

---

*Available at Oriental food stores and some supermarkets

When sauce begins to thicken, add the chicken, red pepper, and pineapple and stir until well coated. If sauce is too thick, add more water, 1 tablespoon at a time.

5 servings
Calories per serving: 203 Total; 21 Fat; 5 Sat-fat

Q HUNAN CHICKEN WITH ONIONS AND PEPPERS

4 boned and skinned chicken breasts
½ cup unbleached white flour
½ teaspoon salt (optional)
¼ teaspoon freshly ground black pepper
2 tablespoons cornstarch
2 tablespoons + 1 cup water
3 tablespoons soy sauce
1 tablespoon dry sherry
3 tablespoons white vinegar

1 can (8 oz) water chestnuts
1 tablespoon olive oil
1 clove garlic, minced
2 medium onions, sliced (about 1½ cups)
1 red pepper and 1 green pepper (or 2 green peppers), seeded and cut into strips
2–3 whole dried chili peppers, crumbled*

Preheat oven to 375°F.

Shake chicken in a plastic bag with flour, salt, and pepper until coated. Place chicken in a single layer in a baking pan and bake until fully cooked, about 20–30 minutes. When chicken is cool enough to handle, cut into bite-size pieces. Set aside.

Combine cornstarch with two tablespoons water. Stir in remaining cup of water. Set aside.

Combine soy sauce, sherry, and vinegar and set aside.

Heat olive oil in large skillet or wok. Sauté garlic, onions, red and green peppers, and water chestnuts on high heat for 1 minute, adding a splash of water as they begin to cook. Lower to medium and cook until soft but not limp. Add chili peppers.

Mix chicken into vegetables. Add sauce. Stir until chicken is well coated. Add cornstarch mixture. Stir until sauce thickens. If sauce is

---

*Do not crumble with bare fingers or you may burn your skin.

too thick, add water, a tablespoon at a time, until it reaches the right consistency.

Serve over rice.

6 servings
Calories per serving: 162 Total; 29 Fat; 5 Sat-fat

▢ BALSAMIC CHICKEN WITH POTATOES AND ONIONS

4 tablespoons balsamic or other flavored vinegar
4 boned and skinned chicken breasts
2 medium-large potatoes
¾ cup sliced onion

1 teaspoon olive oil
¼–½ teaspoon thyme
Salt to taste (optional)
Freshly ground black pepper to taste

Pour 3 tablespoons of vinegar over chicken and marinate for several hours or overnight.

Preheat oven to 350°F.

Wash potatoes thoroughly and cut into ¼-inch slices. (You should have about 2 cups.) Steam in a vegetable steamer for ten minutes (until almost tender).

Meanwhile, in a small skillet sauté onion in olive oil on medium heat. Add a splash of water and cook vegetables until soft.

Mix in remaining tablespoon vinegar.

Mix in potatoes.

Pour the potato mixture into a shallow casserole large enough to accommodate a layer of potatoes covered by chicken breasts. Sprinkle potatoes with about ¼ teaspoon thyme.

Remove chicken from marinade and place on top of potatoes. Season with salt and pepper to taste and sprinkle with remaining thyme.

Bake for 30–45 minutes or until chicken is cooked through.

Makes 4 servings
Calories per serving: 193 Total; 23 Fat; 5 Sat-fat

THAI CHICKEN WITH ASPARAGUS

1 pound asparagus
2 tablespoons cornstarch
2 tablespoons water
1 pound boned and skinned
  chicken breasts
1 tablespoon olive oil
¼–½ teaspoon red pepper
  flakes
½ teaspoon caraway seeds

½ teaspoon coriander
½ teaspoon salt (optional)
¼ teaspoon freshly ground
  black pepper
1 tablespoon minced shallot
1 clove garlic, minced
1 can chicken broth (10¾ oz),
  strained

Snap off and discard the bottoms of asparagus. Cut spears into 1½-inch pieces.

Bring a pot of water to a boil and cook asparagus 3–5 minutes, until tender. Drain, run cool water over asparagus, and set aside.

Mix cornstarch with water until smooth and set aside.

Cut chicken breasts into bite-size pieces and sauté in oil until cooked through.

While chicken is cooking, combine the seasonings, shallot, and garlic (this step is easy to do in a food processor or mini food processor) and mix them together with chicken broth. Add cornstarch mixture. When chicken is cooked through, add seasoned broth. Bring to a boil and let sauce thicken. Lower heat and add asparagus.

4 servings
Calories per serving: 201 Total; 42 Fat; 8 Sat-fat

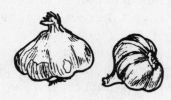

Q̲ # CHICKEN FAJITAS

4 boned and skinned chicken
    breasts

Marinade

2 cloves garlic, minced
1½ teaspoons cumin

½ teaspoon salt (optional)
3 tablespoons fresh lime juice

Tomato Salsa

1 pound tomatoes, chopped
1 small onion, minced

1 fresh chili pepper, sliced thin
1 tablespoon fresh lime juice

Vegetable Mélange

1 large onion, sliced
1 clove garlic, minced
1 green pepper, sliced

1 red or yellow sweet pepper,
    sliced
1 tablespoon olive oil

6 large flour tortillas*

Place chicken breasts in a bowl, combine marinade ingredients, and pour over chicken. Marinate in refrigerator at least 30 minutes.

Combine tomato salsa ingredients and refrigerate until ready to use.

Sauté onion, garlic, and peppers in olive oil until soft. Set aside.

Grill** or broil chicken breasts until cooked through. Slice into strips.

Warm the tortillas as directed on the package. They should be soft. (Don't bake them too long or you will have 6 very large crackers.)

To assemble each tortilla, lay pepper mixture across half, cover with chicken, and top with tomato salsa. Fold over top and serve.

Makes 6 tortillas
Calories per serving: 212 Total; 38 Fat; 6 Sat-fat

*You may find tortillas in your grocery store in a refrigerated case. Look for tortillas with the least amount of fat. Do not use tortillas made with lard.
**Cast-iron griddles make great indoor grills.

Q

ALEX'S CHINESE CHICKEN
WITH ONIONS, MUSHROOMS, AND ZUCCHINI

1–1½ pounds boned and
  skinned chicken breasts
½ cup unbleached flour
½ teaspoon salt (optional)
¼ teaspoon freshly ground
  black pepper
1 medium zucchini
3 tablespoons soy sauce
3 tablespoons white vinegar

1–1½ tablespoons chili paste
  with garlic
¼–1 teaspoon red pepper flakes
  (optional)
2 tablespoons + 1 cup water
2 tablespoons cornstarch
2 large onions, sliced
1 tablespoon olive oil
3 cups mushrooms, sliced

Preheat oven to 375°F.

Shake chicken in a plastic bag with flour, salt, and pepper until coated. Bake chicken in a single layer in a baking pan until it is cooked through. When chicken is cool enough to handle, cut it into bite-size pieces and set them aside.

Quarter zucchini into 4 long sections. Cut these into ½-inch pieces. Steam zucchini 1–3 minutes until tender. Set aside.

Combine soy sauce, vinegar, chili paste, and red pepper flakes and set aside.

Add 2 tablespoons of water to cornstarch and mix until smooth. Add remaining water to cornstarch and set aside.

Sauté onions in the remaining 1 tablespoon olive oil until soft. Add mushrooms and cook for a minute. Stir in chicken.

Add soy sauce and cornstarch mixtures and stir until vegetables and chicken are covered.

Stir in zucchini.

Serve over rice.

6 generous servings
Calories per serving: 192 Total; 31 Fat; 6 Sat-fat

Q

FIFTIES CHICKEN

¼ cup unbleached white flour
1 clove garlic, crushed
4 boned and skinned chicken
   breasts
½ cup chopped onion
½ cup chopped green pepper

2 teaspoons olive oil
¾ cup orange juice
½ cup chili sauce
1 tablespoon Dijon mustard
1 tablespoon soy sauce

Preheat oven to 350°F.

Combine flour and garlic and place on a plate. Roll chicken pieces into flour, covering both sides. Place in shallow baking pan just large enough to hold chicken pieces in one layer. Set aside.

Sauté onion and green pepper in olive oil until tender. Mix in orange juice, chili sauce, Dijon mustard, and soy sauce. Use half the sauce to cover chicken. Reserve the other half in the refrigerator.

Bake chicken for 30–45 minutes or until cooked through. Heat reserved sauce and spoon over chicken.

4 servings
Calories per serving: 200 Total; 33 Fat; 7 Sat-fat

TURKEY

16

URKEY IS the heart of any Thanksgiving dinner, but it makes delicious eating throughout the rest of the year. Turkey can be stuffed and roasted and the leftovers made into numerous interesting dishes. Turkey cutlets can replace veal cutlets with no one being the wiser (but everyone being the healthier).

White meat turkey breast is a must for everyone who wants to consume less saturated fat and who also enjoys eating. One ounce of turkey breast has only ½ calorie of saturated fat!

NOTE: Turkey contains so much protein and so little fat, it tends to cook quickly. Be careful. Overcooking makes turkey tough.

BASIC TURKEY CUTLET

Turkey cutlets provide a quick and extremely elegant meal. In addition, they are low in fat (even lower than chicken), they are inexpensive, and they can be substituted for exorbitantly expensive veal scaloppine. Turkey cutlets can usually be found in the poultry section of your grocery store.

1 pound turkey cutlets
½ cup unbleached white flour
1 tablespoon olive oil*

1 tablespoon margarine*
Salt and freshly ground black
   pepper to taste

*No fat is used in the second cooking method on the next page.

258

Here are two methods to prepare turkey cutlets for any veal scaloppine recipe:

With fat: Place cutlets between two pieces of wax paper and pound with meat mallet or rolling pin until thin.

Place flour on a plate. Dip each cutlet in flour, coating it on both sides, and place it on a large plate. When the plate is completely covered with one layer of cutlets, cover them with a sheet of wax paper to hold the next layer.

Heat olive oil and margarine in a large frying pan or wok.

When very hot (margarine should bubble) place cutlets in frying pan. Do not crowd cutlets.

When the edges turn white, turn the cutlets and cook them until they become light brown and are no longer pink inside. Cutlets cook very quickly. Turn again. Do not overcook or cutlets will be tough.

Remove cutlets to a plate and salt and pepper them liberally.

Do not clean skillet. Now you are ready for any number of scaloppine recipes.

With no fat added: If you wish to reduce the total fat content of turkey cutlets (the sat-fat content is already low), instead of sautéing after you pound and flour them, place them on a cast-iron pancake griddle and cook them with no fat. You will find this method works particularly well in the Turkey with Capers recipe.

4 servings

Calories per serving:	Total	Fat	Sat-fat
	211	60	12
With no added fat	158	8	4

ⵞ TURKEY SCALOPPINE LIMONE

1 pound turkey cutlets
1 teaspoon margarine
½ cup fresh lemon juice
1 teaspoon unbleached white flour

⅓ cup chopped parsley
½ pound mushrooms, sliced (optional)
1 lemon, thinly sliced

Prepare turkey cutlets as in master recipe (page 258).
Melt margarine in skillet. Add lemon juice.

Sprinkle on flour and blend into mixture. Add cutlets. Stir and turn cutlets until they are covered with sauce but do not overcook them.

Add parsley and mushrooms, stirring until mushrooms are covered with sauce.

Garnish with lemon slices and serve immediately.

4 servings

Calories per serving:	Total	Fat	Sat-fat
	246	70	14
With no added fat	194	18	6

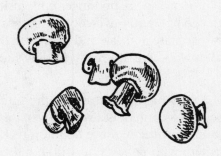

Ⓠ TURKEY SCALOPPINE MARSALA

1 pound turkey cutlets
½–¾ cup Marsala
1 teaspoon margarine

2 teaspoons unbleached white flour
½ pound mushrooms, sliced

Prepare turkey cutlets as in master recipe (page 258).

Add Marsala to pan over high heat. When it begins to boil, add margarine and reduce heat to medium.

Sprinkle on flour and blend.

Add cutlets and stir and turn until covered with sauce.

Add mushrooms and stir until covered with sauce.

Serve immediately.

4 servings

Calories per serving:	Total	Fat	Sat-fat
	268	70	14
With no added fat	216	18	6

Q

TURKEY WITH CAPERS

You may sauté turkey cutlets as in the first method for preparing turkey cutlets (page 259), but this takes a lot of fat. Flouring turkey cutlets, then grilling them on a cast-iron pancake griddle with no added fat, as in the second method (page 259), produces cutlets that are also tender but have almost no fat calories.

1 pound turkey breast cutlets	3 tablespoons red wine vinegar
1 teaspoon olive oil	2 tablespoons Dijon mustard
1 clove garlic, minced	1 cup chicken broth, strained
¼ cup chopped onion	2 tablespoons tomato paste
3 tablespoons capers, drained	⅓ cup chopped parsley

Prepare turkey cutlets as in master recipe (pages 258–59). Set aside.

In a large skillet, sauté garlic and onion in olive oil until soft.

Stir in capers, vinegar, Dijon mustard, chicken broth, and tomato paste. Add parsley.

Add turkey cutlets and mix until they are covered with sauce.

4 servings

Calories per serving:	Total	Fat	Sat-fat
	227	70	13
With no added fat	174	18	5

Q

TURKEY NIÇOISE

1 pound turkey breast cutlets	1 tablespoon capers
¾ cup chopped onion	8 large black olives, halved
3 cloves garlic, minced	¼–½ teaspoon red pepper
1 teaspoon olive oil	flakes
1½ pounds fresh tomatoes,	¼ teaspoon thyme
chopped	¼ teaspoon basil
6 flat anchovies, chopped	¼ teaspoon oregano
½ cup dry vermouth	Salt to taste (optional)

Prepare turkey cutlets as in master recipe (pages 258–59).

In a large skillet, sauté onion and garlic in 1 teaspoon olive oil until soft. Add a splash of water to help cook the vegetables.

Add tomatoes and anchovies and cook for 10–20 minutes until tomato sauce thickens.

Add vermouth, capers, olives, red pepper flakes, thyme, basil, oregano, and salt to taste, and cook for about 5 minutes until sauce thickens.

Mix turkey cutlets into the sauce and serve.

6 servings

Calories per serving:	Total	Fat	Sat-fat
	206	55	11
With no added fat	171	20	6

TURKEY WITH SWEET RED PEPPER SAUCE

The sauce takes about an hour to cook but no time to prepare. You may make this tasty dish in advance and refrigerate it.

Sweet Red Pepper Sauce

2 red peppers, chopped (about 2 cups)
1½ cups sliced tomatoes
1 can chicken broth (10¾ oz), strained
1 cup dry vermouth

Juice of ½ lemon
¼–½ teaspoon red pepper flakes
Salt to taste (optional)
Freshly ground black pepper to taste

½ cup chopped parsley
Peel of ½ lemon

4 cloves garlic

1 pound turkey cutlets

In a medium (about 8-inch) skillet, combine red peppers, tomatoes, chicken broth, vermouth, lemon juice, red pepper flakes, salt, and black pepper.

Bring to a boil, lower heat to medium, and cook until liquid is reduced and sauce is thick, about 50–60 minutes.

Meanwhile, in a food processor or by hand, chop or mince parsley, together with the lemon peel and garlic. Set aside.

Prepare the turkey cutlets as in master recipe (pages 258–59).

Heat red pepper sauce.

Sprinkle parsley mixture over cutlets and cover with sauce.

5 servings

Calories per serving:	Total	Fat	Sat-fat
	237	48	10
With no added fat	185	6	3

Q TURKEY CUTLETS WITH ARTICHOKE-CREAM SAUCE

This turkey dish is so creamy, you would swear it was a no-no! With only 15 sat-fat calories per serving, it is a good choice for keeping your family healthy and impressing your company.

1 pound turkey cutlets
1 tablespoon margarine
3 tablespoons unbleached white
  flour

1 cup skim milk
1 jar (11½ oz) artichoke hearts,
  packed in water
¼ teaspoon salt (optional)

Prepare cutlets as in master recipe (page 258).

In a medium saucepan, melt margarine. Remove from heat and stir in flour to make a smooth paste.

Slowly stir in skim milk and liquid from artichokes. Add salt. Heat until thick.

Mix in artichoke hearts.

Pour sauce over cutlets and serve.

5 servings

Calories per serving:	Total	Fat	Sat-fat
	230	67	15
With no added fat	188	25	9

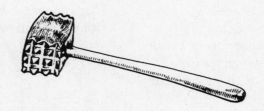

TURKEY VÉRONIQUE

6 turkey cutlets (about 1 pound)
1 teaspoon tarragon
½ cup minced onion
1 cup sliced mushrooms

1 teaspoon olive oil
⅔ cup dry white wine or
  vermouth
2 cups seedless grapes

Preheat oven to 375°F.

Prepare cutlets as in master recipe (page 258), but add tarragon to the flour.

In a large skillet, sauté onions and mushrooms in olive oil. Add a splash of water to help cook the vegetables.

Add wine and heat to boiling. Pour over cutlets.

Cover with foil, place in oven, and bake for 5 minutes.

Add grapes and bake for 5 minutes more.

6 servings

Calories per serving:	*Total*	*Fat*	*Sat-fat*
	234	60	12
With no added fat	145	14	5

TURKEY ROLL-UPS FIRENZE

Avoid commercial bread crumbs. They are high in fat calories (45 per cup) and high in saturated fat calories (14 per cup). Use your food processor or blender to make your own from a few slices of bread (about 9 fat calories and 2 sat-fat calories per slice).

If you forget to thaw the spinach, cook it first until it is no longer frozen.

2 cups bread crumbs made from
  3–4 slices bread
2 cloves garlic, minced
1 teaspoon thyme
1 teaspoon oregano
6 turkey cutlets (about 1 pound)
1 package frozen spinach,
  thawed, or 10 ounces fresh
  spinach

¼ cup low-fat (1%) cottage
  cheese
¼ cup chopped mushrooms
¼ cup chopped onion
2 tablespoons margarine, melted

Preheat oven to 400°F.

Combine bread crumbs, garlic, thyme, and oregano. Or chop garlic in food processor, then add bread slices and spices.

Pound cutlets between two sheets of wax paper until thin.

Squeeze liquid out of spinach.

Combine spinach, cottage cheese, mushrooms, and onions.

Place ⅙ spinach mixture on one side of each cutlet.

Roll up cutlets. Dip in melted margarine. Roll in bread crumbs.

Place rolled cutlets in a shallow casserole greased with margarine.

Bake for 10–20 minutes or until cooked through.

6 servings
Calories per serving: 176 Total; 32 Fat; 10 Sat-fat

Ⓠ TURKEY MEXIQUE

A great dish with a chili taste.

1 cup chopped onion	1½ cups chicken broth, strained
2 teaspoons minced garlic	3 tablespoons tomato paste
1 teaspoon olive oil	3 cups diced turkey breast, raw or cooked
1–2 tablespoons chili powder	1 green pepper, diced
1 tablespoon cumin seed	¼ cup stuffed green olives, sliced
½ teaspoon salt (optional)	½ cup water
1 tablespoon unbleached white flour	

In a large skillet, sauté onion and garlic in olive oil. Add a splash of water and cook until vegetables are soft.

Stir in chili powder, cumin seed, salt, and flour.

Add chicken broth and tomato paste and blend well.

Cook for 5 minutes over low heat.

Stir in turkey, green pepper, and olives and heat through. (If turkey is raw, cook until turkey turns white and is fully cooked.)

If sauce is too thick, add water 2 tablespoons at a time until desired consistency.

Serve over rice.

6 servings
Calories per serving: 146 Total; 16 Fat; 4 Sat-fat

⌨ BREADED TURKEY CUTLET

1 pound turkey cutlets
¼ teaspoon salt (optional)
½ teaspoon basil or oregano

1 cup bread crumbs made from
  2 slices of bread
2 tablespoons olive oil

Pound turkey cutlets between two sheets of wax paper until thin.
Combine salt, herbs, and bread crumbs on a plate.
Coat cutlet on both sides with bread crumbs and shake off excess.
Heat olive oil in large skillet until bubbly.
Cook cutlets a few at a time until golden brown on each side.
Place on paper towels to absorb excess fat and serve immediately.

4 servings
Calories per serving: 228 Total; 72 Fat; 11 Sat-fat

⌨ TURKEY SAUTÉED
WITH ONIONS AND ALMONDS

3 tablespoons slivered almonds
2 cups thinly sliced onion
1 tablespoon olive oil
¼ teaspoon cardamom
½ teaspoon coriander
1 teaspoon salt (optional)

⅓ cup dry sherry
¼ cup raisins
3 cups diced cooked turkey
  breast
¼ cup chopped parsley

Brown almond slivers in a toaster oven and set aside. Watch them
carefully — they burn quickly.
In a large skillet or wok, sauté onion in olive oil until tender.
Stir in cardamom, coriander, salt, sherry, and raisins. Cook until
all excess liquid evaporates.
Stir in turkey, parsley, and almonds and heat through.

6 servings
Calories per serving: 200 Total; 43 Fat; 8 Sat-fat

Q BROCCOLI BAKED TURKEY

1 head broccoli
2 tablespoons margarine
3 tablespoons unbleached white
flour
1 can (10¾ oz) chicken broth,
strained

½ teaspoon salt (optional)
½ pound mushrooms, sliced
2 cups diced cooked turkey
breast

Trim stems and leaves off broccoli and separate flowerets.
Steam flowerets until just tender. Set aside.
In a medium saucepan, melt margarine.
Remove from heat and stir flour into margarine to make a smooth paste.
Return to low heat and blend in chicken broth, stirring constantly until sauce is thick and smooth.
Stir salt and mushrooms into sauce.
Preheat oven to 375°F. Grease a shallow baking pan with margarine.
Place broccoli in baking pan, cover with turkey, and pour mushroom sauce over both.
Bake, uncovered, 15–25 minutes.

6 servings
Calories per serving: 145 Total; 32 Fat; 19 Sat-fat

CREAMY TURKEY CASSEROLE

2 egg whites
2 tablespoons margarine
3 tablespoons unbleached white
flour
1 can (10¾ oz) chicken broth,
strained
1 cup diced celery
2 tablespoons minced green
onion
½ cup (2 oz) chopped pecans

½ teaspoon salt (optional)
¼ teaspoon Worcestershire
sauce
1 egg yolk
1 tablespoon fresh lemon juice
¼ cup reduced-calorie
mayonnaise
3 cups diced cooked turkey
breast

Preheat oven to 400°F. Grease a casserole with margarine.

Whip egg whites until stiff but not dry and set aside.

In a medium saucepan, melt margarine. Remove from heat and stir in flour to make a paste. Gradually blend in chicken broth over low heat. Stir constantly until sauce is thick and smooth.

Stir celery, green onion, pecans, salt, Worcestershire sauce, egg yolk, and lemon juice into sauce.

Fold in egg whites.

Mix mayonnaise with turkey so that turkey is well coated.

Add turkey mixture to sauce and pour into casserole. Bake for 20 minutes.

6 servings
Calories per serving: 255 Total; 49 Fat; 22 Sat-fat

TURKEY WITH SNOW PEAS

1 pound turkey tenderloin	1 tablespoon cornstarch
2 tablespoons white vinegar	¼ cup water
2 tablespoons soy sauce	3 ounces (about 1 cup) snow
1 tablespoon brown sugar	peas
2 slices ginger root	10 water chestnuts, thinly sliced
2 tablespoons dry sherry	

Place turkey in a casserole.

Combine vinegar, soy sauce, brown sugar, ginger, and sherry and pour over turkey.

Simmer for about 20 minutes or until tender. *Do not overcook.*

Remove turkey from casserole and slice into bite-size pieces.

Return sliced turkey to casserole and refrigerate in marinade for several hours or overnight.

Place turkey in a large skillet or wok.

Combine cornstarch and water into a smooth paste. Stir into remaining marinade.

Heat turkey. Pour marinade over turkey and stir until well coated

Stir in snow peas and water chestnuts.

5 servings
Calories per serving: 190 Total; 26 Fat; 9 Sat-fat

FISH AND SHELLFISH

17

FISH IS AN excellent choice for heart-healthy eating. It is a fine source of complete protein. The quality of this protein is about the same as that of red meat. Fish also contains important vitamins and minerals. And, in addition to all this good nutrition, fish contains much less fat than red meat. While 6 ounces of trimmed sirloin steak contains 150 calories of saturated fat, 6 ounces of haddock or flounder contain 6 calories of saturated fat. Fish oils are polyunsaturated and have an unusually potent effect in lowering blood triglyceride levels.

Fish cooks quickly — within minutes — and may be prepared in a multitude of tasty ways: broiled, baked, poached, oven-fried. Fish may be used as the base for soups, salads, pastas, and stews. Even when prepared most simply to enhance its delicacy, fish is delicious. The key is freshness.

Ⓠ BROILED MONKFISH WITH ORANGE SAUCE

Very special and delicious. Skim milk makes a great cream sauce. (And look at the difference in sat-fat calories per cup: 3 for a cup of skim milk versus 335 for a cup of cream.)

2 tablespoons margarine
2 tablespoons unbleached white
   flour
¼ cup orange juice
¾ cup skim milk
Grated peel of 1 orange
1 green onion, sliced
¼ teaspoon salt (optional)

¼ cup flour
½ teaspoon salt (optional)
¼ teaspoon freshly ground
   black pepper
1½ pounds monkfish fillets (or
   any white fish fillets)
2 teaspoons margarine

Preheat broiler and grease broiler pan with oil.

Melt margarine in a small saucepan. Remove from heat and mix in 2 tablespoons flour to make a smooth paste.

Mix in orange juice and skim milk, stirring until smooth.

Cook over medium heat until sauce thickens, stirring constantly.

Stir in 2 tablespoons grated orange rind, green onion, and salt and set aside.

Combine ¼ cup flour, salt, and pepper and place on large plate.

Dredge fillets in flour so both sides are coated.

Lay fillets on broiler pan and dot them with 2 teaspoons margarine.

Sprinkle remaining orange rind on fillets (grate more if needed).

Broil for 5–15 minutes, depending on the thickness of the fish, or until fish flakes easily.

Reheat orange sauce and spoon 1 tablespoon over each serving.

6 servings
Calories per serving: 194 Total; 52 Fat; 13 Sat-fat

◻ MARINATED FISH STEAKS

1½ pounds fish steaks
  (swordfish, cod, halibut, etc.)
2 tablespoons ketchup
1 tablespoon fresh lemon juice
1 clove garlic, minced
1 teaspoon oregano

½ teaspoon salt (optional)
1 teaspoon olive oil
¼ cup orange juice
¼ cup dry vermouth
¼ cup chopped parsley

Place steaks in a shallow casserole.

Combine ketchup, lemon juice, garlic, oregano, salt, olive oil, orange juice, vermouth, and parsley and pour over fish. Marinate several hours or overnight in refrigerator.

Preheat broiler and grease broiler pan with oil.

Broil fish for 5–15 minutes or until it flakes easily.

Heat marinade and spoon over fish.

4 servings

Calories per serving:	Total	Fat	Sat-fat
Swordfish	241	70	17
Cod	175	22	1
Halibut	240	42	7

[Q]
FISH BAKED IN OLIVE,
CHILI PEPPER, AND TOMATO SAUCE

¾ cup chopped onion
2 cloves garlic, minced
1 teaspoon olive oil
1 tablespoon cornstarch
1 can (16 oz) tomatoes,
  chopped, juice reserved
⅓ cup sliced stuffed green olives

1 teaspoon chopped red or
  green chili pepper
1½ pounds flounder fillets (or
  other mild fish)
Salt to taste (optional)
1 tablespoon fresh lemon juice

Preheat oven to 375°F.

In a medium skillet, sauté onion and garlic in olive oil. Add a splash of water and cook vegetables until soft.

Mix in cornstarch.

Add tomatoes and their juice and mix until well blended.

Cook over medium-high heat until sauce thickens.

Stir in olives and chili pepper.

Spoon half the sauce into a baking pan large enough to hold the fillets in one layer. Place fillets over sauce.

Salt fillets and sprinkle them with lemon juice.

Cover fillets with remaining sauce and bake for 10 minutes or until they flake easily.

6 servings
Calories per serving: 150 Total; 18 Fat; 5 Sat-fat

[Q]
SALMON WITH CUCUMBER-GRAPE SAUCE

¼ cup nonfat yogurt
1½ tablespoons reduced-calorie
  mayonnaise
½ tablespoon fresh lemon juice
¼ cup grated cucumber

1 cup seedless grapes
6 salmon steaks* (4 oz each)
1 tablespoon margarine
3 tablespoons fresh lemon juice

Preheat broiler and grease broiler pan.

Combine yogurt, mayonnaise, lemon juice, cucumber, and grapes. Set aside.

---

*Salmon varies greatly in total calories and sat-fat calories depending on the species. This will affect the total calories per serving.

Place salmon steaks on broiler pan.
Melt margarine and combine it with lemon juice.
Baste salmon with lemon-margarine sauce.
Broil 3–5 minutes, turn salmon, and baste again.
Broil 3–5 minutes more or until fish flakes easily.
Spoon cucumber-grape sauce over salmon steaks and serve.

6 servings

Calories per serving:	Total	Fat	Sat-fat
Atlantic	202	58	17
Coho	206	82	17
Pink	174	86	9

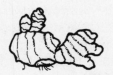

Q ## BROILED GINGER FISH

1 cup flour
1 teaspoon salt (optional)
½ teaspoon freshly ground
   black pepper
4 six-ounce fish fillets
   (monkfish, haddock, etc.)

2 teaspoons margarine
4 teaspoons diced ginger root
Lemon slices to cover fillets

Set oven to broil and grease broiler pan with oil.
Combine flour, salt, and pepper on a large plate.
Dredge fillets in flour, covering both sides.
Dot fillets with margarine, sprinkle them with ginger, and cover with lemon slices.
Broil for 5–15 minutes or until fish flakes easily.

4 servings
Calories per serving: 194 Total; 35 Fat; 4 Sat-fat

[Q]   # CURRY FISH

A simple but impressive dish, which tastes as good as it looks. Fun for company.

1 pound any white fish fillets	Raisins
Salt to taste	Peanuts
2 teaspoons olive oil	Crushed pineapple
½–1 tablespoon curry powder	Scallions
2½ cups cooked long-grain rice	Chutney
2 hard-boiled egg whites, chopped	

Preheat oven to 425°F. Grease a baking dish with margarine.
Place fillets in baking dish, salt lightly, and bake for 20 minutes.
Flake the fish. (If you wish to serve it later, you can refrigerate the fish now.)
Heat olive oil in a large skillet and mix in curry powder.
Add fish and stir until it is covered with curry sauce.
Mix cooked rice and fish together gently.
Place egg whites, raisins, peanuts, crushed pineapple, scallions, and chutney in small dishes and pass with main dish.

4 servings

Calories per serving:	*Total*	*Fat*	*Sat-fat*
Without condiments	283	28	5
With teaspoon of each	349	41	7

[Q]   # DILL FISH

1½ pounds fish fillets (flounder, sole, turbot, etc.)	1 clove garlic, minced
¼ cup fresh lime juice	Salt and freshly ground black pepper to taste
1 teaspoon dillweed	

Preheat oven to 350°F.
Squeeze lime juice over fillets and marinate for at least 30 minutes in refrigerator.
Grease a shallow baking pan with margarine.

Place fillets in baking pan and sprinkle with dill, garlic, salt, and pepper.

Bake for 5–10 minutes or until fish flakes easily.

6 servings
Calories per serving: 115 Total; 12 Fat; 4 Sat-fat

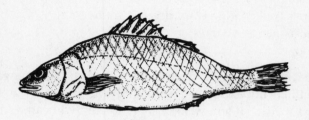

FLOUNDER FILLETS STUFFED WITH FENNEL RICE

Raw fennel, or *finocchio,* as the Italians call it, tastes of licorice or anise. The taste of cooked fennel is more subtle and sweet. Cook sliced fennel bulb with margarine and water to cover for a delicious vegetable dish. You may substitute celery in this recipe, but try to find fennel at your grocery store or an Italian market for a more unusual dish. Despite its lack of cream or whole milk, this dish is quite creamy.

⅓ cup sliced fennel stalks	1½ cups cooked long-grain rice
⅓ cup sliced mushrooms	2 tablespoons margarine
1 teaspoon fennel seeds	3 tablespoons fresh lemon juice
1 teapoon olive oil	8 flounder fillets

Preheat oven to 375°F. Grease a shallow baking pan with margarine.

In a medium skillet, sauté fennel and mushrooms in olive oil until just tender.

Add fennel seeds and cooked rice. Stir for a minute and set aside.

Melt 2 tablespoons margarine in a small saucepan. Add lemon juice and set aside.

Lay out fillets on waxed paper.

Place several tablespoons of rice mixture in the middle of each fillet.

Roll up the fillets and place them seam-side down in the baking dish. (The sides may barely reach each other, but that is okay.)

Pour margarine-lemon mixture over fish and bake for about 20 minutes or until fish flake easily. (Measure thickness of rolled fish and allow 10 minutes per inch.)

If you have any rice mixture left over, reheat and serve with the fish.

8 servings
Calories per serving: 130 Total; 22 Fat; 9 Sat-fat

PHYLLO-WRAPPED FISH AND MUSHROOM SAUCE

Fish wrapped in phyllo dough is an elegant company dish. If you want a simpler (as in less work) dish, just ignore the phyllo part of the recipe. The fish with the mushroom sauce is still luscious.

NOTE: If you are using phyllo dough, the directions on the box usually recommend that you thaw it in the refrigerator overnight and 2–3 hours at room temperature before you use it.

Fish

8 fillets (6 oz each) pollack, monkfish, or other white fish
Salt and freshly ground black pepper

1 pound phyllo leaves
1/4 cup melted margarine

Mushroom Sauce

2 tablespoons margarine
1/4 cup unbleached white flour
3 cups sliced mushrooms
1/4 cup dry sherry
1 1/4 cups skim milk

1/4 teaspoon salt
1/8 teaspoon freshly ground black pepper
Grated nutmeg to taste

The Fish

Preheat oven to 350°F. Grease a baking sheet with margarine.
Check fillets for small bones and remove them.

Lightly salt and pepper fish.

Unroll phyllo dough and cover it with plastic wrap or a towel to keep it from drying out and becoming brittle.

Place one sheet of phyllo dough on the counter with a narrow end toward you. Brush phyllo with melted margarine. Cover with a second sheet of phyllo and brush it with melted margarine. Repeat process for third sheet.

Place fillet on the phyllo edge nearest you. (If fillet is long and narrow, you may have to fold the fillet in half.) Fold left side, then right side of phyllo over fillet and roll it up.

Place seam-side down on baking sheet.

Wrap each fillet in phyllo dough and place on baking sheet.

Bake for 20 minutes. Make a small slit in phyllo to see if fish is done. Bake until fish flakes easily and is opaque.

While fish is baking, make mushroom sauce.

The Mushroom Sauce

In a medium saucepan, melt margarine.

Lower heat and mix in flour. Remove pan from heat.

In a medium skillet, cook mushrooms in sherry until all but ¼ cup liquid is evaporated. Drain liquid from mushrooms and set it aside. Set mushrooms aside.

In a small saucepan, heat milk until steaming but *not boiling*. Slowly pour milk into flour mixture, blending until sauce is smooth. Stir in mushroom liquid.

Return saucepan to burner and slowly heat sauce to boiling.

Add mushrooms, salt, pepper, and nutmeg to thickened sauce.

Serve over phyllo-wrapped fish.

8 servings

Calories per serving:	Total	Fat	Sat-fat
With mushroom sauce	397	85	17
Without mushroom sauce	342	61	12

Q   # FISH WITH MUSHROOM SAUCE

8 fillets (6 oz each) pollack,
    monkfish, or other white fish

Make mushroom sauce (see page 276).
Preheat oven to 350°F. Grease a shallow baking pan with margarine.
Place fish in baking pan.
Bake for 5–10 minutes or until fish flakes easily and is opaque.
Spoon mushroom sauce over fish and serve.

8 servings
Calories per serving: 254 Total; 40 Fat; 8 Sat-fat

Q   # ORIENTAL FISH KEBABS

1¼ pounds swordfish steaks
½ cup fresh lime juice
1 tablespoon soy sauce
1 tablespoon brown sugar
2 cloves garlic, minced
2 tablespoons sliced green onion

1 medium onion, cut into
    eighths
1 green pepper, cut into 1½-
    inch pieces
8 cherry tomatoes

Cut fish into 1½-inch cubes.
Combine lime juice, soy sauce, brown sugar, garlic, and green onion and pour over fish. Marinate for at least 2 hours in refrigerator.
Arrange fish, onion chunks, green pepper, and tomatoes on skewers. Rotate skewers in marinade to cover vegetables and let sit for several minutes so the vegetables can absorb the flavor.
Broil for 10 minutes per inch of thickness of fish or until it flakes easily.
Heat remaining marinade and spoon over fish.

4 servings
Calories per serving: 243 Total; 51 Fat; 10 Sat-fat

Q

SHANGHAI FISH

1½ pounds white fish fillets

2 tablespoons soy sauce

1 clove garlic, minced

2 tablespoons dry sherry

3 green onions, sliced

1 tablespoon hoisin sauce*

Marinate fish in soy sauce, garlic, sherry, green onions, and hoisin sauce for several hours in refrigerator.

Broil for 5–10 minutes or until fish flakes easily and is opaque.

Heat marinade to boiling and serve over fish.

6 servings
Calories per serving: 117 Total; 12 Fat; 4 Sat-fat

Q

FISH WITH PEPPERCORNS, THYME, AND MUSTARD

¼–½ teaspoon black
  peppercorns

4 teaspoons Dijon mustard

1 teaspoon thyme

2 tablespoons vermouth

½ teaspoon olive oil

1 pound fish fillets (sole,
  flounder, etc.)

Preheat oven to 450°F. With margarine, grease shallow glass casserole or baking pan large enough to hold fish.

Crush peppercorns coarsely in food processor or mortar and pestle.

Combine and mix with mustard, thyme, vermouth, and oil.

Make several diagonal slashes across the fillets.

Place fish in baking pan and spread mustard mixture over it.

Bake for 5–20 minutes, until fish flakes easily.

3 servings
Calories per serving: 70 Total; 23 Fat; 5 Sat-fat

---

*Available at Oriental food stores and some supermarkets

⌑ SALMON SOUFFLÉ

1 can (8 oz) salmon
1 cup skim milk
1 cup fine bread crumbs made
from 2 slices whole-wheat
bread

3 egg whites

Preheat oven to 350°F. Grease a small casserole with margarine.

Prepare salmon by carefully rinsing it with water and removing any bones. Set aside.

Heat skim milk and bread crumbs slowly in a double boiler until thick.

Meanwhile, whip egg whites until stiff but not dry. Set aside.

Flake salmon with a fork and add it to the thickened milk mixture. Remove from heat.

Fold salmon mixture into egg whites.

Pour into casserole and bake for 30 minutes.

4 servings
Calories per serving: 149 Total; 32 Fat; 9 Sat-fat

⌑ CAJUN FISH

This spicy fish will wake up your taste buds.

Seasoning Mix

1 teaspoon paprika
¼ teaspoon white pepper
¼ teaspoon cayenne pepper
½ teaspoon freshly ground
black pepper

½ teaspoon oregano
½ teaspoon thyme
½ teaspoon basil
½ teaspoon salt (optional)

1 clove garlic, minced

1¼ pound skinned fish fillets

Preheat broiler.

Combine seasonings and garlic in a small bowl.

Spread garlic mixture over both sides of fillets.

Sprinkle remaining herbs over fillets and rub into each side. (For a milder version, use seasonings more sparingly.)

Broil fillets until cooked through (5–20 minutes depending on thickness of fish).

4 servings

Calories per serving	Total	Fat	Sat-fat
Sole	140	15	5

To determine the total calories, fat calories, or sat-fat calories for this recipe, find the total calories per ounce, fat calories per ounce, or sat-fat calories per ounce of your chosen fish in the Food Tables and multiply by 5.

Q FENNEL FISH

1¼ pound thick fish fillets, such as grouper
1 tablespoon olive oil

3 tablespoons fennel seed
2 tablespoons water

Cut fish crosswise into ½-inch-thick slices. Set aside.

Pour oil into a skillet large enough to hold the fish pieces in one layer. Add fennel and sauté for a few seconds.

Add fish. Let cook for about 2 minutes on medium heat.

Add 1 tablespoon of the water and cover skillet. In about 2 more minutes, add the second tablespoon of water and replace cover to finish steaming the fish. Cook until fish is cooked through.

Serve immediately.

4 servings
Calories per serving: 134 Total; 42 Fat; 4 Sat-fat

Q FISH IN WINE SAUCE

This delicate fish dish takes no time to make.

¾ pound of white fish fillets, such as flounder or sole
¼–½ cup white wine or vermouth

3 tablespoons minced shallot
Freshly ground black pepper to taste

Preheat oven to 400°F. Place the fillets in one layer so they fill a shallow baking pan and pour the wine over them. The wine should *not* cover them.

Sprinkle shallots over fish.

Depending on the thickness of the fish, bake for 5–20 minutes until it flakes easily.

Pepper liberally and serve.

3 servings
Calories per serving: 119 Total; 12 Fat; 4 Sat-fat

SCALLOPS AND SHRIMP

Both scallops and shrimp are low-sat-fat gems. They take only 3–5 minutes to cook, may be added to innumerable sauces with no fuss or bother, are extremely low in saturated fat (1 ounce of either contains only 1 sat-fat calorie), and are delicious.

You may have been told to avoid shrimp because it is higher in cholesterol than other shellfish. Don't worry. Shrimp contains only slightly more cholesterol than other meats, but is extremely low in saturated fat. It also contains risk-reducing omega-3 polyunsaturated fats. We recommend that you eat as much shrimp as you can afford unless you are wealthy or a shrimp fisherman.

☑ SCALLOP OR SHRIMP CURRY

Delight your guests or family with this unusual curry. The apples and lime create a unique combination of sweet and sour tastes.

1 cup chopped onion
1 apple, peeled, cored, and diced
2 cloves garlic, minced
1–3 teaspoons curry powder
1 tablespoon olive oil
¼ cup unbleached white flour
½ teaspoon salt (optional)
¼ teaspoon cardamom
¼ teaspoon freshly ground black pepper

1 can chicken broth (10¾ oz), strained
1 tablespoon fresh lime juice
1¼ pounds bay scallops or shrimp, shelled and deveined
1 cup sliced mushrooms
10–15 snow peas (optional)
½–1 cup water

In a large skillet, sauté onion, apple, garlic, and curry powder in olive oil until tender.

Remove skillet from heat and blend in flour, salt, cardamom, and pepper.

Stir in chicken broth and lime juice until curry sauce is well blended.

Bring curry sauce to a boil, reduce heat, and simmer, uncovered, for about 5 minutes. Stir occasionally.

Meanwhile, place scallops or shrimp in a pot of boiling water and cook until just tender (5–10 minutes). Drain and set aside.

When curry sauce is finished cooking, add shellfish, mushrooms, and snow peas. If sauce is too thick, add water, ¼ cup at a time until desired consistency is achieved. Serve curry over rice.

6 servings

Calories per serving:	Total	Fat	Sat-fat
Scallops	187	25	7
Shrimp	187	35	7

Q ## SCALLOPS PROVENÇAL

It takes only about 15 minutes and very little effort to create this delightful combination of color, texture, and taste.

1 pound bay scallops
¼ cup unbleached white flour
3 cloves garlic, minced
2 tablespoons olive oil

2 cups snow peas (about ½ pound)
2 cups sliced red pepper
1 cup sliced mushrooms

Rinse scallops, dry with a paper towel, and roll scallops in flour.

In a wok or large skillet, sauté scallops and garlic in olive oil until tender (about 5–10 minutes).

Add snow peas, red peppers, and mushrooms and mix until heated through.

Serve over rice.

5 servings
Calories per serving: 190 Total; 55 Fat; 8 Sat-fat

⌷ SCALLOP OR SHRIMP CARIBBEAN

¼ cup sugar
2 tablespoons cornstarch
⅛ teaspoon salt (optional)
½ cup orange juice
⅓ cup white vinegar
½ cup water
1 pound bay scallops or shrimp,
  shelled and deveined

2 teaspoons grated orange peel
½ pound mushrooms, sliced
1 medium orange, peeled and
  cut into bite-size pieces
¼ pound snow peas
¼ cup sliced green onions
3 cups cooked long-grain rice
3 tablespoons sliced almonds

In a large skillet, combine sugar, cornstarch, and salt. Slowly stir in orange juice, vinegar, and water.

Stir constantly over medium heat until mixture thickens.

Add scallops or shrimp and orange peel.

When shellfish is cooked through (5–10 minutes), add mushrooms, orange pieces, snow peas, and green onions.

Serve over rice, topped with almonds.

6 servings

Calories per serving:	Total	Fat	Sat-fat
Scallops	170	26	3
Shrimp	170	35	3

⌷ SCALLOP OR SHRIMP CREOLE

2 green peppers, chopped
1 cup chopped onion
2 cloves garlic, minced
2 teaspoons olive oil
1 teaspoon brown sugar
¼ teaspoon freshly ground
  black pepper
½ teaspoon thyme
¼ teaspoon cayenne pepper
1 bay leaf

½ teaspoon salt (optional)
2 large cans (28 oz each)
  tomatoes, drained, juiced, and
  chopped
½ cup sliced celery
1½ cups sliced mushrooms
3 tablespoons chopped parsley
1 pound bay scallops or shrimp,
  shelled and deveined

Sauté green peppers, onion, and garlic in olive oil. Add a splash of water and cook vegetables until soft.

Add brown sugar, pepper, thyme, cayenne pepper, bay leaf, and salt and stir well.

Stir in tomatoes and cook over low heat for 30 minutes or until sauce is thick.

Add celery and mushrooms and cook for a few minutes more.

Mix in parsley and scallops or shrimp and cook for 5–10 minutes or until shellfish is cooked through.

Serve immediately so shellfish will not overcook.

Serve over rice.

6 servings

Calories per serving:	Total	Fat	Sat-fat
Scallops	177	18	6
Shrimp	177	28	6

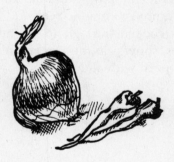

SPICY SHRIMP LOUISIANA

1–1¼ pounds shrimp
¼ teaspoon ground white
  pepper
⅛ teaspoon freshly ground
  black pepper
¼ teaspoon cayenne pepper
½ teaspoon basil
¼ teaspoon thyme
¼ teaspoon salt (optional)
¼ cup water

¼ cup unbleached white flour
2 teaspoons olive oil
½ cup chopped onion
1 green pepper, chopped
2 stalks celery, chopped
2 cloves garlic, minced
1 can (10¾ oz) chicken broth,
  strained
1 tablespoon tomato paste
¼ cup chopped green onions

Shell, devein, and clean shrimp. Cook in boiling water for about 3 minutes. Discard water. Set shrimp aside.

Combine the white, black, and cayenne pepper, basil, thyme, and salt. Set aside.

Slowly add water to flour and mix into a paste. Set aside.

Heat oil in wok or large frying pan until hot.

Stir in onion, green pepper, celery, and garlic, and cook until soft.

Mix in spice mixture.

Stir in broth and tomato paste.

Stir in flour mixture and cook until sauce thickens.

Add shrimp and green onions and serve over rice.

6 servings
Calories per serving: 88 Total; 28 Fat; 2 Sat-fat

Q   SHRIMP WITH GREEN PEPPERS

1 pound shrimp, shelled and deveined

2 tablespoons soy sauce

2 tablespoons dry sherry

1–2 teaspoons chili paste with garlic*

2 tablespoons tomato paste

½ teaspoon sugar

1 tablespoon cornstarch

2 tablespoons + 1 cup water

1–2 teaspoons chopped ginger root

2 green onions, sliced

2 teaspoons olive oil

1 large green pepper, sliced

¼ cup water

Put shrimp in a pot of boiling water and cook for 2–5 minutes until no longer raw. Drain and set aside. (Shrimp may be made a day in advance and refrigerated.)

Combine soy sauce, sherry, chili paste, tomato paste, and sugar. Set aside.

Combine cornstarch with 2 tablespoons water. Then stir in 1 cup water. Set aside.

In a large skillet or wok, sauté ginger and green onions in olive oil for a few seconds.

Remove skillet from heat and stir in soy sauce and cornstarch mixtures. Return skillet to high heat. When sauce begins to thicken, mix in cooked shrimp and green pepper until well coated. If sauce is too thick add more water, 1 tablespoon at a time.

4 servings
Calories per serving: 174 Total; 36 Fat; 6 Sat-fat

---

*Available at Oriental food stores and some supermarkets

Q

HONEY-CURRY SCALLOPS

2 tablespoons honey
½–1 teaspoon curry powder
2 tablespoons Dijon mustard

1 teaspoon fresh lemon juice
1 pound sea scallops

Preheat broiler.

Mix honey, curry powder, Dijon mustard, and lemon juice in a medium bowl. Add scallops and mix until they are well coated with sauce.

Lay scallops on broiler pan and place about 5 inches from source of heat. Broil for 5–10 minutes or until scallops are no longer pink inside. Don't overcook or scallops will be rubbery.

4 servings (about 5 scallops each)
Calories per serving: 140 Total; 8 Fat; 4 Sat-fat

VEGETABLES

18

HOORAY FOR vegetables! Vegetables provide meals with texture, color, dietary fiber, vitamins, and minerals. They score high in a cancer-prevention eating plan as well as a heart-healthy eating plan. And, in addition, they are delicious! They fill you up without filling you out.

One of the best ways to cook vegetables is also the easiest. Cook fresh vegetables in a steamer until they are just tender (a few minutes at most). Perhaps add some melted margarine or oil, vinegar, and herbs. Or, for a nonfat treat, sprinkle on vinegar or minced garlic. Steaming vegetables minimizes loss of vitamins. It also brings out the unique taste of each vegetable.

In addition to steaming, vegetables may be prepared in a variety of enticing ways, as you will find in the recipes below.

Q SWEET VEGETABLE MÉLANGE

2 large onions, sliced (about 2 cups)

2 teaspoons olive oil

2 cups sliced carrot

2 small sweet potatoes, cubed (about 2 cups)

1½ tablespoons brown sugar

1 teaspoon cinnamon

¼ cup raisins

½ cup water

In a medium casserole, sauté onions in olive oil until soft.

Cover with carrots, then sweet potatoes.

Mix brown sugar, cinnamon, and raisins and sprinkle over vegetables.

Pour water over vegetables.

Cover and bake at 400°F for 45 minutes or until vegetables are tender.

8 servings
Calories per serving: 85 Total; 10 Fat; 1 Sat-fat

INDIAN VEGETABLES

Indian Vegetables is one of our all-time favorite recipes. This large pot of colorful, tasty vegetables may be eaten warm or cold. Try it as a main dish served over rice.

2 teaspoons olive oil
1 teaspoon black mustard seeds*
3 cloves garlic, chopped
1 medium onion, chopped
1 green pepper, chopped
2–3 potatoes, peeled and cubed
1 small eggplant, peeled and
  cubed
1½ teaspoons turmeric
1 teaspoon salt (optional)
¼ cup water
1 teaspoon cumin
1 teaspoon coriander

1 teaspoon garam masala*
Any vegetables, for example:
1 head broccoli, cut into
  flowerets (about 3 cups)
1 cup or more cauliflower
  flowerets
6 carrots, sliced
1 cup or more green beans,
  cut in half
1 cup sliced celery
1 zucchini, sliced
1 cup water

In a large pot, heat olive oil and add black mustard seeds.

When the mustard seeds begin to pop, add garlic, onion, and green pepper and cook until soft.

Stir in potatoes and eggplant.

Add turmeric and salt and mix until vegetables are covered with turmeric sauce.

Add ¼ cup water, reduce heat to low, cover the pot, and cook for 10 minutes.

Stir in cumin, coriander, garam masala, and vegetables.

Add 1 cup water and increase heat to medium.

*Available at Indian or Mideast food stores

After 10 minutes, lower heat and cook until vegetables are tender.

12 servings
Calories per serving: 72 Total; 7 Fat; 1 Sat-fat

VEGETABLE SOUFFLÉ
WITH TAHINI SAUCE

This recipe is a lot of work, but it's worth it. You may prepare the vegetable purée one or two days before serving and refrigerate it.

1 turnip, peeled and grated
6 carrots, peeled and grated
3 cups broccoli flowerets (about 1 head)
2 tablespoons margarine
2 tablespoons firmly packed brown sugar

1 tablespoon curry powder
½ teaspoon salt (optional)
¼ teaspoon freshly ground black pepper
⅛ teaspoon grated nutmeg

Tahini Sauce

1 clove garlic
1 tablespoon parsley
3 tablespoons tahini (sesame seed paste)*

1 cup nonfat yogurt
1 tablespoon fresh lemon juice
½ tablespoon fresh dill, or ½ teaspoon dried dillweed

4 egg whites

The Vegetable Purée

Steam turnip and carrot 2–3 minutes or until tender. Set aside.
Steam broccoli flowerets about 5 minutes or until tender.
Purée turnip, carrot, and broccoli in food processor or blender until smooth. Set aside.
Melt margarine in a large skillet over low heat.
Stir in brown sugar until well blended.
Stir in curry powder, salt, pepper, and nutmeg.
Add puréed vegetables and mix well, stirring frequently until most moisture has evaporated.

_____

*Available at Mideast food stores and many supermarkets

Cool. (Cover and refrigerate if you wish to finish dish later.)
While vegetable purée is cooling, make tahini sauce.

The Tahini Sauce

Chop garlic and parsley in food processor or blender.
Add tahini, yogurt, lemon juice, and dill.
Blend until smooth. Chill.

The Soufflé

Preheat oven to 450°F. Grease a 1- or 2-quart casserole with margarine.
Beat egg whites until stiff but not dry.
Fold vegetable purée into egg whites, ⅓ at a time. Place in baking dish and bake at 450°F for 15 minutes.
Reduce heat to 350°F and bake for 30 minutes more or until puffed and golden brown.
Serve with tahini sauce.

8 servings

Calories per serving:	Total	Fat	Sat-fat
	75	22	5
Tahini sauce per tablespoon	20	11	1

Ⓠ MURIEL'S CHINESE VEGETABLES

2 ounces cellophane noodles*
3 cups broccoli flowerets (about 1 head)
2 cups cauliflower flowerets
2 cloves garlic, minced
1 red pepper, sliced

1 teaspoon olive oil
1 teaspoon sesame oil
2 tablespoons dry white wine or vermouth
1 teaspoon five-spice powder*
2 tablespoons soy sauce

Pour boiling water over cellophane noodles and let them soak for 15–30 minutes.
Steam broccoli and cauliflower in steamer until just tender. Set aside.
Sauté garlic and red pepper in oils for a few seconds.
Mix in broccoli and cauliflower.

---

*Available in Oriental food stores and some supermarkets

Stir in wine and five-spice powder.

Drain cellophane noodles and stir into vegetables.

Stir in soy sauce until vegetables are well coated with sauce.

9 servings
Calories per serving: 54 Total; 9 Fat; 1 Sat-fat

Q ## ITALIAN MIXED VEGETABLES

1 clove garlic, minced
1 onion, sliced
2 teaspoons olive oil
3 cups combined red and/or yellow and/or green sweet peppers, sliced

2 zucchini, sliced (about 2 cups)
Salt to taste
1 teaspoon thyme, oregano, or basil, or combination

In a large skillet, sauté garlic and onion in olive oil. Add a splash of water and cook vegetables until tender.

Stir in peppers, zucchini, salt, and herbs.

Cover. Cook until tender.

8 servings
Calories per serving: 27 Total; 10 Fat; 1 Sat-fat

RATATOUILLE

Add eggplant, bay leaf, and tomatoes to Italian mixed vegetables and you have a French dish — ratatouille.

2 cloves garlic, minced
1 onion, sliced
2 teaspoons olive oil
3 cups combined red and/or yellow and/or green sweet peppers, sliced
2 zucchini, sliced (about 2 cups)
4 fresh tomatoes, cubed, or 1 large can (28 oz) Italian plum tomatoes, drained

Salt to taste
1 bay leaf
1 teaspoon dried basil, or 2 tablespoons fresh basil, chopped
1 small eggplant, cubed and steamed (about 2 cups)*

*See page 298 for eggplant preparation.

Sauté garlic and onion in olive oil in a medium-large casserole.
Add peppers, zucchini, tomatoes, salt, bay leaf, and basil.

Cover and simmer until vegetables are tender (about 15–20
minutes).

Add steamed eggplant and cook for 5 minutes more.

10 servings
Calories per serving: 32 Total; 8 Fat; 2 Sat-fat

Q # ARTICHOKES

Artichokes make a great appetizer. Watch your family gobble
them up and then fight for the delectable hearts.

1 artichoke for two people   Margarine

Trim the stem and pull off the small leaves at the base of the
artichoke.

With scissors, cut off the tips of the bottom leaves.

Drop artichoke into a large pot of boiling water and boil slowly
for 40–45 minutes or until a leaf will pull off easily.

To eat an artichoke, pull off a leaf, dip the bottom in a small bowl
of melted margarine, and scrape the leaf between your teeth to extract the "meat." Discard the leaf.

When no more edible leaves are left, you have reached the heart.
Remove excess leaves and scrape off the hairy fibers above the heart.
Dip the heart in margarine.

Calories per serving:	Total	Fat	Sat-fat
Artichoke	26	0	0
Margarine per tablespoon	90	90	18

BEANS

If you have been avoiding beans because eating them produces more gas than you care to discuss, here is a way to prepare dried beans (except lentil and split peas) that reduces their gas-producing potential.

1. Rinse beans and pick out foreign matter.
2. Pour boiling water over beans and let them soak for four hours.
3. Drain beans and cook them in fresh water.

CURRIED BEANS

2 cups dried beans (½ cup each chickpeas, black-eyed peas, pinto beans, small red chili beans, or any combination)
1 teaspoon minced ginger root
1 cup chopped onion
1 teaspoon olive oil

1 cup chopped tomato
1 teaspoon coriander
2 teaspoons cumin
1 teaspoon turmeric
¼ teaspoon cayenne pepper
1 teaspoon salt (optional)
2 tablespoons tomato paste

Place dried beans in a large bowl or casserole. Rinse and remove any foreign matter.

Cover beans with boiling water and let them soak for at least 4 hours.

Drain water. Cover beans with fresh water and simmer for 40–60 minutes or until tender.

In a skillet, sauté ginger and onion in olive oil until soft.

Stir in tomato, coriander, cumin, turmeric, cayenne pepper, salt, and tomato paste.

Stir periodically for about 5 minutes. If beans become too dry, add a few tablespoons of water.

11 half-cup servings
Calories per serving: 137 Total; 7 Fat; 1 Sat-fat

CHICKPEAS WITH LEMON AND HERBS

This dish also tastes good when made with black-eyed peas instead of chickpeas, and parsley instead of oregano.

1 cup dried chickpeas	½ teaspoon salt (optional)
¼ cup fresh lemon juice	1 teaspoon oregano
1 tablespoon olive oil	2 green onions, sliced

Place chickpeas in a large bowl or casserole. Rinse and remove any foreign matter.

Cover chickpeas with boiling water and let them soak for at least 4 hours.

Drain water. Cover chickpeas with fresh water and simmer for 40–60 minutes or until tender.

Combine lemon juice, olive oil, salt, oregano, and green onions and pour over chickpeas. Mix thoroughly.

5 half-cup servings
Calories per serving: 170 Total; 46 Fat; 5 Sat-fat

Ⓠ GREEN BEANS BASILICO

3 cups green beans, trimmed, and cut in half	2 teaspoons olive oil
1 clove garlic, minced	1 teaspoon basil
½ cup chopped onion	½ teaspoon oregano
½ cup chopped green pepper	½ teaspoon salt (optional)

In a pot of boiling water, cook green beans 5–10 minutes until tender but still crisp and bright green. Drain and set aside.

In a large skillet, sauté garlic, onion, and green pepper in olive oil until soft.

Stir in basil, oregano, and salt.

Stir in green beans.

6 servings
Calories per serving: 42 Total; 13 Fat; 2 Sat-fat

Q # BROCCOLI AND MUSHROOMS

Because broccoli is a cruciferous vegetable, it is highly recommended for both heart health and cancer prevention. Even if it were not so healthy it would still be a pleasure to eat.

2 cloves garlic, minced
1 teaspoon olive oil
2 heads broccoli, cut into
   flowerets

½ pound mushrooms, sliced

In a large skillet or wok, sauté garlic in olive oil.
Add broccoli and mushrooms and stir for about 1 minute.
Add 2 tablespoons of water, cover, and cook over low heat until broccoli is just tender (about 5–10 minutes).

6 servings
Calories per serving: 51 Total; 7 Fat; 1 Sat-fat

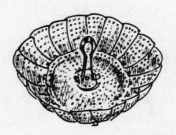

Q # SESAME BROCCOLI

1 tablespoon soy sauce
1 tablespoon sesame oil
¼ cup dry sake or vermouth
2 teaspoons honey

2 heads broccoli, cut into
   flowerets
1 tablespoon sesame seeds,
   toasted

Combine soy sauce, sesame oil, wine, and honey in bowl. Set aside.
Steam broccoli until tender.
Toss broccoli and dressing together.
Sprinkle sesame seeds over broccoli and serve.

8 servings
Calories per serving: 50 Total; 20 Fat; 3 Sat-fat

Q   CARAWAY CARROTS

Carrots are an excellent source of vitamin A. They keep well in the refrigerator and make great snacks. They are perfect for last-minute chefs because they cook quickly and taste wonderful with very little embellishment.

6 carrots, sliced (about 3 cups)   2 teaspoons caraway seeds
1 teaspoon margarine

Place sliced carrots in a small saucepan with water to cover.
Gently simmer until carrots are soft. Drain.
Add margarine and mix until carrots are covered.
Stir in caraway seeds.

6 servings
Calories per serving: 35 Total; 5 Fat; 2 Sat-fat

Q   CARROTS AND LEEKS

1 leek, cleaned thoroughly and   2 cups sliced carrots
   the white bulb sliced   ¼ teaspoon thyme
1 teaspoon olive oil

In a small saucepan, sauté leeks in olive oil. Add a splash of water and cook until tender.
Add carrots and thyme.
Cover and cook over low heat until carrots are tender.

4 servings
Calories per serving: 51 Total; 10 Fat; 1 Sat-fat

Q   CAULIFLOWER SAUTÉ

2 cups cauliflower flowerets   1 cup snow peas
2 cloves garlic, minced   1 red pepper, sliced
1 small onion, sliced (about ¼   1 cup sliced mushrooms
   cup)   1 teaspoon oregano
1 tablespoon olive oil

Steam cauliflower until just tender. Set aside.
In large skillet or wok, sauté garlic and onion in olive oil until soft.

Add steamed cauliflower, snow peas, red pepper, mushrooms, and oregano and stir until heated through.

6 servings
Calories per serving: 47 Total; 20 Fat; 3 Sat-fat

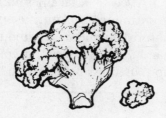

Q   # CELERY-MUSHROOMS

3 cups sliced celery	1 cup sliced onions
½ teaspoon salt (optional)	1 cup sliced mushrooms
2 teaspoons olive oil	

Place celery and salt in a medium saucepan with water to cover.
Bring to a boil, reduce heat, and simmer for 8–10 minutes or until celery is tender.
Sauté onions in olive oil until golden.
Add mushrooms and stir for several minutes to blend flavors.
Drain celery and stir it into onion-mushroom mixture.

6 servings
Calories per serving: 27 Total; 13 Fat; 2 Sat-fat

Cooking with Eggplant

Choose the blackest eggplant you can find. Peel it, cut it into bite-size pieces, and salt them heavily. Place a heavy plate on top of the pieces to help squeeze out the bitter juices. In 30–60 minutes, wash off the salt and gently squeeze eggplant pieces to rid them of bitter juices.

Steam eggplant in a vegetable steamer until tender. There are two advantages to steaming eggplant: steamed eggplant needs no oil (eggplant absorbs an enormous amount of oil) and thus has fewer sat-fat and total calories; and you can test the pre-cooked eggplant for bitterness before using it in a recipe.

Q KEEMA EGGPLANT

1 medium eggplant, cubed
(about 4 cups)
1 cup sliced onion
1 teaspoon olive oil
2 teaspoons curry powder

3 tablespoons fresh lemon juice
1 tablespoon brown sugar
1 tablespoon ketchup
¼ cup water
1 cup canned chickpeas

Prepare eggplant as explained above.

Meanwhile, sauté onion slices in olive oil until tender.

Stir in curry powder. Add to eggplant.

Combine lemon juice, brown sugar, ketchup, and water and stir into eggplant mixture. Cook for 5 minutes.

Add chickpeas and cook for 2 minutes more.

6 servings
Calories per serving: 86 Total; 7 Fat; 1 Sat-fat

⧉ HOT AND GARLICKY EGGPLANT

1 medium eggplant (about 1 pound)

5 small, dried black Chinese mushrooms*

1 tablespoon chili paste with garlic*

1 tablespoon vinegar

½ tablespoon soy sauce

½ tablespoon double black soy sauce*

2 tablespoons dry sherry

½ teaspoon sugar

1 large green pepper, chopped

1 teaspoon olive oil

½ cup water

Prepare eggplant as explained on page 298.

Place mushrooms in a small bowl and cover with boiling water.

After about 15 minutes remove mushrooms. Squeeze out the excess water and discard stems. Slice mushrooms. Set aside.

Combine chili paste with garlic, vinegar, soy sauces, sherry, and sugar and set aside.

In a large skillet, sauté green pepper and mushrooms in oil. Add a splash of water and cook vegetables until tender.

Stir in eggplant.

Mix in soy sauce mixture until vegetables are covered and then stir in water.

Simmer for about 5 minutes.

8 half-cup servings
Calories per serving: 25 Total; 5 Fat; 1 Sat-fat

⧉ EGGPLANT WITH A GREEK INFLUENCE

1 large or 2 small eggplants

2 teaspoons olive oil

¼ cup fresh lemon juice

12 pitted black olives

1 teaspoon capers

½ teaspoon oregano

Prepare eggplant as explained on page 298. Taste steamed eggplant. If not bitter, proceed.

In a saucepan, combine eggplant, olive oil, lemon juice, olives, capers, and oregano.

*Available at Oriental food stores

Cook over low heat for 10 minutes or until heated through.

6 servings
Calories per serving: 44 Total; 28 Fat; 4 Sat-fat

Q   # LENTILS AND POTATOES

Lentils, a type of legume, are both delicious and nutritious. They are rich in vitamin C, folic acid, and many minerals, including iron and calcium. They are a good source of soluble fiber, which has been shown to lower blood cholesterol.

Lentils and Potatoes may be served at room temperature on a bed of lettuce or warm as a side dish.

1 cup lentils	2 cloves garlic, minced
1 cup peeled and cubed potato	⅓ cup chopped onion
(about 1 medium potato)	2 teaspoons olive oil
½ teaspoon salt (optional)	

Wash lentils and place them in a medium saucepan with potatoes, salt, and water to cover.

Bring to a boil. Reduce heat, cover, and simmer for about 20–25 minutes or until vegetables are tender.

Drain and set aside.

In a large skillet, sauté garlic and onion in olive oil.

Stir in cooked lentils and potatoes and serve or refrigerate.

6 servings
Calories per serving: 48 Total; 16 Fat; 3 Sat-fat

Q   # BRAISED MUSHROOMS ORIENTAL

These mushrooms make a tasty hors d'oeuvre or side dish.

1 pound mushrooms, sliced	4 teaspoons soy sauce
2 teaspoons olive oil	1 cup water
2 teaspoons sugar	1 teaspoon sesame oil

Sauté mushrooms in olive oil until tender.

Stir in sugar, soy sauce, and water.

Cover and simmer for 25 minutes or until water is absorbed. Add sesame oil.

6 side-dish servings
Calories per serving: 50 Total; 22 Fat; 2 Sat-fat

POTATOES

Of all vegetables, potatoes are probably the most maligned. Many people consider them highly caloric and devoid of nutritional value. What injustice! Potatoes are filled with vitamins (particularly vitamin C), minerals, and protein. Eaten plain they have no fat and are extremely filling and delicious.

Q

POTATO SKINS

Leslie Goodman-Malamuth of the Center for Science in the Public Interest devised this recipe as a substitute for the highly saturated potato skins you often find in restaurants. Not only is this recipe quick and easy, the resulting potatoes are scrumptious.

4 large potatoes
1 teaspoon olive oil (optional)

Paprika to taste

Preheat oven to 450°F.

Scrub potatoes well, cut them lengthwise into six wedges the size and shape of dill pickle spears, and dry them on a paper towel.

In a large bowl, toss potato spears with olive oil until they are well covered.

Spread potatoes on a baking sheet, dust them with paprika, and bake for 20–30 minutes or until fork-tender.

6 servings (So good, 2 people can easily finish them off!)
Calories per serving: 66 Total; 7 Fat; 1 Sat-fat

POTATOES LYONNAISE

2 pounds boiling or all-purpose
    potatoes (about 4 large)
½ tablespoon margarine
½ teaspoon salt (optional)
¼ teaspoon freshly ground
    black pepper

1½ cups sliced onion (about 2
    onions)
1 teaspoon olive oil
¼ cup chopped parsley

Peel and halve potatoes. Cut them into ¼-inch-thick slices. Then steam or boil them until just tender (about 10 minutes).

Melt margarine in a large skillet. Add potato slices and cook for 15 minutes, shaking pan periodically. After 10 minutes, add salt and pepper and turn potatoes.

In a small skillet, sauté onions in olive oil until browned.

Add onions and parsley to potatoes and cook for 5 minutes more.

8 servings
Calories per serving: 63 Total; 11 Fat; 2 Sat-fat

Q   BOUILLON POTATOES

4 medium potatoes, peeled and
    cut into ⅜-inch-thick slices
½ cup canned beef broth or beef
    stock, strained
1 teaspoon vinegar
1 tablespoon minced carrot
1 small onion, quartered

2 cloves garlic, peeled
2 sprigs parsley
1 bay leaf
½ teaspoon thyme
3 sprigs parsley chopped
1 teaspoon garlic minced

Line the bottom of a large skillet with the sliced potatoes.

Combine the broth, vinegar, carrot, onion, whole garlic, cloves, parsley sprigs, bay leaf, and thyme, and pour over potatoes. Add water just to cover potatoes.

Bring to a boil and continue to boil until the liquid is completely evaporated (about 20 minutes). Check frequently, as the liquid's final evaporation occurs suddenly.

Sprinkle with chopped parsley and minced garlic and serve.

4 servings
Calories per serving: 106 Total; 0 Fat; 0 Sat-fat

Ｑ CURRIED WHIPPED POTATOES

You need not add butter or margarine to make delectable whipped potatoes. In this recipe, sautéed onions, mustard seed, and cumin make them special and exotic. Leave the onions out of this recipe and you have plain but scrumptious whipped potatoes at 0 fat calories per serving.

4 potatoes (about 2 pounds)
¾ cup chopped onions
1 teaspoon olive oil
½ teaspoon mustard seed

½ teaspoon cumin
1–4 tablespoons skim milk
Salt and freshly ground black
    pepper to taste

Peel potatoes, slice thinly, and place in a medium saucepan with water to cover. Bring to a boil and boil until tender.

Meanwhile, sauté onions in olive oil. Lower heat to medium and stir in mustard seed and cumin. Cook a few moments until onions are soft.

Drain potatoes. Beat potatoes with an electric mixer. Add milk, one tablespoon at a time, until potatoes are whipped.

Mix in onions and salt and pepper to taste.

4 servings
Calories per serving: 168 Total; 10 Fat; 1 Sat-fat

SWEET POTATOES

Sweet potatoes are often considered a fattening treat. They are a healthy treat, but not fattening. One sweet potato has no fat and is chock-full of vitamins A and C and many minerals.

Q SWEET POTATOES WITH ORANGES, APPLES, AND SWEET WINE

4 cups sweet potatoes cut into
 ½-inch slices
1 cup diced apple
1 orange, peeled and cut into
 bite-size pieces

2–3 tablespoons brown sugar
¼ cup plum wine or other
 sweet wine
3 whole cloves

Preheat oven to 375°F.

Place sweet potato slices in a saucepan with water to cover. Bring to a boil. Reduce heat, cover, and simmer until just tender when pierced with a fork.

Drain sweet potatoes and place in a casserole.

Mix apple, orange, brown sugar, wine, and cloves.

Pour mixture over sweet potatoes.

Bake, covered, for 30 minutes or until apples are tender.

6 servings
Calories per serving: 125 Total; 0 Fat; 0 Sat-fat

FLUFFY SWEET POTATOES

3 sweet potatoes (to make 2
 cups mashed)
⅔ cup orange juice
½ teaspoon grated orange peel

2 tablespoons brown sugar
1 tablespoon margarine, melted
1 egg yolk
2 egg whites

Peel sweet potatoes, cut into chunks, place in a medium saucepan, and cover with water.

Bring to a boil, then reduce heat and simmer until tender (about 10–15 minutes).

Preheat oven to 375°F. Grease a casserole with margarine.

Drain potatoes and mash in a large bowl.

Mix in juice, peel, sugar, melted margarine, and egg yolk.

Whip egg whites until stiff but not dry. Fold into sweet potato.

Pour sweet potato mixture into casserole and bake for 30 minutes.

6 servings
Calories per serving: 118 Total; 23 Fat; 8 Sat-fat

[Q]
SPICED SWEET POTATOES

This sweet potato recipe needs no fat to make it delicious.

2 large sweet potatoes
1 tablespoon brown sugar
¼ teaspoon ground cloves

¼–½ teaspoon cinnamon
¼–½ teaspoon salt (optional)
2–4 tablespoons nonfat
    buttermilk

Peel and thinly slice sweet potatoes. Place in saucepan, cover with water, and boil until tender (about 10–20 minutes).

Drain and place in the bowl of an electric mixer.

Add sugar, spices, salt, and 2 tablespoons of the buttermilk. Beat until fluffy.

Add more buttermilk if necessary for puréed consistency.

4 servings
Calories per serving: 78 Total; 0 Fat; 0 Sat-fat

[Q]
SPINACH AND TOMATOES

Spinach is an excellent source of vitamin A. It is also rich in vitamin C and iron. It may be eaten raw in a salad or cooked in many interesting ways.

10 ounces fresh spinach,
    washed and shredded
2 cloves garlic, minced

1 teaspoon olive oil
1 tomato, diced
1 tablespoon raisins

In a medium saucepan, cook spinach in boiling water to cover until tender (about 2 minutes). Drain well and chop coarsely.

Sauté garlic in olive oil.

Mix in spinach.

Add tomatoes and raisins and heat through.

4 servings
Calories per serving: 40 Total; 9 Fat; 1 Sat-fat

Q

SPINACH ORIENTAL

10 ounces fresh spinach, washed and shredded
1 teaspoon olive oil

1 teaspoon chopped ginger root
1 teaspoon double black soy sauce*

In a large skillet, lightly sauté spinach in oil until soft.
Stir in ginger and soy sauce.

4 servings
Calories per serving: 30 Total; 10 Fat; 1 Sat-fat

SQUASH

Squash, both winter and summer varieties, is rich in vitamin A, vitamin C, niacin, and iron. Squash is delicious when simply baked, boiled, or steamed and enhanced with a little margarine and freshly ground pepper. Or it may be prepared in a variety of other interesting ways.

Q

ACORN SQUASH

3 medium acorn squash**
1 cup boiling water
3 teaspoons margarine (optional)

Freshly ground black pepper to taste

Preheat oven to 400°F.
Cut each squash in half and scoop out seeds and fibers.
Slice a small piece off the bottom of each half so that they will not roll over.
Place squash halves, cut-side down, in a shallow casserole.
Pour boiling water into the casserole and cover it tightly with aluminum foil.

---

*Available at Oriental food stores and some supermarkets
**Butternut squash may also be cooked this way and is delicious. Its dull cream exterior conceals a beautiful, deep orange interior.

Bake for 45 minutes or until squash is soft when pierced with a fork.

Turn squash cut-side up and fill each half with ½ teaspoon margarine.

Bake for 5 minutes more.

Grind pepper over squash and serve.

6 servings

Calories per serving:	Total	Fat	Sat-fat
	40	0	0
With margarine	55	15	3

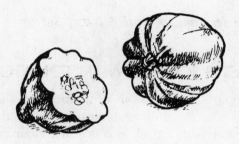

Ⓠ GLAZED ACORN SQUASH

2 acorn squash   ¾ cup orange juice
2 tablespoons brown sugar

Cut squash crosswise (not through the stem) into ½-inch slices. Clean out fibers and seeds and peel.

Place squash in a large skillet.

Combine brown sugar and orange juice and pour over squash.

Cover and cook over medium heat for 15 minutes. Turn squash.

Raise heat and cook, uncovered, for 10 minutes more or until squash is tender and sauce is reduced.

6 servings
Calories per serving: 58 Total; 0 Fat; 0 Sat-fat

Ⓠ

AFGHAN SQUASH

½ cup sliced onion
1 teaspoon olive oil
½ teaspoon salt
½ teaspoon cumin
½ teaspoon coriander

¼ teaspoon cardamom
¼ teaspoon ground cloves
1 butternut squash, peeled and
    cubed (about 3 cups)

Sauté onion in olive oil in a small casserole.
Stir in salt, cumin, coriander, cardamom, and cloves.
Add squash and 1 cup water.
Cook until tender (about 25 minutes).

8 servings
Calories per serving: 25 Total; 5 Fat; 1 Sat-fat

SPAGHETTI SQUASH WITH TOMATO SAUCE

Spaghetti squash looks like an ordinary yellow squash — until you bake it. Inside, the pulp separates into long, thin strands like spaghetti. Use spaghetti squash as a healthy, vitamin-rich, delicious pasta. Top the squash with the tasty sauce below or Sweet Red Pepper Sauce (page 262).

1 spaghetti squash (about 3 pounds)

Tomato Sauce

¼ cup sliced onion
1–2 teaspoons minced garlic
1 teaspoon olive oil
¼ cup chopped parsley
2 cups chopped cherry tomatoes
    (or regular tomatoes)
¼ teaspoon oregano

¼ teaspoon basil
¼ teaspoon cumin
¼–½ teaspoon red pepper
    flakes
¼–½ freshly ground black
    pepper
Salt to taste (optional)

The Squash

Preheat oven to 350°F.
Cut squash in half lengthwise and scoop out seeds.
Place halves face down in shallow baking pan.
Bake for 45 minutes or until tender when poked with a fork.

The Sauce

Meanwhile, in an 8-inch skillet, sauté onion and garlic in olive oil until soft. Lower heat to medium and stir in parsley.

Stir in tomatoes. Add oregano, basil, cumin, red pepper flakes, black pepper, and salt. Cook on medium heat, stirring occasionally, for about 10 minutes. Turn to low and let flavors blend for about 5–10 minutes. Set aside.

When squash is cooked, scrape inside with a fork to release spaghetti strands. Pile onto a plate (as you would spaghetti) and top with tomato sauce.

4 servings
Calories per serving: 117 Total; 10 Fat; 2 Sat-fat

Q   STEAMED ZUCCHINI MATCHSTICKS

So light, so tasty — you don't even need to add salt, spices, or fat. But you may want to crush garlic into one teaspoon of melted margarine and combine it with the vegetables.

2 small zucchini (or ½ small zucchini per person)
1 thick carrot, peeled

1 teaspoon margarine (optional)
1 clove garlic (optional)

Cut zucchini and carrot into 2-inch lengths.

Place a zucchini section on a cutting surface, skin-side down.

Holding the sides of the section, slice lengthwise at ⅛-inch intervals. Hold the slices together.

Roll the section one-quarter turn, making sure the slices stay together.

Again, make parallel slices, ⅛-inch apart lengthwise.

Result: zucchini matchsticks.

Repeat for remaining sections of zucchini and carrot.

Place zucchini sticks on top of carrot sticks in a vegetable steamer and steam until just tender (about 1 or 2 minutes).

4 servings

Calories per serving:	Total	Fat	Sat-fat
	17	0	0
With margarine	24	7	2

Q # CURRIED ZUCCHINI

You can use this basic recipe for any vegetable.

1 clove garlic, minced
½ cup chopped onion
1 teaspoon olive oil
½ teaspoon salt
½–1 teaspoon turmeric

¼–½ teaspoon cumin
½ teaspoon red pepper flakes
  (optional)
3 zucchini, sliced (about 3 cups)
2 tomatoes, chopped

In a large skillet, sauté garlic and onion in olive oil until soft.
Add salt, turmeric, cumin, and red peppers. Blend well.
Stir in zucchini and cook until tender.
Stir in tomatoes and serve.

8 servings
Calories per serving: 23 Total; 5 Fat; 1 Sat-fat

PIZZA, QUICHE, CHILI, AND TORTILLAS

19

"**O**H, WOE IS ME," says the sat-fat counter. "How can I go on without pizza and chili? Life will be bare." STOP! The following recipes for pizza, chili, quiche, and tortillas are delectable. The only thing they lack is saturated fat. So don't feel sorry for yourself. You *can* have your cake — or pizza — and eat it too!

PIZZA

You might think that a low-sat-fat diet would eliminate pizza, but the following recipes will prove to you how fabulous low-sat-fat pizzas can be. They make good snacks as well as main courses for lunch or dinner. Freeze leftovers (if there are any!). Then, in the future when you want a treat, heat the frozen slices in your toaster oven.

To make pizza with a crisper crust, buy four inexpensive unglazed quarry tiles (each about a 5-inch square) at a tile store or purchase a pizza tile at a store that sells kitchen supplies. Pizza baked directly on hot tiles has a crunchier crust.

To slide the pizza onto the tiles it helps to have a pizza peel. It looks like this:

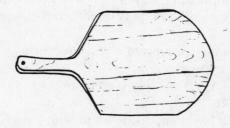

You may devise other gizmos to slide the pizza onto the tiles if you wish, but a pizza peel really works well. Of course, you may forgo both the tiles and the pizza peel and use a metal pizza pan or cookie sheet instead.

PIZZA

Dough

1 tablespoon active dry yeast
¼ cup warm water
Pinch of sugar
4 cups unbleached white flour

1 teaspoon salt (optional)
1 cup warm water
2 tablespoons olive oil

Topping

2 cloves garlic
Salt to taste
1½ cups tomato sauce (page 314)
2 cups sliced mushrooms
1½ sliced green peppers (about 1½ cups)

1 cup sliced onion
1⅓ cups low-fat (1%) cottage cheese
3 teaspoons oregano

The Dough

Place yeast, the ¼ cup warm (but not hot) water, and sugar in a large bowl or the work bowl of your food processor. Let proof (become bubbly).

Mix in flour and salt.

Mix in the 1 cup warm (but not hot) water and olive oil.

Knead or process until dough is smooth and elastic, adding more flour if needed.

Place dough in a large greased bowl, cover with a towel, and let rise for about 45 minutes.

While the dough is rising, place tiles (see page 311) in oven and heat oven to 450°F.

After the dough has risen, divide it into four parts, form each into a smooth ball, and cover for 10 minutes.

Roll the dough into four small circles, 10 to 12 inches each. Wait 10 minutes more. Roll the dough thinner.

To Make Each Pizza

Cover pizza peel with a thin layer of cornmeal or grease pizza pan with oil.

Place one rolled circle of dough on the pizza peel or in the pizza pan.

Crush garlic. Spread it over the surface of the dough and sprinkle with salt.

Spoon about ¼ cup tomato sauce over the dough.

Arrange mushrooms, green peppers, and onions over tomato sauce.

Put cottage cheese on top (as if it were mozzarella).

Sprinkle with ¾ teaspoon oregano.

Bake for 10–20 minutes or until crust is golden brown.

4 pizzas, 4 slices per pizza
Calories per slice: 116 Total; 4 Fat; 1 Sat-fat

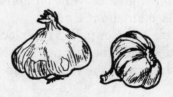

CALZONE

A recipe that you can enjoy with no pangs of remorse. This seems like a lot of work, but once you do it, it goes quickly and is quite delicious.

Dough

1 tablespoon active dry yeast
pinch of sugar
½ cup warm water
3–4½ cups unbleached white
  flour

1–1½ teaspoons salt (optional)
1 cup skim milk
1 tablespoon olive oil

Tomato Sauce*

1 teaspoon olive oil
1 cup chopped onion
4 large cans (28 oz each)
  tomatoes

1 can (6 oz) tomato paste
2 teaspoons basil
1 teaspoon salt

Filling

1 clove garlic
Salt to taste
1 cup low-fat (1%) cottage
  cheese

1 green pepper, sliced
1 cup sliced mushrooms
1 cup sliced onion

The Dough

Place yeast, sugar, and warm water in food processor or large bowl and let proof.

Add 3 cups flour and salt and mix.

Add skim milk and olive oil and process until dough masses into a ball or knead until smooth and elastic. Add more flour if dough is too sticky.

Place dough in a bowl greased with oil and cover with a towel. Let rise in a warm place for about 1 hour.

If you are using pizza tiles (see page 311), place them in preheated 450°F oven 30 minutes before baking pizza.

While dough is rising, make the tomato sauce.

The Tomato Sauce

Place olive oil in large saucepan.

Add onion and a splash of water and cook over low heat until tender.

Strain juice from canned tomatoes. (Freeze juice for soups.) Chop tomatoes (easily done in food processor).

Mix tomato paste into tomatoes. Add tomato mixture to saucepan.

Add basil and salt and cook until thick (about 45 minutes).

To Make the Calzone

When dough has risen, divide it into 8 parts and form each part into a smooth ball. Cover with a towel or plastic wrap for about 10

---

*This recipe makes 8 cups of tomato sauce. You will need only about one cup for calzone. Freeze the rest for future use in other recipes or as spaghetti sauce.

minutes. It is important that you let the dough "rest" or it will be difficult to roll flat.

Roll each ball into a flat circle. Wait 10 minutes more.

Make each circle thinner. Place dough on floured surface or pizza peel sprinkled with cornmeal (see page 311).

Crush garlic and spread it over the dough, then sprinkle it with salt.

Spread about 2 tablespoons of tomato sauce over half the dough, leaving a border of ½ inch.

Spread 2 tablespoons cottage cheese evenly over tomato sauce.

Top with a few slices of green pepper, mushroom, and onion.

Fold the top half of the dough over and pinch the top and bottom edges together.

Slide calzone onto hot tiles or onto cookie sheet.

Bake for about 10–20 minutes or until browned.

Makes 8 calzone
Calories per calzone: 296 Total; 24 Fat; 4 Sat-fat

FOCACCIA

The whole-wheat flour in this pizza not only makes it healthier but also gives it a toasty taste and crunchy texture. Try it! It is easy and makes great snacks. Freeze it in snack-size slices.

Dough

1½ teaspoons dry active yeast
½ teaspoon honey
1 cup warm water

2½ cups whole-wheat flour
¾ teaspoon salt (optional)
1 tablespoon olive oil

Tomato Sauce

1 large can (28 oz) tomatoes, or
   3 large tomatoes
2 cloves garlic, minced
1 small onion, chopped
1 teaspoon olive oil

½ teaspoon oregano
¼ teaspoon basil
Ground hot cherry peppers
   (optional)

The Dough

Place yeast, honey, and warm water in food processor or large bowl. Let proof.

Add flour, salt, and olive oil and process or knead until smooth and elastic, adding flour if needed.

Place dough in an oiled bowl, cover with a towel, and let rise in a warm place for about 1 hour.

Punch down dough and let it rest on floured counter for 10 minutes.

Grease a 10 × 15-inch cookie sheet with oil. Roll out dough (or press with your hands) onto the cookie sheet.

Pinch a rim around the edge. Cover with a towel and let rise for 30 minutes.

Meanwhile, make the tomato sauce.

The Tomato Sauce

If using canned tomatoes, drain liquid and chop tomatoes. If using whole tomatoes, chop fine.

In a medium skillet, sauté garlic and onion in olive oil until tender.

Stir in tomatoes, oregano, and basil and let simmer until thick (about 10–15 minutes).

Let cool.

Preheat oven to 400°F.
Spread the sauce over the dough.
Add hot cherry peppers, if desired.
Bake for 20–25 minutes.

Makes 12 pieces
Calories per piece: 113 Total; 18 Fat; 3 Sat-fat

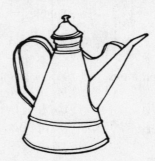

PISSALADIÈRE

An onion pizza of Provence. Pissaladière makes a perfect luncheon dish, snack, or light dinner. Although it looks as if it took a lot of work, it is quite simple to make. Cook the onions ahead to save time later.

Filling

3 cups chopped onion
2 cloves garlic, minced

2 teaspoons olive oil

Dough

1 teaspoon dry yeast
Pinch of sugar
¼ cup water
1–1½ cups unbleached white
   flour

½ teaspoon salt (optional)
¼ cup warm water
1 teaspoon olive oil

12 pitted black olives, halved

6 anchovies

The Filling

In a small covered skillet, slowly cook onion and garlic in olive oil. Add a splash of water and cook vegetables until soft (about 30 minutes). Stir occasionally. Set aside. (You can refrigerate cooked onions for a few days.)

The Dough

About 1 hour before serving, place yeast, sugar, and ¼ cup warm water in bowl or food processor. Let proof.

Mix in 1 cup of flour and salt.

Add ¼ cup warm water and olive oil and knead or process for 15 seconds.

Add more flour until dough is smooth and elastic.

Place dough in oiled bowl, cover with towel, and let rise for about 45 minutes.

After 35 minutes, preheat oven to 450°F.

On a greased round pizza pan or cookie sheet, roll out or push the dough into a 10-inch circle.

Spoon onions evenly over dough.

Starting from the center of the circle, place olives in lines like the spokes of a wheel.

Place anchovies between the lines of olives.

Bake for 20 minutes or until dough is slightly golden brown.

Makes 8 slices
Calories per slice: 196 Total; 29 Fat; 5 Sat-fat

QUICHE

The word *quiche* conjures up images of dozens of eggs and tons of cream, ham, and cheese. The following wonderful lower-fat (but *not* low-fat) versions will expand your definition. They are made with only low-sat-fat ingredients and make perfect appetizers or light meals.

SPINACH QUICHE

Partially baked nonsweet quiche
  crust (page 398)
1 tablespoon chopped parsley
1 teaspoon basil
1 package (10 oz) fresh spinach
  (or frozen spinach, thawed)
1 cup low-fat (1%) cottage
  cheese
1 cup buttermilk

1 egg
1 egg white
1 tablespoon unbleached flour
½ teaspoon salt (optional)
¼ teaspoon freshly ground
  black pepper
¼ teaspoon grated nutmeg
2 tablespoons sliced green onion

Preheat oven to 375°F.

Combine parsley with basil (easily done in food processor) and set aside.

If using fresh spinach, wash leaves and tear off stems.

In a medium saucepan, cook fresh or thawed spinach for about 3 minutes in ½ cup boiling water. Drain. Squeeze all liquid out of spinach or quiche will be watery.

Combine cottage cheese, buttermilk, egg, egg white, flour, salt, pepper, and nutmeg in food processor or bowl.

If using processor, add spinach and process. If mixing in bowl, chop spinach finely and add to cottage cheese mixture.

Stir in green onion and parsley-basil mixture and pour into partially baked pie crust.

Bake for about 30 minutes.

Makes 9 slices
Calories per slice: 177 Total; 47 Fat; 10 Sat-fat

TOMATO QUICHE

Here is another quiche you can eat with no qualms. It has an absolutely delicious Mediterranean flavor. If you are an anchovy-hater, do not avoid this recipe. The anchovies enhance the flavor but are not discernible.

Partially baked nonsweet quiche crust (page 398)
⅓ cup chopped onion
1 teaspoon olive oil
1 large can (28 oz) + 1 small can (16 oz) tomatoes
1 clove garlic, minced
¼ teaspoon basil
½ teaspoon oregano

½ teaspoon salt (optional)
6 sprigs parsley, stems removed
1 tin (2 oz) anchovies
1 egg
1 egg white
3 tablespoons tomato paste
12 large pitted black olives, cut in half

In a medium skillet, sauté onion in olive oil until tender.

Meanwhile, drain the juice from the tomatoes. (Freeze the liquid for future use.) Chop tomatoes and add to onion.

Mix in garlic, basil, oregano, and salt.

Increase heat to high. When tomato mixture begins to bubble, reduce heat to medium.

Cook tomatoes for about 50 minutes or until thick, stirring occasionally. You may have to reduce heat if mixture begins to boil. Make sure there is no excess liquid.

When sauce is very thick, remove skillet from heat. Cool sauce slightly.

Preheat oven to 375°F.

In a food processor or blender, mix parsley, anchovies, egg, egg white, and tomato paste.

Fold anchovy mixture into tomato sauce and pour into partially baked pie crust.

Artistically arrange olive halves on top of tomato mixture.

Bake quiche for 25–30 minutes or until puffy and browned on top.

Makes 9 slices
Calories per slice: 183 Total; 63 Fat; 12 Sat-fat

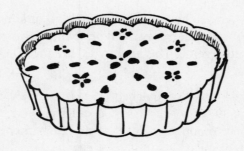

Q TOMATO TART

Wonderful! So light and tasty.

Biscuit Crust

1 cup unbleached white flour
1½ teaspoons baking powder
½ teaspoon salt (optional)

3 tablespoons olive oil
¼ cup nonfat skim milk

Tomato Filling

1 pound fresh whole or cherry
   tomatoes or 1 large can
   tomatoes (28 oz)
¾ cup nonfat plain yogurt
1 small jar pimientos (2 oz),
   drained
2 teaspoons unbleached white
   flour

¾ teaspoon sugar
½ teaspoon salt
⅛–¼ teaspoon red pepper
   flakes
Freshly ground black pepper to
   taste
2 green onions, thinly sliced

The Crust
Preheat oven to 425°F and lightly oil a 9-inch tart pan.*

Combine flour, baking powder, and salt in a mixing bowl or food processor bowl.

Add oil and milk and mix until a ball of soft dough forms.

Place the dough on a floured piece of wax paper and roll into a ⅛-inch-thick circle, about 12 inches in diameter.

Flip the paper and dough onto the tart pan. Peel off the wax paper and press the dough into the pan. If there is excess, roll it over the edge into a ridge.

Press a sheet of aluminum foil into the dough to keep it from forming large bubbles during baking.

Bake 5 minutes and remove foil.

Bake 5–10 more minutes until crust is evenly browned. Set aside.

The Filling
Meanwhile, slice the tomatoes in half and squeeze out their juices, or drain the canned tomatoes and squeeze out their juices.

Chop the tomatoes into small pieces (preferably by hand — you don't want a purée). Set aside.

Combine yogurt, pimientos, flour, sugar, salt, red pepper flakes, and black pepper. Mix in green onions and tomatoes.

Spread tomato filling evenly over crust.

Place metal rim of tart pan upside down so it covers the edges of the crust and prevents it from burning. Broil for about 4 minutes or until warmed.

Makes 6 slices
Calories per slice: 173 Total; 63 Fat; 8 Sat-fat

---

*A 9-inch tart pan with a removable bottom makes a very pretty crust that is easy to pop out. If you don't have a tart pan, a 9-inch pie plate will also work.

CHILI

Chili is traditionally made with beef. You will not miss the beef in the following vegetarian recipes. They are delicious and filling — wonderful for a fall or winter day.

Q ## CHILI NON CARNE

This is one of the best chili recipes we have ever tasted. It is filled with nutritious vegetables that provide texture but do not interfere with the delicious chili taste. Eat it hot in a bowl mixed with chopped onions, tomatoes, and lettuce, or spoon it into pita bread with chopped onion, lettuce, and tomatoes. Dried beans such as kidney beans and navy beans have been shown to have a modest effect in lowering blood cholesterol.

¾ cup chopped onion
2 cloves garlic, minced
1 teaspoon olive oil
2 tablespoons chili powder
¼ teaspoon basil
¼ teaspoon oregano
¼ teaspoon cumin
2 cups finely chopped zucchini
1 cup finely chopped carrot
1 large can (28 oz) tomatoes +
    1 small can (14½ oz) toma-
    toes, drained and chopped

1 can (15 oz) kidney beans,
    undrained
2 cans (15 oz each) kidney
    beans, *drained* and thoroughly
    rinsed
Chopped onions, tomatoes,
    lettuce, green peppers, for
    garnish

In a large pot, sauté onion and garlic in olive oil. Add a splash of water and cook vegetables until soft.

Mix in chili powder, basil, oregano, and cumin.

Stir in zucchini and carrots until well blended. Cook for about 1 minute over low heat, stirring occasionally.

Stir in chopped tomatoes, undrained and drained kidney beans.

Bring to a boil. Reduce heat and simmer for 30–45 minutes or until thick.

Top with chopped onions, tomatoes, lettuce, or green peppers.

Makes 8 one-cup servings
Calories per serving: 117 Total; 5 Fat; 1 Sat-fat

Q

PAWTUCKET CHILI

1 large can (40 oz) kidney beans
1 can (15 oz) chickpeas
2 cloves garlic, minced
1 medium onion, chopped
1 teaspoon olive oil
1 can (8 oz) tomato sauce

1 large can (28 oz) whole
   tomatoes, drained and
   chopped
1–3 teaspoons oregano
½ teaspoon thyme
1 teaspoon cumin
½ teaspoon basil
1–2 tablespoons chili powder

Rinse kidney beans and chickpeas to remove salt. Set aside.
Sauté garlic and onion in olive oil.
Add beans, chickpeas, and remaining ingredients and bring to a boil.
Simmer for 20 minutes (or longer) until thick.

Makes 8 one-cup servings
Calories per serving: 105 Total; 9 Fat; 1 Sat-fat

TORTILLAS

Who says you can't have tortillas on a low-sat-fat diet? Admittedly, these tortillas contain no meat or cheese, but they are spicy and great tasting, just like their Mexican counterparts. As a bonus, your arteries will be happier with these than with beef or cheese.

Filling

Corn tortillas*
1 cup dried lentils
2 cups water
2½ tablespoons raisins
3 cloves garlic, minced
¼ teaspoon red pepper flakes

2 teaspoons chili powder
½ teaspoon cumin
¼ teaspoon basil
7 tablespoons tomato paste
2 cups water

Toppings

Shredded zucchini

Nonfat yogurt

---

*Look for corn tortillas in the refrigerator section of your supermarket. Be sure they contain only corn, water, and lime — no lard or other saturated fat.

The Filling

In a large pot, combine lentils and 2 cups water and simmer for 10 minutes.

Add raisins, garlic, red pepper flakes, chili powder, cumin, basil, tomato paste, and 1 cup of the remaining 2 cups water and mix well.

Cook slowly for 15 minutes, adding additional 1 cup water when lentil mixture becomes too thick. Stir periodically.

Continue cooking, stirring occasionally (15–30 minutes more) until lentil mixture is thick.

Makes filling for 16 tortillas. Freeze half for future use.

Meanwhile, wrap tortillas completely in aluminum foil and bake at 350°F for 10–15 minutes.

Assembling the Tortillas

Place about 3 tablespoons lentil mixture in center of each tortilla.
Cover with about 1 tablespoon shredded zucchini.
Top with about 1 tablespoon yogurt. Serve.

Makes 8 tortillas
Calories per tortilla: 90 Total; 11 Fat; 0 Sat-fat

PASTA, RICE, AND OTHER GRAINS

20

P ASTA, BARLEY, rice, and bulgur are filling and low in saturated fat. As side dishes or complete meals, they add texture and variety to your eating.

Q   ## ASPARAGUS PASTA

Asparagus Pasta makes a delightful luncheon dish, first course for an elegant meal, or light dinner. No one consuming this dish will believe how incredibly simple it is to make.

1 pound asparagus, sliced into
    1–2-inch pieces
3 tablespoons Dijon mustard
1 tablespoon olive oil
¼ cup thinly sliced shallots
1 clove garlic, minced
2 anchovy fillets

¼ teaspoon thyme
2 tablespoons chopped parsley
¾ pound very thin spaghetti or
    pasta of your choice
Salt and freshly ground black
    pepper to taste
1 cup sliced mushrooms

In a large pot of boiling water, cook asparagus until tender and still bright green (about 3 minutes).

Combine mustard, olive oil, shallots, garlic, anchovies, thyme, and parsley. Set aside.

Cook pasta. Drain, but reserve 1 cup of the cooking water.

Combine pasta with dressing. Add asparagus and mushrooms. Mix well. Add some of the cooking water if pasta is too dry. Add salt and pepper to taste.

325

Variation: Follow the original recipe but add two boned and skinned chicken breasts that have been steamed and cut into bite-size pieces.

4 servings

Calories per serving:	Total	Fat	Sat-fat
	253	26	4
With chicken	296	30	5

Q   ## SALMON PASTA NIÇOISE

This delicious pasta may be eaten warm or cold. It is a meal in itself. (Beware: Although the dish is not high in sat-fat, it is very high in total fat.)

3 large fresh tomatoes
1 egg or 1 egg white
1 tablespoon olive oil
4 tablespoons wine vinegar
1 tin anchovy fillets
1 large clove garlic, minced
6 large black pitted olives,
   halved

Salt to taste (optional)
Freshly ground black pepper to
   taste
8 ounces thin spaghetti
1 can pink salmon (7½ oz)*
1–2 slices red onion, coarsely
   chopped

Cut tomatoes into slices about ¼–⅜-inch thick. Cut these in half or smaller.

Place egg in small pot, cover with water, and bring to boil. Let boil 1 minute or so. Cover pot, turn off heat, and let sit for 10 minutes until hard-boiled. Set aside or refrigerate. (You can do this step anytime during the day.)

Combine olive oil, vinegar, 4 smashed anchovy fillets, and garlic and pour over tomatoes. Mix in olives. Season with salt and pepper. Set aside to marinate for about 30 minutes or more.

Cook spaghetti, drain it, and place it in a large bowl. Stir tomato mixture into pasta. Break up salmon with a fork and add to pasta.

_____

*You may also substitute canned tuna in water for many fewer total fat calories.

Slice egg (or remove egg yolk and slice white) and add along with onion and remaining anchovies.

4 servings

Calories per serving:	Total	Fat	Sat-fat
With salmon	378	86	19
With tuna	359	67	13

PEASANT PASTA

Any combination of vegetables will do. Try these:

2 cups broccoli flowerets
1 cup cauliflower flowerets
1 zucchini, sliced
5 spears asparagus
20 green beans
½ pound very thin spaghetti
¼ cup chopped fresh parsley
2 cloves garlic
8 anchovy fillets

2 tablespoons olive oil
1 large tomato, coarsely chopped
1 sweet red pepper, coarsely chopped
10–15 snow peas
2 dried chili peppers or ½ teaspoon red pepper flakes

Steam broccoli, cauliflower, and zucchini until tender, and set aside.

Snap off the bottoms of the asparagus and boil for 1–2 minutes, until just tender. Set aside.

Submerge green beans in boiling water for 1–3 minutes, until just tender. Set aside.

While spaghetti is boiling (6 minutes), blend together parsley, garlic, anchovy fillets, and olive oil in a blender or food processor.

Drain spaghetti. Reserve 1 cup of water.

Stir anchovy sauce into spaghetti. If spaghetti is too dry, add a little water.

Stir in cooked vegetables, tomato, red pepper, and snow peas, until well covered with sauce.

Stir in red pepper flakes.

6 servings
Calories per serving: 240 Total; 41 Fat; 6 Sat-fat

PASTA MEXICALI

½ pound fancy pasta (fusilli, rigatoni, shells, etc.)
1 zucchini
½ cup chopped onion
1 teaspoon olive oil
1 teaspoon cumin
1 teaspoon chili powder
¼ teaspoon salt (optional)
1 red pepper, sliced
¼ cup tomato juice

Cook pasta according to package directions. Set aside.
Cut zucchini in quarters lengthwise. Slice into bite-size chunks.
Steam zucchini until just tender. Set aside.
In a small skillet, sauté onion in olive oil until soft.
Stir in cumin, chili powder, and salt.
Add onion mixture to pasta and mix well.
Add zucchini and red pepper. Add tomato juice and mix well.
Serve warm or at room temperature.

6 servings
Calories per serving: 161 Total; 7 Fat; 1 Sat-fat

DAN-DAN NOODLES

½ pound fettuccine or linguine
1 teaspoon natural all-peanut peanut butter
2 teaspoons sesame oil
½ teaspoon minced garlic
½ teaspoon minced ginger root
½ teaspoon hot chili oil
2½ tablespoons white vinegar
1 teaspoon sugar
4 teaspoons soy sauce
2 green onions, chopped

Cook noodles according to package directions. Drain and refrigerate.
Combine peanut butter and sesame oil until mixture is completely smooth.
Mix in garlic, ginger, chili oil, vinegar, sugar, and soy sauce. Pour sauce over noodles. Sprinkle green onions over the noodles and serve.

4 servings
Calories per serving: 252 Total; 32 Fat; 5 Sat-fat

Q
PASTA WITH PESTO

Pesto hails from Genoa, Italy, where the salty soil makes the basil particularly wonderful. Even in the United States, pesto can be superb. It is easy to make and freezes well. This is the only recipe in this book that calls for hard cheese. If you don't have a food processor or blender, you can use a mortar and pestle.

2 cups fresh basil
3 cloves garlic
1 teaspoon salt
2 tablespoons olive oil
1 tablespoon margarine

2 tablespoons Parmesan cheese
1 tablespoon Romano cheese
1 package (16 oz) very thin
    spaghetti

Prepare basil by rinsing it and tearing off the leaves. Discard the stems.

Chop garlic in a food processor or blender.

Add basil and salt. Process.

Add olive oil. Process until smooth. At this point you can put pesto aside for later use or freeze.

When ready to serve, mix margarine into pesto with a fork and blend well.

Blend in cheeses. Set aside.

Make spaghetti according to package directions.

Drain, but reserve 1 cup of the cooking water.

Mix pesto into pasta. If pesto is too dry, carefully stir in a small amount of spaghetti water.

8 servings
Calories per serving: 287 Total; 54 Fat; 14 Sat-fat

Q
SPAGHETTI SAUCE À LA SICILIA

Make a basic tomato sauce and add steamed eggplant and mushrooms for an appetizing spaghetti sauce that needs no ground meat.

1 small eggplant, peeled and
    cubed
6 cups Basic Tomato Sauce
    (page 330) or Zesty Fresh
    Tomato Sauce (page 330)

2 cups sliced mushrooms
12 ounces spaghetti

Prepare eggplant (see page 298) and steam until tender. Set aside.
In a medium saucepan, heat 6 cups of tomato sauce.
Stir in eggplant and mushrooms, cook 5 minutes more.
While spaghetti sauce is cooking, prepare spaghetti according to package directions.
Pour tomato sauce over spaghetti and serve.

6 servings
Calories per serving: 275 Total; 10 Fat; 1 Sat-fat

BASIC TOMATO SAUCE

1 cup chopped onion
2 teaspoons olive oil
4 large cans (28 oz each)
  tomatoes, drained

1 can (6 oz) tomato paste
2 teaspoons basil
1 teaspoon salt

In a large saucepan, cook onion in olive oil until soft.
Chop tomatoes and add to onion.
Stir in tomato paste. (Tomatoes can easily be chopped and tomato paste blended in food processor.)
Stir in basil and salt.
Simmer until thick (at least 1 hour).
This tomato sauce freezes well.

Makes 16 half-cup servings
Calories per serving: 32 Total; 5 Fat; 0 Sat-fat

ZESTY FRESH TOMATO SAUCE

Fresh tomatoes make this sauce special. It's fragrant, tasty, and simple to make.

1 medium onion, sliced
2–3 cloves garlic, minced
1 teaspoon olive oil
½ cup chopped parsley
4 cups chopped cherry tomatoes
  (or regular tomatoes)
½ teaspoon oregano

½ teaspoon basil
½ teaspoon cumin
½–1 teaspoon red pepper flakes
¼–½ freshly ground black
  pepper
Salt to taste (optional)

In a large skillet, sauté onion and garlic in olive oil until soft. Lower heat to medium and stir in parsley.

Stir in tomatoes. Add oregano, basil, cumin, red pepper flakes, black pepper, and salt. Cook at medium heat, stirring occasionally, for about 10 minutes. Turn to low and let flavors blend for about 5–10 more minutes.

Makes 5 half-cup servings (approximately)
Calories per serving: 48 Total; 8 Fat; 1 Sat-fat

SPAGHETTI TOURAINE

1¼ pounds fresh tomatoes
4 cloves garlic, peeled
1 tablespoon + 1 teaspoon olive oil
Salt to taste
1 tablespoon minced carrot
1 tablespoon minced celery
1 tablespoon minced leek
1 tablespoon minced shallot
1 cup dry white wine or vermouth

Bouquet garni (2 parsley sprigs, ⅓ bay leaf, and ⅛ teaspoon thyme wrapped in cheese-cloth)
½ cup + 2 tablespoons evaporated skim milk
¼ teaspoon salt (optional)
1 tablespoon dried tarragon (or fresh, if available)
10 ounces spaghetti

Place tomatoes in a large saucepan of boiling water. Immediately pour out hot water and pour in cold water.

Peel tomatoes, cut them in half crosswise (not across the stem), squeeze out the seeds and juice, and coarsely chop.

In a medium skillet, cook tomatoes and garlic in 1 tablespoon olive oil until reduced to a thick sauce (about 20 minutes). Stir occasionally. Add salt.

Meanwhile, heat 1 teaspoon olive oil in a small saucepan. Stir in carrot, celery, leek, and shallot.

Add wine and bouquet garni.

Reduce until thick and stir in evaporated skim milk.

Remove bouquet garni and pour mixture through a sieve to strain out the vegetables. Add tarragon.

Mix with tomato sauce and pour over pasta.

4 servings
Calories per serving: 165 Total; 40 Fat; 5 Sat-fat

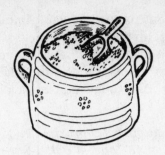

Q   RICE PILAU WITH APRICOTS AND RAISINS

3 tablespoons slivered almonds
1 teaspoon olive oil
1 teaspoon minced ginger root
1 clove garlic, minced
¼ cup chopped onion
1 teaspoon salt (optional)
2 whole cloves

½ cinnamon stick
1 teaspoon turmeric
1½ cups long-grain rice
3¾ cups water
¼ cup apricots, sliced
2 tablespoons raisins

In a medium casserole, sauté slivered almonds in olive oil over medium heat until golden.

Add ginger, garlic, and onion and sauté until soft.

Mix in salt, cloves, cinnamon stick, and turmeric.

Add rice and stir until well coated.

Add water and bring to a boil. Cover, reduce heat to low (or off), and cook until water is absorbed (about 25 minutes).

Mix in apricots and raisins.

Makes 14 half-cup servings
Calories per serving: 96 Total; 11 Fat; 1 Sat-fat

Q

OLIVE-ARTICHOKE RICE

3¾ cups water
1½ cups long-grain rice
½ teaspoon salt (optional)
1 tablespoon olive oil
1 tin (2 oz) anchovies (omit if
 you hate anchovies)

1 red pepper, sliced
½ cup artichoke hearts, diced
12 pitted black olives, sliced

In a medium saucepan, bring water to a boil.

Add rice and salt, cover, reduce heat to low, and cook for 25 minutes or until all water is absorbed.

Mix in remaining ingredients and cool to lukewarm.

Makes 14 half-cup servings
Calories per serving: 88 Total; 16 Fat; 3 Sat-fat

Q

INDIAN RICE

1 teaspoon olive oil
2 cloves garlic, minced
1 tablespoon minced ginger root
¾ cup chopped onion
¼ teaspoon cardamom
¼ teaspoon caraway seeds

1 teaspoon coriander
¼ teaspoon cinnamon
¼ teaspoon ground cloves
¼ teaspoon salt (optional)
1½ cups long-grain rice
3¾ cups water

In a medium saucepan, heat olive oil.

Add garlic, ginger, onion, and a splash of water and cook until soft.

Mix in cardamom, caraway seeds, coriander, cinnamon, cloves, salt, and rice and blend well.

Add water, cover, and bring to a boil. Reduce heat and cook until all water is absorbed (about 25 minutes).

Makes 12 half-cup servings
Calories per serving: 91 Total; 5 Fat; 1 Sat-fat

Q
LEMON RICE WITH SPINACH AND RED PEPPER

⅓ cup chopped onion
1 teaspoon olive oil
1 cup long-grain rice
½ teaspoon salt (optional)
2½ cups water

1 cup chopped spinach
2 tablespoons fresh lemon juice
1 red pepper, chopped (about ½ cup)

In a medium saucepan, sauté onion in olive oil until soft.

Mix in the rice and salt. Add water and bring to a boil. Reduce heat to low or off and cover saucepan.

After 15 minutes, stir spinach and lemon juice into rice.

Cook for 10 minutes more or until liquid is completely absorbed.

Mix in red pepper and serve.

Makes 8 half-cup servings
Calories per serving: 90 Total; 5 Fat; 0 Sat-fat

Q
FRIED RICE

2 egg whites
½ egg yolk
1 teaspoon + 1 teaspoon olive oil
3 green onions, cut into ¼-inch pieces

3 cups boiled rice (cold)
1 tablespoon soy sauce
¼ teaspoon sugar
¼ cup cooked diced chicken, shrimp, turkey, or combination

Beat egg whites and yolk together.

In a small skillet, scramble eggs in 1 teaspoon of the olive oil. Set aside.

In a large skillet, sauté green onions in the remaining teaspoon oil.

Add rice and mix thoroughly.

Stir in soy sauce and sugar.

Stir in eggs and meat.

Makes 6 half cup servings
Calories per serving: 154 Total; 20 Fat; 4 Sat-fat

Q   BULGUR WITH TOMATOES AND OLIVES

1 cup bulgur (cracked wheat)	1 tomato, chopped
2 teaspoons olive oil	¼ cup sliced green olives
1 cup tomato juice	2 stalks celery, chopped
1 cup water	3 green onions, sliced

In a large skillet, sauté bulgur in olive oil until bulgur begins to color and crackle.

Add tomato juice, water, and tomato and simmer until most liquid is absorbed (about 35 minutes).

Add olives, celery, and green onions and mix until heated through.

Makes 9 half-cup servings
Calories per serving: 68 Total; 12 Fat; 1 Sat-fat

Q   BARLEY PLUS

An interesting alternative to rice.

¾ cup chopped onion	1 can (10¾ oz) chicken broth,
½ cup chopped mushrooms	strained
2 teaspoons olive oil	½ teaspoon salt (optional)
1 cup pearl barley, rinsed	

Sauté onion and mushrooms in olive oil until tender. Stir in barley.

Add 1 cup of the chicken broth plus salt and bring to a boil. Cover and simmer for 25 minutes.

Add remaining broth plus water to equal 1 cup. Cook 25 more minutes until liquid is absorbed.

Fluff barley with a fork before serving.

6 servings
Calories per serving: 150 Total; 13 Fat; 3 Sat-fat

21 SALADS

S ALADS ARE refreshing. They can be quite nutritious and add texture and bulk to a meal. Salads by themselves generally contain very little fat. But beware of high-fat salad dressings! These culprits turn many a healthy salad into a fat-calorie extravaganza.

Gourmet food shops specialize in a variety of salads — pasta salad, rice salad, chicken, turkey, and fish salads. Here are a few you can make yourself and eat without hesitation.

Ⓠ TARRAGON-RAISIN CHICKEN SALAD

4 boned and skinned chicken
  breasts
¼ cup unbleached white flour
½ teaspoon salt (optional)
¼ teaspoon freshly ground
  black pepper

2 tablespoons reduced-calorie
  mayonnaise
2 tablespoons nonfat yogurt
2 teaspoons tarragon
2 tablespoons golden raisins

Preheat oven to 375°F.

Shake chicken in a plastic bag with flour, salt, and pepper to coat. Place chicken in a single layer in a shallow pan and bake until fully cooked, about 20–30 minutes.

When chicken is cool enough to handle, cut it into large chunks and set aside.

Combine mayonnaise, yogurt, tarragon, and raisins.

Add to chicken and mix until chicken is well coated.

4 servings
Calories per serving: 180 Total; 36 Fat; 12 Sat-fat

▣ CORIANDER CHICKEN SALAD

6 boned and skinned chicken
breasts
½ cup unbleached white flour
½ teaspoon salt (optional)
¼ teaspoon freshly ground
black pepper

¼ teaspoon coriander
2 cups broccoli flowerets
2 tablespoons reduced-calorie
mayonnaise
2 tablespoons nonfat yogurt
2 teaspoons Dijon mustard

Cook chicken as in Tarragon-Raisin Chicken Salad (page 336).
Cut chicken into large chunks, mix with coriander, and set aside
to cool.
Steam broccoli until just tender.
Combine salad dressing, yogurt, and mustard.
Mix mustard-yogurt dressing with chicken.
Stir in broccoli until coated with dressing.

8 servings
Calories per serving: 90 Total; 21 Fat; 12 Sat-fat

▣ CHICKEN SALAD WITH SHALLOTS
AND MUSHROOMS

3 boned and skinned chicken
breasts
¼ cup unbleached white flour
½ teaspoon salt (optional)
¼ teaspoon freshly ground
black pepper

1 teaspoon olive oil
2 tablespoons white vinegar
2 teaspoons minced shallot
1 cup sliced mushrooms
1 teaspoon thyme
¼ teaspoon salt (optional)

Cook chicken as in Tarragon-Raisin Chicken Salad (page 336).
When chicken is cool enough to handle, cut it into bite-size pieces.
Combine remaining ingredients and pour over chicken.
Mix until chicken is well coated.

4 servings
Calories per serving: 113 Total; 20 Fat; 4 Sat-fat

Ⓠ DIJON CHICKEN-RICE SALAD

3¾ cups water
1½ cups long-grain rice
½ teaspoon salt (optional)
3 tablespoons Dijon mustard
3 tablespoons white vinegar
1 tablespoon olive oil

1½–2 cups diced green and/or
  red pepper
¼ cup pitted black olives, sliced
¼ cup sliced green onion
3 cooked chicken breasts, diced

In a medium saucepan, bring water to a boil.

Add rice and salt, reduce heat, cover, and simmer for 20–25 minutes or until water is absorbed.

Place rice in a bowl.

Combine mustard, vinegar, and olive oil and mix into rice.

Add green pepper, olives, green onion, and chicken and mix well.

Tastes best when tepid. If too dry, mix in a little water, 1 tablespoon at a time.

6 one-and-a-half-cup servings
Calories per serving: 267 Total; 34 Fat; 7 Sat-fat

Ⓠ ORIENTAL CHICKEN SALAD

4 boned and skinned chicken
  breasts
¼ cup unbleached white flour
½ teaspoon salt (optional)
¼ teaspoon freshly ground
  black pepper
1 head broccoli, cut into
  flowerets (about 3 cups)

1 teaspoon walnut oil
3 tablespoons soy sauce
2 tablespoons dry vermouth
2 teaspoons minced ginger root
2 teaspoons chopped walnuts
2 cups mushrooms, sliced
1 head red-leaf or Boston
  lettuce

Cook chicken as in Tarragon-Raisin Chicken Salad (page 336).

When chicken is cool enough to handle, cut it into bite-size pieces. Set aside.

Steam broccoli flowerets until *just* tender.

Combine walnut oil, soy sauce, and ginger in a large bowl.

Add walnuts, mushrooms, and chicken and mix until all are coated with sauce. Stir in broccoli.

Place some lettuce on each salad plate. Top with chicken salad.

6 servings
Calories per serving: 140 Total; 29 Fat; 6 Sat-fat

▢ CURRIED TUNA SALAD WITH PEARS

1½ tablespoons reduced-calorie mayonnaise

2 tablespoons nonfat yogurt

¼–½ teaspoon curry powder

2 cans (6½ oz each) water-packed tuna, drained

¼ cup diced pear

Lettuce

Combine mayonnaise, yogurt, and curry powder.
Mix into tuna fish.
Stir in pear.
Serve over lettuce.

3 servings
Calories per serving: 175 Total; 23 Fat; 7 Sat-fat

SALADE NICOISE

A salad that is a meal in itself. Our Salade Niçoise is just like those served on the Riviera, but the egg yolks have been removed.

Dressing

1 clove garlic, minced

1 tablespoon lemon juice

1 tablespoon white vinegar

½ tablespoon Dijon mustard

½ teaspoon basil

¼ teaspoon salt (optional)

1½ tablespoons olive oil

Salad

2 potatoes

1½ cups green beans, tips removed and cut in half

1 small head red-leaf or Boston lettuce, shredded

2 tomatoes, cut into eighths

Whites from 2 hard-boiled eggs

2 tablespoons pitted black olives

1 tablespoon capers

1 oz anchovy fillets

3 oz water-packed solid white tuna, drained

Combine all dressing ingredients in a jar and shake vigorously. Set aside.
Steam potatoes until tender, peel, and cut into bite-size pieces.
Mix potatoes with 1 teaspoon dressing and set aside.
Cook green beans in boiling water for 5 minutes or until just tender and bright green.

Put lettuce and tomatoes in a large salad bowl and toss them with the remaining dressing.

Add potatoes, green beans, egg whites, olives, capers, anchovies, and drained tuna and mix until well coated with dressing. Traditionally each vegetable is segregated on a plate. We prefer them mixed into the salad.

5 servings
Calories per serving: 128 Total; 43 Fat; 6 Sat-fat

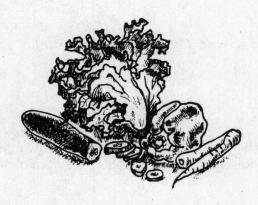

INDONESIAN VEGETABLE SALAD

2 cups shredded lettuce or
  Chinese celery cabbage
1 cup sliced carrot
1 cup green beans, cooked in
  boiling water until just tender

2 tomatoes, sliced
1 cucumber, peeled and sliced

Dressing

1 tablespoon sliced green onion
½ tablespoon olive oil
4 tablespoons natural all-peanut
  peanut butter
1 clove garlic, minced
½ teaspoon red pepper flakes

1 bay leaf
1 slice lemon
1 teaspoon sugar
½ teaspoon salt
¾ cup skim milk
2 tablespoons water

Place lettuce on a platter.

Artistically arrange carrots, green beans, tomatoes, and cucumber over lettuce. Cover with plastic wrap and chill in refrigerator.

In a small saucepan, sauté green onion in olive oil.

Mix in peanut butter, garlic, red pepper flakes, bay leaf, lemon, sugar, and salt until peanut butter starts to melt.

Gradually blend in skim milk. Cook over low heat, stirring constantly, until thick. Chill dressing.

Before serving, dilute dressing with water, if necessary.

Pass platter and dressing separately so everyone can take what they want.

Salad
6 servings
Calories per serving: 32 Total; 0 Fat; 0 Sat-fat

Dressing
Makes ¾ cup
Calories per tablespoon: 43 Total; 30 Fat; 5 Sat-fat

TABBOULI

1 cup bulgur (cracked wheat)	2 cloves garlic, minced
3 cups boiling water	1 small onion, chopped
1 can (15 oz) chickpeas, drained	1 green pepper, chopped
¼ cup fresh mint, minced, or 1 teaspoon dried mint	2 medium tomatoes, chopped
2 teaspoons oregano	1 tablespoon olive oil
½ teaspoon salt (optional)	3 tablespoons fresh lemon juice
¼ teaspoon freshly ground black pepper	¼ cup chopped parsley

Place bulgur in a large bowl and cover with boiling water.

Let stand for about 1 hour or until fluffy. Squeeze out excess water.

Combine bulgur with remaining ingredients.

Chill for at least 1 hour.

Makes 14 half-cup servings
Calories per serving: 87 Total; 10 Fat; 2 Sat-fat

Q

CUCUMBER SALAD

2 cucumbers, peeled and sliced
   thin
1 medium onion, sliced thin
½ teaspoon salt (optional)

1 teaspoon sugar
1 teaspoon dill weed
1 cup white vinegar

Mix cucumbers and onion together in a ceramic or glass bowl.
Add salt, sugar, and dill weed to vinegar and pour over cucumbers
and onion.
Chill 1 hour.

6 servings
Calories per serving: 20 Total; 0 Fat; 0 Sat-fat

Q

EASTERN SPINACH SALAD

1 package (10 oz) fresh spinach,
   washed and shredded
10 water chestnuts, sliced
3 green onions, sliced
1 cup sliced mushrooms
1 cucumber, peeled and sliced
   thin

1 tablespoon olive oil
2 tablespoons soy sauce
3 tablespoons fresh lemon juice
1½ tablespoons honey
1 tablespoon sesame seeds,
   toasted

In a salad bowl, combine spinach, water chestnuts, green onions,
mushrooms, and cucumber slices.
Mix together olive oil, soy sauce, lemon juice, and honey and pour
over salad.
Sprinkle with sesame seeds.

8 servings
Calories per serving: 55 Total; 20 Fat; 3 Sat-fat

Q

POTATO SALAD

4–5 red potatoes
½ cup nonfat yogurt
3 tablespoons reduced-calorie
   mayonnaise

1 teaspoon tarragon
1 tablespoon white vinegar
1 teaspoon Dijon mustard
½ teaspoon salt (optional)

Scrub potatoes thoroughly. Steam until tender.
Meanwhile, combine remaining ingredients. Set aside.
Cut potatoes into chunks (do not remove skin).
Pour sauce over potatoes so they are thoroughly coated.
Serve warm or cold.

6 servings
Calories per serving: 105 Total; 14 Fat; 5 Sat-fat

▣ FRUIT SALAD WITH COTTAGE CHEESE OR YOGURT

This high-protein, low-fat dish makes a filling lunch. Round it off with a piece of homemade bread and, for dessert, air-popped pop-corn.

Spring or Summer Fruits

¼ cantaloupe   1 peach
½ cup blueberries   ⅙ honeydew melon

Fall or Winter Fruits

½ Golden Delicious apple   ½ Bosc pear
1 kiwi fruit   ½ orange

½ cup low-fat (1%) cottage
   cheese or nonfat yogurt

Cut fruit into bite-size pieces and place in bowl.
Mix in cottage cheese or yogurt.

Serves 1

	Total	Fat	Sat-fat
Spring or summer salad:			
with cottage cheese	280	10	7
with nonfat yogurt	250	0	0
Fall or winter salad:			
with cottage cheese	270	10	7
with nonfat yogurt	245	0	0

22 SANDWICHES, DIPS, AND A DRINK

S OUR CREAM need not be the basis for your dips and sandwich spreads. Sour cream has 270 sat-fat calories per cup. In its place, use nonfat or low-fat yogurt, eggplant, chickpeas, or cottage cheese for delicious, low-fat dips and spreads.

Q CREAMY GINGER-CURRY DIP

A good substitution for sour cream or cream cheese is yogurt cheese (see page 347). Made with nonfat yogurt, it adds 0 sat-fat and 0 total fat to your dish. Remember: In this recipe, allow 12–24 hours to make the yogurt cheese.

2 cups nonfat yogurt	2 tablespoons cider vinegar
1/3 cup orange marmalade	1/4 teaspoon salt (optional)
2 teaspoons brown sugar	1/4 teaspoon curry powder
1 1/2 teaspoons granulated sugar	1/4 teaspoon powdered ginger

Make yogurt cheese (page 347). Let yogurt drain in the refrigerator for about 12–24 hours.

When yogurt has become yogurt cheese, combine it with the remaining ingredients. Chill.

Makes about 1 1/2 cups
Calories per tablespoon: 24 Total; 0 Fat; 0 Sat-fat

Q   BABA GHANOUSH

1 medium eggplant
¼ cup or more fresh lemon
   juice
3 tablespoons tahini (sesame
   seed paste)*

1–2 cloves garlic
¼ cup chopped parsley
Salt to taste

Peel eggplant, cut into bite-size pieces, and salt heavily. Set aside for 15 minutes. Rinse and squeeze eggplant and steam in vegetable steamer until soft.

Purée eggplant in food processor or blender.

Blend in lemon juice and tahini.

Just before you serve, crush garlic into purée and mix in parsley and salt.

Taste. Add more lemon juice if you wish.

Serve with whole-wheat or plain pita bread cut into pieces.

Makes about 2 cups
Calories per tablespoon: 12 Total; 7 Fat; 1 Sat-fat

Q   CHICKPEA SANDWICH OR DIP

1 can chickpeas
2 cloves garlic
⅓ cup parsley
1 tablespoon tahini (sesame
   seed paste)*
Juice of 1 lemon (about ¼ cup)

4 six-inch whole-wheat pita
   bread pockets
Chopped tomatoes, green
   onions, and lettuce, for
   garnish

Drain chickpeas. Reserve liquid. In blender or food processor, chop garlic and parsley.

Add chickpeas, tahini, and lemon juice.

Blend until smooth, adding more chickpea liquid if spread is too stiff.

*Available at Mideast food shops and many supermarkets

Make sandwiches by spooning chickpea spread into pita bread pockets.

Garnish with chopped tomatoes, green onions, and lettuce.

Makes 4 sandwiches

Use as a dip for vegetables, crackers, squares of pita, etc.

Makes about 1½ cups

Calories	Total	Fat	Sat-fat
Per sandwich	195	35	4
Per tablespoon	20	4	1

EGGPLANT APPETIZER

A tasty appetizer. Eat with quartered pita bread or crackers or heat and serve as a vegetable.

4 cups peeled, cubed eggplant	½ cup Spanish olives
½ cup chopped onion	½ cup black olives
4 cloves garlic, minced	2 teaspoons capers
2 stalks celery, sliced	2 teaspoons brown sugar
1 teaspoon olive oil	2 tablespoons white vinegar

Salt eggplant heavily and set aside for 15 minutes.

Rinse salt off eggplant under running water while squeezing out bitter juices.

Steam eggplant until tender.

Taste. If not bitter, set aside. If bitter, find a recipe without eggplant!

Sauté onion, garlic, and celery in olive oil until soft.

Mix in eggplant, olives, capers, brown sugar, and vinegar and heat until warm.

Eat hot, at room temperature, or chilled.

10 servings
Calories per serving: 38 Total; 24 Fat; 5 Sat-fat

YOGURT CHEESE

Yogurt cheese made with nonfat yogurt may be substituted for sour cream and cream cheese in some recipes, greatly reducing the sat-fat and total fat calories. It is easy to make. Place nonfat yogurt (without gelatin) in a coffee filter (or cheesecloth) in a coffeepot or in a strainer over a bowl. Cover and refrigerate overnight. As the yogurt drains, it condenses. About half the yogurt will become cheese. Pour off whey and keep cheese in a covered container in the refrigerator. Add herbs, green onions, or Dijon mustard to make a flavored cheese.

Calories per tablespoon: 7 Total; 0 Fat; 0 Sat-fat

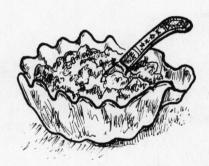

FAUX GUACAMOLE

Your guests will never imagine that the dip they are eagerly devouring was made with asparagus. What a buy. A great-tasting treat at a cost of 0 sat-fat and 0 total fat calories.

2 tablespoons yogurt cheese*
1 pound asparagus
1 clove garlic, crushed
¼ teaspoon cayenne pepper
¼ teaspoon chili powder
1 tablespoon fresh lemon juice

2 ounces diced green chili peppers**
1 cup chopped tomatoes
1 tablespoon chopped onion
Whole-wheat pita bread

*See box above.
**Available in small cans in most supermarkets

Prepare yogurt cheese a day in advance (see box).

Snap off the bottom ends of the asparagus and discard. Find a frying pan that will hold the asparagus in one layer and fill it with an inch of water. Bring the water to a boil and add the asparagus. Cook until soft. Drain asparagus and purée with garlic in blender or food processor.

Mix in cayenne pepper, chili powder, lemon juice, yogurt cheese, chili peppers, tomatoes, and onion. Chill for several hours.

Serve with toasted whole-wheat pita pockets divided into quarters or Bagel Chips (recipe follows).

Makes 1½ cups (approximately)

Calories	Total	Fat	Sat-fat
Per tablespoon	7	0	0
With pita bread quarter	33	2	0

BAGEL CHIPS

A great crunchy snack — eat them alone or with dips.

Bagels (plain, onion, garlic, etc.)

Flavor Options

1 clove garlic
Chili powder

Cajun Seasoning Mix (page 243)
Cinnamon and sugar

Preheat oven to 200°F.

Cut bagel into ¼–⅜-inch-thick slices. They will look like very thin bagels. (Halve or quarter slices if you want smaller bagel chips.) Place pieces on cookie sheet in one layer.

Either press garlic and spread over bagel slices, sprinkle chili powder or spice mix over them, leave them plain, or for a sweet treat, sprinkle on a mix of cinnamon and sugar.

Bake for 1–2 hours.

Calories per bagel chip: 38 Total; 2 Fat; 0 Sat-fat

TED MUMMERY'S TURKEY BARBECUE

We discovered a most wonderful turkey barbecue while at a health conference in Steven's Point, Wisconsin. Ted Mummery, the owner of La Claire's Frozen Yogurt, Inc., has kindly allowed us to share his recipe with you. It's delicious in a whole-wheat pita pocket, on an onion bagel, or any other bread.

5–6 lbs turkey breast
4 cans (14½ oz each) stewed
   tomatoes
2 large cans (12 oz each) tomato
   paste
1 cup water
½ cup brown sugar
⅓ cup dark molasses
½ cup apple cider vinegar
1 teaspoon hickory salt*
   (optional) or 1 teaspoon salt

1 heaping teaspoon garlic
   powder
1½ heaping teaspoons onion
   powder
1 heaping teaspoon basil
1½ heaping teaspoons oregano
1 heaping teaspoon cayenne
1 teaspoon all-purpose
   seasoning
½ teaspoon white pepper

Preheat oven to 350°F.

Remove skin and fat from turkey breast.

Bake turkey with breast down until fully cooked, about 1½–2½ hours. (You may do this the night before.) Refrigerate.

Mix tomatoes, tomato paste, and water in blender or food processor for a few moments. You want to chop the tomatoes, not purée them.

Place in 5-quart Crockpot or slow cooker. (You may also cook barbecue in a large pot on the stove.) Stir in remaining ingredients. Set Crockpot on automatic or cook at low heat for about 2 hours.

Pull turkey from bones and cut into bite-size pieces. Add turkey to sauce and cook for about another hour.

Makes 30 half-cup servings
Calories per serving: 131 Total; 5 Fat; 1 Sat-fat

---

*Ted recommends 3 teaspoons of hickory salt. If you are eating this barbecue often, I suggest eliminating the hickory salt as it contains an unhealthy ingredient — smoke (charcoal).

FROTHY FRUIT SHAKE

Use your imagination and the fruit you have in the house to create refreshing fruit shakes of different flavors. Here's one example:

1 cup strawberries
1 ripe banana, peeled and
    quartered
1 orange, peeled and halved

Dash of salt (optional)
½ cup crushed ice or 4–5 ice
    cubes

Place fruit and salt in a blender and purée.

Combine purée with ½ cup of finely crushed ice. You can make crushed ice by placing ice cubes in a plastic bag and smashing them with a meat-tenderizing mallet or hammer until crushed evenly. You can also crush ice in an electric ice-crusher. You may add ice cubes to the purée in the blender and blend until cubes are crushed.

Makes 2 one-cup servings
Calories per serving: 105 Total; 2 Fat; 0 Sat-fat

BREADS

STARCHES HAVE received bad press over the years. Bread, rice, pasta, and potatoes have been associated with weight gain. Weight problems begin not with starch but with the fat that is put on the starch: bread slathered with margarine, potatoes stuffed with sour cream. An ounce of carbohydrate has less than *half* as many calories as an ounce of fat. An average piece of bread has 9 fat calories. Cover it with margarine and the fat calorie value goes up to 109. And, of course, the saturated fat content also rises.

You can cut down on saturated fats and cholesterol by replacing fatty meats and high-fat dairy products with grains, potatoes, breads, and pasta. Many starchy foods (such as whole grains and potatoes with skin) provide fiber, bulk, vitamins, and minerals.

Many of the following recipes are for 1 loaf so that you can make them in your food processor. Double ingredients for 2 loaves.

You can make any loaf into baguettes by following the recipe for French Bread, page 354, beginning with "Divide dough in half."

We have chosen to use olive oil in baking most of our breads because olive oil lowers LDL-cholesterol without lowering HDL-cholesterol, as well as preventing the oxidation of LDL-cholesterol — the first step in the process of atherosclerosis. Choose a mild-tasting olive oil, and your taste buds won't notice the difference.

NOTE: The instruction "Let proof" means to wait for the yeast to ferment, swell, and get bubbly. This takes only a few minutes at most.

SHAKER DAILY LOAF

1 tablespoon active dry yeast
Pinch of sugar
¼ cup warm water
6 cups unbleached white flour
  (approximately)

2¼ cups skim milk
2 tablespoons margarine
2 tablespoons maple syrup or
  honey
2 teaspoons salt

Dissolve yeast and sugar in the warm water in a large bowl or a food processor. Let proof (become bubbly).

Mix in 3 cups of the flour.

In a small saucepan, scald skim milk. Remove from heat.

Add margarine, maple syrup, and salt to milk and mix until margarine melts.

When liquid has cooled to lukewarm, add to flour in bowl.

Stir in more flour, ½ cup at a time, until dough is fairly stiff.

Knead dough 10 minutes or process 15 seconds or until dough is smooth and elastic.

Place dough in a large oiled bowl, cover with a towel, and let rise in a warm place for 1 hour or until doubled in bulk.

Remove dough from bowl and divide it in half.

Let dough rest, covered, for 10 minutes.

Roll into two loaves and place in loaf pans greased with margarine.

Cover and let rise until doubled (1–2 hours).

Preheat oven to 350°F.

Bake loaves for 35–40 minutes or until they are golden brown and sound hollow when tapped.

Makes 2 loaves

Calories	Total	Fat	Sat-fat
Per ½-inch slice	90	7	2
Per loaf	1512	117	28

CARDAMOM BREAD

1 tablespoon active dry yeast	1 teaspoon salt
2 tablespoons brown sugar	¼–½ teaspoon cardamom*
¼ cup warm water	2 tablespoons olive oil
2–4 cups unbleached white flour	1 cup skim milk

Combine yeast, brown sugar, and water in a large bowl or a food processor. Let proof.

Add 2 cups flour, salt, and cardamom and mix.

Mix in olive oil and skim milk. Add more flour until you produce a stiff dough.

Knead dough 10 minutes or process 15 seconds or until dough is smooth and elastic, adding more flour if necessary.

Place dough in a large oiled bowl, cover with a towel, and let rise in warm place for 1 hour or until doubled in bulk.

Roll into loaf and place in loaf pan greased with margarine.

Cover with a towel and let rise for 1 hour or until doubled in bulk.

Preheat oven to 425°F.

Bake loaf for 10 minutes.

Reduce heat to 350°F and bake for 30 minutes more or until loaf is golden brown and sounds hollow when tapped.

Makes 1 loaf

Calories	Total	Fat	Sat-fat
Per ½-inch slice	98	15	2
Per loaf	1663	255	41

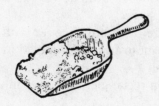

*For a totally different taste, substitute 1 teaspoon cinnamon.

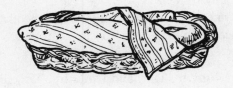

FRENCH BREAD I

A French bread of peasant stock. Give yourself a treat and eat it warm, straight from the oven. It also freezes well. Make smaller loaves for submarine sandwiches. Any bread is an impressive gift to bring to friends. And this bread is so easy you'll be embarrassed to answer yes when asked if you made it yourself.

1½ tablespoons active dry yeast   1 teaspoon salt
½ teaspoon sugar   2 tablespoons olive oil
¼ cup warm water   1 cup water
2–3 cups unbleached white
   flour

Place yeast, sugar, and ¼ cup very warm, but *not hot*, water in a large bowl or a food processor. Let proof.

Mix in 2 cups flour and the salt.

Add olive oil and 1 cup water to flour and knead dough 10 minutes or process 15 seconds or until dough is smooth and elastic, adding more flour if necessary.

Place dough in large oiled bowl, cover with a towel, and let rise in a warm place for 1 hour or until doubled in bulk.

Divide dough in half.

Roll each half into a rectangle. Fold over in thirds like this:

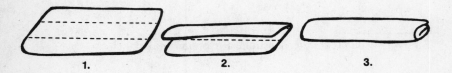

1.   2.   3.

Press the edge into the dough after each fold.

Put into greased (with margarine) French bread pan that looks like this:

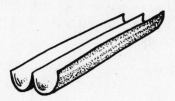

Cover and let rise for about 1 hour, or until doubled in bulk.

After 50 minutes, preheat oven to 450°F.

Uncover bread and slash with parallel or diagonal lines like this:

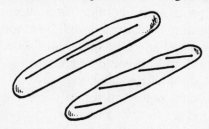

Place bread pan in oven on a diagonal to the right. Put 4 ice cubes in the bottom of the oven to create steam for crustier loaves.

In 5 minutes, add 4 more ice cubes.

In 10 minutes, shift pan so it is on a diagonal to the left, like this:

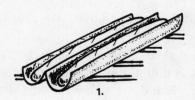 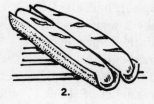

Reduce heat to 400°F and bake for 10 minutes more or until golden brown. Take loaves out of pan and cool or eat immediately.

Freezes nicely. If thawed, slice *before* reheating. Thawed French bread flakes like crazy when cut after reheating.

Makes 2 baguettes

Calories	Total	Fat	Sat-fat
Per ½-inch slice	87	13	2
Per baguette	874	133	19

FRENCH BREAD II

There is almost nothing more satisfying and delicious than eating freshly baked bread hot from the oven — particularly French Bread II. This French bread is lighter than French Bread I. It takes a long time to rise, but it's worth the wait.

1 tablespoon active dry yeast	4 + cups unbleached white flour
1 tablespoon sugar	1–1½ teaspoons salt
⅓ cup warm water	1¼ cups water

Place yeast, sugar, and ⅓ cup warm water in large bowl or bowl of food processor and let proof.

Mix in 4 cups of flour and salt.

Add 1¼ cups water and knead dough 10 minutes or process about 15 seconds. Keep adding flour until dough is smooth and elastic.

Make dough into a ball and place in an oiled bowl approximately twice the size of the dough so you'll be able to see when the dough is doubled in size. Cover with a damp dish towel.

Place bowl in a warm place (on top of the refrigerator is often a nice, warm spot) and let rise until doubled in size. The dough will swell above the edge of the bowl. This will take at least 1½ hours.

When the dough has doubled in bulk, punch it down and knead it a few times. Let it rest a few minutes. If you have two French bread pans, which together hold 4 loaves, divide the bread into 4 equal pieces. If you have one French bread pan that holds 2 loaves, divide the dough in half, then divide one of the halves in half again. You will make 2 baguettes with the smaller pieces of dough and 1 round loaf with the larger piece.

For the baguettes: Grease the bread pan with margarine. Flatten the dough into an oval. Squeeze the dough into a long, thin rope with a diameter of about 1½ inches. Roll the dough with the palms of both of your hands (to resemble the clay coils you made as a kid) to lengthen and smooth it. Place in bread pan.

For the round bread: Grease the bottom of an 8-inch cake pan with margarine. Form a ball by folding the edges of the dough under itself. Place in cake pan.

Cover bread with towel and let rise until baguette dough fills out the bread pan.

When bread has completed its second rise (about 1½ hours), pre-heat oven to 450°F. Make 3 diagonal slashes in the baguettes, about

⅛–⅜ inches deep. In the round bread, make a 4-inch slash through the center of the top. Make another slash through the center perpendicular to the first slash.

Place bread pans in the oven. You will probably have to use 2 shelves or 2 ovens. Put 4 ice cubes on the oven floor to make the loaves crusty. Bake for 5 minutes. Add 4 more ice cubes. Bake for 5 more minutes. Shift the direction of the bread pans (see drawings on page 355) and bake for 10 more minutes or until golden brown.

Makes 4 baguettes or 2 baguettes and 1 round loaf

Calories	Total	Fat	Sat-fat
Per baguette	471	12	2
Per 1½-inch slice	52	1	0
Per round loaf	942	24	4
Per ½-inch slice	94	2	0

BUTTERMILK HERB BREAD

1 tablespoon active dry yeast
2 tablespoons sugar
¼ cup warm water
2–3 cups unbleached white
    flour
1 teaspoon salt

¼ teaspoon marjoram
¼ teaspoon oregano
¼ teaspoon thyme
½ cup buttermilk
2 tablespoons olive oil
1 egg

Place yeast, sugar, and water in a large bowl or in your food processor. Let proof.

Mix in 2 cups flour, salt, marjoram, oregano, and thyme.

Mix in buttermilk and olive oil. (If using a food processor, process at least 15 seconds.)

Mix in enough flour to make a stiff but soft dough.

Add egg. Knead dough 10 minutes or process 15 seconds or until dough is smooth and elastic.

Put dough in a large oiled bowl, cover with a towel, and let rise in a warm place for 1 hour or until doubled in bulk.

Form loaf and place in loaf pan greased with margarine. Cover and let rise 1 hour or until doubled in bulk.

Preheat oven to 375°F.

Bake loaf for about 35 minutes or until it is golden brown and sounds hollow when tapped.

Makes 1 loaf

Calories	Total	Fat	Sat-fat
Per ½-inch slice	108	18	5
Per loaf	1842	306	80

GINGER-ORANGE BREAD

A very subtle taste of ginger pervades this whole-wheat bread.

1 tablespoon active dry yeast
2 tablespoons brown sugar
¼ cup warm water
1½ cups whole-wheat flour
1½ cups unbleached white flour
    (approximately)

1 teaspoon salt
2 teaspoons ground ginger
2 tablespoons olive oil
½ cup buttermilk
½ cup orange juice

Combine yeast, brown sugar, and warm water in a large bowl or a food processor. Let proof.

Mix in whole-wheat flour, white flour, salt, and ginger.

Add olive oil, buttermilk, and orange juice. Knead 10 minutes or process 15 seconds or until dough is smooth and elastic, adding more flour if necessary.

Place dough in a large oiled bowl, cover with a towel, and let rise in a warm place for 1 hour or until doubled in bulk.

Shape into a loaf and place in a loaf pan greased with margarine.

Cover with a towel and let rise in warm place for about 1 hour or until doubled in bulk.

Preheat oven to 400°F.

Bake loaf for 10 minutes.

Reduce heat to 350°F and bake for 30 minutes more or until golden brown.

Makes 1 loaf

Calories	Total	Fat	Sat-fat
Per ½-inch slice	99	16	3
Per loaf	1678	279	46

CHALLAH

A delicious bread for the Jewish Sabbath or just for enjoyable eating.

1 tablespoon active dry yeast	½ teaspoon salt
2 tablespoons sugar	2 tablespoons olive oil
1 cup warm water	1 egg
2–4 cups unbleached white flour	

Place yeast, sugar, and ¼ cup warm water in a large bowl or a food processor. Let proof.

Mix in 2 cups flour and salt.

Add ¾ cup warm water, oil, and egg and mix or process for 15 seconds.

Knead dough 10 minutes or process 15 seconds or until dough is smooth and elastic, adding more flour if necessary.

Place dough in a large oiled bowl, cover with a towel, and let rise in warm place for 1 hour or until doubled in bulk.

Divide dough into two unequal portions, one-third and two-thirds.

Divide the smaller portion of the dough into three pieces. Roll each into a rope.

Divide the larger portion into three pieces. Roll each into a rope.

Braid the three larger ropes and place them on a greased cookie sheet.

Braid the three smaller ropes and place them on top of the larger braided pieces. Pinch the two together.

Cover with a towel and let rise for 1 hour or until doubled in bulk.

Preheat oven to 400°F.

Bake bread for 10 minutes.

Reduce heat to 375°F and bake for 30 minutes more or until golden brown.

Makes 1 large loaf or 2 small loaves

Calories	Total	Fat	Sat-fat
Per ½-inch slice	70	13	2
Per loaf	1670	317	47

ANADAMA BREAD

This version of the New England bread has whole-wheat flour added to it to make it healthier while retaining its wonderful taste and texture.

1 tablespoon active dry yeast
Pinch of sugar
¼ cup warm water
¾ cup cornmeal
1½ cups whole-wheat flour
1½ cups unbleached white flour
   (approximately)

1–1½ teaspoons salt
2 tablespoons olive oil
1 cup water
3 tablespoons molasses

Dissolve yeast with pinch of sugar in ¼ cup warm water in a large bowl or a food processor. Let proof.

Mix in cornmeal, whole-wheat flour, 1 cup of the white flour, and salt.

Stir in olive oil, 1 cup water, and molasses.

Knead dough 10 minutes or process 15 seconds or until dough is smooth and elastic, adding more white flour if necessary.

Place dough in a large oiled bowl, cover with a towel, and let rise in a warm place for 1 hour or until doubled in bulk.

Form into a loaf and place in a loaf pan greased with margarine. Cover and let rise for 1 hour or until doubled in bulk.

Preheat oven to 400°F.

Bake loaf for 15 minutes.

Reduce heat to 350°F and bake about 30 minutes more or until loaf is golden brown and sounds hollow when tapped.

Makes 1 loaf

Calories	Total	Fat	Sat-fat
Per ½-inch slice	113	15	2
Per loaf	1919	257	42

PEANUT BUTTER BREAD

A bread with a subtle peanut buttery taste and aroma.

1 tablespoon active dry yeast
2 tablespoons sugar
¼ cup warm water
2 cups whole-wheat flour
2½ cups unbleached white flour (approximately)

2 teaspoons salt
2 tablespoons olive oil
¼ cup natural all-peanut peanut butter
1 cup buttermilk

Place yeast, sugar, and warm water in a large bowl or a food processor. Let proof.

Mix in whole-wheat flour, white flour, and salt.

Stir in olive oil, peanut butter, and buttermilk. Knead 10 minutes or process 15 seconds or until dough is smooth and elastic, adding more white flour if necessary.

Place dough in a large oiled bowl, cover with a towel, and let rise in a warm place for about 1 hour or until doubled in bulk.

Divide dough in half and form loaves.

Place in loaf pans greased with margarine, cover, and let rise for about 1 hour or until doubled in bulk.

Preheat oven to 350°F.

Bake for 45–60 minutes or until loaves are golden brown and sound hollow when tapped.

Makes 2 small loaves

Calories	Total	Fat	Sat-fat
Per ½-inch slice	78	18	3
Per loaf	1358	321	50

PUMPERNICKEL BREAD

1 tablespoon yeast	1 teaspoon salt
¼ cup warm water	2 tablespoons olive oil
Pinch of sugar	2 tablespoons molasses
1 cup rye flour	1¼ cups warm water
2 cups whole-wheat flour	1 tablespoon caraway seeds
(approximately)	Corn flour
2 cups unbleached white flour	

Place yeast in a large bowl or a food processor. Add ¼ cup warm water and sugar. Let proof.

Mix in rye flour, whole-wheat flour, 1½ cups white flour, and salt.

Add olive oil, molasses, and 1¼ cups warm water. Knead 10 minutes or process 15 seconds or until dough is smooth and elastic, adding more white flour if necessary.

Knead in caraway seeds.

Place dough in a large oiled bowl, cover with a towel, and let rise in a warm place for 1 hour or until doubled in bulk.

Sprinkle corn flour on a baking sheet.

Form dough into a round or loaf, place on baking sheet, cover, and let rise 1 hour or until doubled in bulk.

Preheat oven to 450°F.

Bake loaf for 10 minutes.

Reduce heat to 350°F and bake for 35 minutes more or until loaf sounds hollow when tapped.

Makes 1 large loaf

Calories	Total	Fat	Sat-fat
Per ½-inch slice	92	12	2
Per loaf	2273	301	39

HONEY WHOLE-WHEAT BREAD

Whole-grain breads are much more nutritious than breads made with white flour. In whole-grain flours, the entire kernel is ground into flour so that vitamins, minerals, and fiber are not lost.

Honey Whole-Wheat Bread makes wonderful toast. Top it with bananas and cottage cheese and you have a filling, nutritious, and scrumptious breakfast. Honey Whole-Wheat Bread freezes well.

This recipe makes 4 loaves of bread. Freeze the ones you are not using.

2 tablespoons active dry yeast	½ cup honey
2 tablespoons salt	½ cup olive oil
1 quart-size package nonfat dry milk	2 teaspoons cinnamon
	½ teaspoon grated nutmeg
1 five-pound bag whole-wheat flour (about 16 cups)	1½ cups rolled oats
	½ cup raisins
6½ cups water	

In a mixing bowl, combine yeast, salt, nonfat dry milk, and 2 cups flour.

In a large saucepan, combine water, honey, and oil and heat until quite warm (about 115°F) but *not too hot* or you will kill the yeast.

Add liquid to dry ingredients in mixing bowl and beat for 4 minutes.

Mix in 4 cups flour.

Mix in the cinnamon, nutmeg, oats, and raisins.

Keep adding flour until you produce a stiff dough. Your mixer probably will not be large enough to handle all the dough. When the mixer reaches its limit, remove the dough to a pastry board or counter and add flour until the dough is stiff enough to knead.

Knead dough for 8–10 minutes or until smooth and elastic.

Place dough in large oiled bowl, cover with a towel, and let rise in warm place for about 1 hour or until doubled in bulk.

Form 4 loaves, place in loaf pans greased with margarine, cover with a towel, and let rise 1 hour or until doubled in bulk.

Preheat oven to 350°F.

Bake loaves for 45 minutes to 1 hour or until they are golden brown and sound hollow when tapped.

Makes 4 loaves

Calories	Total	Fat	Sat-fat
Per ½-inch slice	130	17	2
Per loaf	2222	342	39

CUMIN WHEAT BREAD

Although this is a totally whole-wheat bread, it is not the least bit heavy. It is a favorite with young children as well as adults.

1 tablespoon dry yeast	1 teaspoon salt
¼ cup warm water	½ teaspoon whole cumin seeds
2 tablespoons honey	1½ tablespoons olive oil
3½ cups whole-wheat flour	1 cup skim milk

In a large mixing bowl or the bowl of a food processor, combine yeast, water, and honey. Let proof.

Mix in 2 cups of the flour, the salt, and cumin seeds.

Add oil and milk and mix or process well, adding more flour until dough is fairly stiff.

Knead dough 10 minutes or process for 15 seconds or until dough is smooth and elastic, adding more flour if necessary.

Form dough into a ball. Place in an oiled bowl. Cover and let rise for about 1 hour.

Roll dough into a loaf and place in loaf pan greased with margarine. Cover with towel and let rise for 1 hour.

Preheat oven to 375°F and bake for 50–60 minutes or until bread is golden and sounds hollow when tapped.

Makes 1 loaf

Calories	Total	Fat	Sat-fat
Per ½-inch slice	107	15	2
Per loaf	1814	252	35

CINNAMON APPLESAUCE BREAD

1 tablespoon active dry yeast	1 teaspoon cinnamon
2 tablespoons brown sugar	⅔ cup applesauce
1 cup warm water	1 tablespoon olive oil
1½ cups whole-wheat flour	½ apple, peeled, cored, and
2 cups unbleached white flour	chopped (about ½ cup)
1 teaspoon salt	¼ cup raisins (optional)

Combine yeast, sugar, and water in a large bowl or a food processor. Let proof.

Mix in whole-wheat flour, 1 cup of white flour, salt, and cinnamon.

Mix in applesauce and olive oil.

Add remaining cup of white flour and more of either or both flours until dough is fairly stiff. Knead dough 10 minutes or process for 15 seconds or until dough is smooth and elastic, adding more flour if necessary.

Mix in apple and raisins.

Form dough into a ball. Place in an oiled bowl. Cover with towel and let rise for about 1 hour.

Roll dough into a loaf and place in loaf pan greased with margarine. Cover and let rise for an hour.

Preheat oven to 350°F. Bake for 50–60 minutes or until loaf sounds hollow when tapped.

Makes 1 large loaf

Calories	Total	Fat	Sat-fat
Per ½-inch slice	119	10	1
Per loaf	2025	177	24

WHOLE-WHEAT BANANA RAISIN BREAD

This is a banana bread, not a banana cake. It is dense and delicious.

1 tablespoon yeast
Pinch of sugar
¼ cup warm water
1 cup unbleached white flour
2½ cups whole-wheat flour
1 teaspoon salt

2 ripe bananas, mashed
2 tablespoons molasses
1 tablespoon olive oil
1 cup nonfat buttermilk
¼ cup raisins (optional)

Combine yeast, sugar, and water in a large bowl or the bowl of a food processor. Let proof.

Mix in white flour, 2 cups of whole-wheat flour, and salt.

Mix bananas, molasses, oil, and buttermilk together and add to the flours. Add more whole-wheat flour to make a dough you can knead.

Knead 10 minutes or process 15 seconds or until dough is smooth and elastic, adding more whole-wheat flour if necessary.

Add raisins.

Place dough in a large oiled bowl. Rotate dough to cover surface with a film of olive oil. Cover bowl with a towel and let rise in a warm place for about 1 hour or until doubled in bulk.

Form loaf and place in a loaf pan greased with margarine. Cover with a towel and let rise in a warm place for about 1 hour or until doubled in bulk.

Preheat oven to 350°F.

Bake for 45–55 minutes or until golden brown and hollow when tapped.

Makes 1 large loaf

Calories	Total	Fat	Sat-fat
Per ½-inch slice	123	11	2
Per loaf	2099	195	30

OATMEAL BREAD

1 cup water	1 tablespoon active dry yeast
1 cup rolled oats	Pinch of sugar
2 tablespoons honey	⅓ cup warm water
1 tablespoon olive oil	2½ cups unbleached white flour
1 teaspoon salt	(approximately)

In a small saucepan, boil 1 cup water and add oats, honey, oil, and salt. Let cool.

Combine yeast, sugar, and ⅓ cup warm water in a large bowl or a food processor. Let proof.

Add 2 cups flour to the yeast mixture.

When oat mixture is warm, but *not hot*, add it to the flour mixture and knead dough 10 minutes or process 15 seconds or until dough is smooth and elastic, adding more flour if necessary.

Place dough in a large oiled bowl, cover with a towel, and let rise in a warm place for 1 hour or until doubled in bulk.

Form dough into a loaf and place in a loaf pan greased with margarine. Cover and let rise about 1 hour or until doubled in bulk.

Preheat oven to 350°F.

Bake for 45 minutes or until golden brown.

Makes 1 loaf

Calories	Total	Fat	Sat-fat
Per ½-inch slice	96	11	2
Per loaf	1630	196	31

CRANBERRY BREAD

This tart but sweet loaf lies somewhere between bread and cake. To make sure you can bake it all year round, buy extra packages of cranberries at Thanksgiving and freeze them.

1½ cups cranberries
2 cups unbleached white flour
1½ teaspoons baking powder
½ teaspoon baking soda
1 teaspoon salt

¾ cup sugar
¾ cup orange juice
1 tablespoon grated orange peel
2 tablespoons margarine
1 egg

Preheat oven to 350°F and grease a loaf pan with margarine.

Chop cranberries in a food processor or hand chopper. Set aside.

In a large bowl, or the bowl of your electric mixer, combine flour, baking powder, baking soda, salt, and sugar.

Add orange juice, orange rind, margarine, and egg and mix until well blended.

Mix in cranberries.

Pour batter into loaf pan and bake for 45–55 minutes or until cake tester comes out clean.

Makes 1 loaf

Calories	Total	Fat	Sat-fat
Per ½-inch slice	112	15	3
Per loaf	1899	254	55

ONION FLAT BREAD

1 tablespoon active dry yeast
1 pinch sugar
1 cup warm water
2½–3 cups unbleached white
   flour*

1 teaspoon + a few shakes salt
1 teaspoon margarine
1 cup chopped onions
1 teaspoon paprika

Place yeast, sugar, and water in large bowl or a food processor. Let proof.

Mix in 2 cups flour and salt. Knead for 10 minutes or process for 15 seconds, until smooth and elastic, adding flour if necessary.

Place dough in an oiled bowl, cover with a towel, and let rise in a warm place for an hour or until doubled in bulk.

Punch dough down and split in half. Let rest for 5 minutes.

Meanwhile, grease two 9-inch cake pans with margarine.

Melt margarine.

Press dough into cake pans.

Spread margarine over the tops and press onion into the surface.

Let rise about 45 minutes or until doubled in bulk.

Preheat oven to 450°F.

Sprinkle tops with paprika and a few shakes of salt.

Bake 20–25 minutes, until lightly browned.

Makes 2 loaves, 8 slices per loaf

Calories	Total	Fat	Sat-fat
Per slice	83	7	1
Per loaf	667	56	7

FOCACCIA GENOVESE

1 package active dry yeast
Pinch of sugar
1 cup warm water
2 teaspoons olive oil
1 teaspoon salt

2¾ cups unbleached white flour
1 teaspoon olive oil
1 teaspoon or more garlic slivers
1 teaspoon rosemary
¼ teaspoon salt

In a large bowl or food processor mix yeast, sugar, and water. Let proof.

---

*For a slightly different taste, use 1 cup of whole-wheat flour, along with 1½–2 cups unbleached white flour.

Stir in 2 teaspoons olive oil, 1 teaspoon salt, and 2 cups flour. Process 15 seconds or mix until smooth, adding more flour until dough is smooth and firm. Place in bowl lightly oiled with olive oil and cover with towel for about 1 hour or until doubled in size.

Grease 12-inch-round pizza pan with olive oil. Punch down dough and spread evenly over pan. Cover with towel and let rise 30 minutes.

Preheat oven to 375°F.

Brush dough with 1 teaspoon olive oil. Distribute garlic slivers evenly over surface and push them into the dough. Sprinkle dough evenly with rosemary and ¼ teaspoon salt.

Bake dough 30 minutes or until golden.

Makes 1 large flat loaf, 12 slices per loaf

Calories	Total	Fat	Sat-fat
Per slice	116	13	2
Per loaf	1390	156	22

WHOLE-WHEAT BAGELS

1 tablespoon active dry yeast
3 tablespoons sugar
1 cup warm water
1½ cups whole-wheat flour

1½ cups unbleached white flour
1 teaspoon salt
2 tablespoons olive oil

Mix yeast, sugar, and warm water in a large bowl or a food processor. Let proof.

Mix in whole-wheat flour, white flour, and salt.

Knead 8–10 minutes or process 15 seconds or until dough is smooth and elastic, adding more flour if necessary.

Place dough in a large oiled bowl, cover with a towel, and let rise in a warm place for 40 minutes. Punch down.

Roll into lengths about 5 inches long and ¾ inch wide. Pinch each into a circle to make a bagel.

Preheat oven to 350°F and grease cookie sheet with oil.

Fill a medium saucepan with water. Add oil and bring to a boil.

Drop a bagel into the boiling water.

When it rises to the top, remove it with a slotted spoon or spatula so the excess water can drip off.

Repeat this process with all the bagels.

Place bagels on cookie sheet and bake for 10 minutes.
Raise heat to 400°F and bake for 10 minutes more.

Makes 12 bagels
Calories per bagel: 115 Total; 23 Fat; 1 Sat-fat

PEPPERY BREADSTICKS

1 teaspoon peppercorns or
   freshly ground black pepper
1 tablespoon yeast
Pinch of sugar
¼ cup warm water
3 + cups unbleached white flour

1 teaspoon salt
1 cup warm water
1 teaspoon olive oil
1 egg white
1 tablespoon water

Place 1 teaspoon of peppercorns in food processor and process until coarsely ground or grind 1 teaspoon of freshly ground black pepper in large bowl.

Add yeast, sugar, and ¼ cup warm water. Let proof.

Mix in 3 cups of flour and salt.

Add oil and 1 cup warm water and knead about 10 minutes or process 15 seconds until dough is smooth and elastic, adding more flour if necessary.

Place dough in large oiled bowl, cover with a towel, and let rise for 1 hour or until doubled in bulk.

Push down dough. Let rest 5 minutes.

Preheat oven to 400°F.

Divide dough into 16 equal pieces.

Roll each piece into a long stick thickness and then divide into three breadsticks. Lay them on baking sheet. Let rest 15 minutes.

Beat egg white with a fork and mix with 1 tablespoon water. Paint breadsticks with egg white mixture.

Bake for 20–30 minutes or until browned.

Makes about 35 six-inch sticks
Calories per breadstick: 41 Total; 2 Fat; 0 Sat-fat

SESAME BREADSTICKS

Beware! These breadsticks are habit-forming.

1 teaspoon active dry yeast	⅔ cup nonfat skim milk
¼ cup warm water	1 tablespoon olive oil
⅔ cup whole-wheat flour	1 egg white
2 or more cups unbleached white flour	2 teaspoons water
1 teaspoon salt, optional	1 tablespoon sesame seeds

Place yeast and warm water in large bowl or a food processor. Let proof.

Mix in flours and salt.

Add milk and olive oil, and knead for 10 minutes or process until dough is smooth and elastic, adding more flour if necessary.

Place dough in ungreased bowl, cover with a towel, and let rise 1 hour.

Preheat oven to 400°F.

On a lightly floured surface, roll the dough into a ¼-inch-thick rectangle. One dimension of the rectangle should be the length of your breadsticks.

Cut the dough into ½-inch strips. (If you prefer thicker breadsticks, cut the dough into one-inch strips.)

Roll each strip in your palms to make a breadstick and lay it on an ungreased baking sheet. Place the sticks in a line, about a ½-inch apart.

Beat the egg white and water together and brush onto breadsticks.

Sprinkle sesame seeds evenly over breadsticks.

Count the breadsticks so you can calculate their sat-fat calories.

Bake for 20–30 minutes or until golden brown. Cool on a rack.

Makes about 35 six-inch sticks

To determine the total, fat, and sat-fat calories for each breadstick, divide the number of breadsticks you made into the following numbers:

Total calories: 1423   Total fat calories: 196   Total sat-fat calories: 30

For example, 30 sat-fat calories divided by 35 breadsticks = 0.86 sat-fat calories each.

OAT BRAN MUFFINS

Oat bran, a food rich in soluble fiber, has a modest effect on lowering blood cholesterol levels.

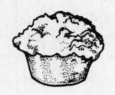

APPLE OAT MUFFINS

1½ cups oat bran
½ cup whole-wheat flour
3 tablespoons brown sugar
2 teaspoons baking powder
½ teaspoon salt
1 teaspoon cinnamon
½ cup apple juice

¼ cup skim milk
1 egg
2 tablespoons olive oil
2 tablespoons honey
1 cup apples, peeled, cored, and diced
2 tablespoons raisins

Preheat oven to 400°F. Grease a 12-cup muffin tin with margarine.

Combine oat bran, flour, brown sugar, baking powder, salt, and cinnamon and set aside.

In a large mixing bowl, combine apple juice, skim milk, egg, oil, and honey.

Add flour mixture, apples, and raisins and combine until just moistened.

Fill muffin tin and bake at 400°F for about 20 minutes or until golden brown and a cake tester comes out clean.

Makes 12 muffins
Calories per muffin: 125 Total; 32 Fat; 4 Sat-fat

Q MOTHER'S OAT BRAN MUFFINS

2¼ cups oat bran
¼ cup brown sugar
¼ cup chopped walnuts
¼ cup raisins
1 tablespoon baking powder

½ teaspoon salt
¾ cup skim milk
1 egg + 1 egg white, beaten
¼ cup honey
2 tablespoons olive oil

Preheat oven to 425°F. Grease a 12-cup muffin tin with margarine.

Combine oat bran, brown sugar, walnuts, raisins, baking powder, and salt.

Add skim milk, eggs, honey, and oil. Mix until ingredients are just moistened.

Fill muffin tin and bake for 15 minutes or until golden brown and a cake tester comes out clean.

Makes 12 muffins

Calories	Total	Fat	Sat-fat
Per muffin	160	49	6
Without walnuts	144	36	5

Q ORANGE OAT MUFFINS

Can you believe it? Another oat bran muffin.

1 cup oat bran
½ cup wheat germ
½ cup whole-wheat flour
3 tablespoons brown sugar
2 tablespoons grated orange
    peel

2 teaspoons baking powder
1 egg
2 tablespoons olive oil
½ cup orange juice
¼ cup skim milk
2 tablespoons raisins

Preheat oven to 400°F. Grease a 12-cup muffin tin with margarine.

Combine oat bran, wheat germ, whole-wheat flour, brown sugar, orange peel, and baking powder. Set aside.

In a mixing bowl, mix egg, oil, orange juice, and skim milk.

Mix in dry ingredients until just moistened.

Carefully mix in raisins.

Fill muffin tin and bake for 15 minutes or until golden brown and a cake tester comes out clean.

Makes 12 muffins
Calories per muffin: 110 Total; 34 Fat; 4 Sat-fat

Ⓠ APRICOT OAT MUFFINS

Yet another oat muffin. Healthy and delicious — a good snack or breakfast on the run.

½ cup orange juice
1 cup dried apricots, chopped (easily done in food processor)
¼ cup brown sugar
1 cup oat bran

¼ cup wheat germ
¾ cup whole-wheat flour
2 teaspoons baking powder
2 tablespoons olive oil
½ cup skim milk
1 egg

Preheat oven to 400°F. Grease a 12-cup muffin tin with margarine.

In a small saucepan, heat orange juice until boiling. Mix in apricots and brown sugar.

Remove saucepan from heat and cool apricot mixture slightly.

In a medium bowl, combine oat bran, wheat germ, whole-wheat flour, and baking powder. Set aside.

In a mixing bowl, beat together oil, skim milk, and egg.

Add dry ingredients and apricot–orange juice mixture to milk mixture and mix until just moistened.

Fill muffin tin and bake for 15 minutes or until golden brown and a cake tester comes out clean.

Makes 12 muffins
Calories per muffin: 135 Total; 32 Fat; 4 Sat-fat

BRAN MUFFINS

Wheat bran, made from the outer coverings of wheat kernels, is rich in vitamins, minerals, and insoluble dietary fiber. Insoluble dietary fiber promotes regularity and is believed to protect against colon cancer.

1 cup whole-wheat flour	1 cup buttermilk
1 cup wheat bran	1 egg, beaten
3 tablespoons brown sugar	3 tablespoons molasses
¼ teaspoon salt	2 tablespoons olive oil
1 teaspoon baking soda	⅓ cup raisins
½ teaspoon baking powder	

Preheat oven to 400°F. Grease a 12-cup muffin tin with margarine.
Combine whole-wheat flour, wheat bran, brown sugar, salt, baking soda, and baking powder. Set aside.
In a mixing bowl, mix buttermilk, egg, molasses, and oil.
Add dry ingredients and mix until just moistened.
Fold in raisins.
Fill muffin tin and bake for about 15 minutes or until golden brown and a cake tester comes out clean.

Makes 12 muffins
Calories per muffin: 116 Total; 23 Fat; 4 Sat-fat

BANANA-CARROT MUFFINS

Not an oat bran muffin but tasty anyway. Eat as a snack or for a light breakfast.

3 medium carrots	2 teaspoons double-acting
2 medium bananas	baking powder
¼ cup margarine	¼ teaspoon salt
½ cup brown sugar	¼ teaspoon baking soda
1 large egg	1 teaspoon vanilla
2 cups whole-wheat flour	½ cup chopped walnuts

Preheat oven to 350°F. Grease a 12-cup muffin tin with margarine.
Grate carrots (a food processor does this well) and set aside.
Mash bananas with a fork and set aside.

In a mixing bowl, cream the margarine and brown sugar until fluffy. Add egg and beat well.

Stir in the mashed bananas.

In a small bowl, mix together flour, baking powder, salt, and baking soda.

Add flour mixture to banana mixture. Do not overmix.

Add grated carrots, vanilla, and nuts and combine carefully.

Fill muffin tin and bake for 20–25 minutes or until a cake tester comes out clean.

Makes 12 muffins
Calories per muffin: 195 Total; 64 Fat; 11 Sat-fat

As an alternative, try substituting 1 cup oat bran + ½ cup wheat germ + ½ cup whole-wheat flour for the 2 cups of whole-wheat flour. Use only 2 tablespoons margarine and ¼ cup brown sugar.

Calories per muffin: 155 Total; 51 Fat; 8 Sat-fat

GINGERBREAD MUFFINS

These muffins taste like cake because they are cake. Use self-control! One muffin has only 9 sat-fat calories, but it has 59 calories of total fat.

1 cup unbleached white flour	¼ teaspoon allspice
¾ cup whole-wheat flour	¼ teaspoon grated nutmeg
¼ cup sugar	¾ cup buttermilk
¼ cup brown sugar	⅓ cup olive oil
1 teaspoon baking soda	1 egg
¼ teaspoon salt	1 egg white
1 teaspoon ginger	¼ cup light unsulphured
1 teaspoon cinnamon	molasses
¼ teaspoon cloves	

Preheat oven to 400°F and grease a 12-cup muffin tin with margarine.

Combine flours, sugars, baking soda, salt, and spices in a large bowl. Set aside.

In a large mixing bowl, combine buttermilk, oil, egg, egg white, and molasses.

Add flour mixture to buttermilk mixture. Do not overmix.

Pour into cups of muffin pan and bake for 15 minutes, or until cake tester comes out clean.

Makes 12 muffins
Calories per muffin: 177 Total; 59 Fat; 9 Sat-fat

BUTTERMILK PANCAKES

Breakfast need not be a problem for those watching their sat-fat intake. In addition to the preceding bread and muffin recipes, try these pancakes, waffles, and the French toast that follows.

Instead of using sour cream (270 sat-fat calories per cup) or whole milk (45 sat-fat calories per cup), make your pancakes with buttermilk (0–12 sat-fat calories per cup). Buttermilk enhances the taste of waffles and pancakes. These delicious buttermilk pancakes will hardly make a dent in your sat-fat budget.

Use maple syrup or powdered sugar to sweeten pancakes and waffles. Butter adds only unneeded sat-fat calories.

HINT: Use a cast-iron griddle, and you will need little or no margarine to keep your pancakes from sticking to the surface.

½ cup unbleached white flour
¼ cup whole-wheat flour
½ teaspoon baking powder
½ teaspoon baking soda
½ cup nonfat buttermilk*

¼–½ cup skim milk*
1 egg white, lightly beaten
2 teaspoons olive oil (optional)
Margarine to grease grill

In a large bowl, combine the flours, baking powder, and baking soda.

Mix in buttermilk and skim milk, egg white, and oil. Do not overmix.

Lightly grease a hot griddle or skillet with margarine, making sure you keep track of the amount you use.

For each pancake, spread a tablespoon of batter on the griddle. When the pancake solidifies and the edges come away from the grid-

*For equally delicious pancakes, substitute ½ cup nonfat yogurt + ½ cup skim milk for the ½ cup nonfat buttermilk + ¼ cup skim milk.

dle, turn the pancake. The bottom should be golden brown. Cook until other side is also golden.

Makes about 16 pancakes

Calories	Total	Fat	Sat-fat
Total batter	495	90	13
Per pancake	31	13	1
With no added oil			
Total batter	415	10	1
Per pancake	26	1	0

If you used more than 1 teaspoon of margarine to grease your griddle, for each pancake add 6 total calories, 6 fat calories, and 1 sat-fat calorie for each additional teaspoon.

BUTTERMILK WAFFLES

1 egg white at room
  temperature
1 cup whole-wheat flour
1 cup unbleached white flour
2 teaspoons baking powder

½ teaspoon salt
1 cup buttermilk
1 cup skim milk
2 teaspoons olive oil

Preheat waffle iron.

Beat egg white until stiff but not dry. Set aside.

In a medium bowl, combine whole-wheat flour, white flour, baking powder, and salt.

Add buttermilk and skim milk. *Do not overmix.*

Fold in egg white. Fold in oil.

---

*Because waffle irons come in many sizes, this recipe may make more or less than 8 waffle squares. Divide 1102 by the number of waffle squares you make to figure out the total calories per square (for example, 1102 ÷ 8 = 138). Divide 16 by the number of waffle squares to figure out the sat-fat calories per square (for example, 16 ÷ 8 = 2). Divide 107 by the number of waffle squares to figure out the fat calories per square (for example, 107 ÷ 16 = 13).

Place batter on waffle iron in amounts specified by your waffle-iron instructions. Cook accordingly.

Makes 8 Belgian waffles

Calories	Total	Fat	Sat-fat
Total batter	1102	107	16
Per square*	138	13	2

CINNAMON FRENCH TOAST

2 egg whites
3 tablespoons skim milk
½ teaspoon vanilla
½ teaspoon ground cinnamon
Pinch of grated nutmeg

3 slices whole-wheat bread or
 French bread
2 teaspoons margarine
 (optional)

In a shallow dish, mix egg whites, skim milk, vanilla, cinnamon, and nutmeg.

Soak both sides of bread in mixture.

Heat a large frying pan or cast-iron griddle.* Spread margarine over it if necessary.

Add bread. Reduce heat to medium.

Turn bread after 2 minutes. Cook until golden brown and crispy.

3 servings

Calories per serving:	Total	Fat	Sat-fat
	106	29	8
Without margarine	86	9	4

---

*Use a cast-iron griddle, which requires little or no margarine to keep the French toast from sticking, to reduce the sat-fat and total fat even more.

24 DESSERTS

YOU MIGHT think dessert would be the most difficult part of the meal to make low in saturated fat. This is not true. There are many desserts that not only are scrumptious and beautiful but fit perfectly into a low-sat-fat diet. (That is not to say they are necessarily low in total fat — so go easy.)

The trick to keeping desserts low in saturated fat is to substitute nonfat yogurt, buttermilk, or skim milk for sour cream, sweet cream, or whole milk and margarine or oil for butter; never to use lard, shortening, palm, or coconut oil; and to reduce eggs to no more than one and substitute egg whites for additional eggs.

You may be surprised that we use olive oil in making these desserts. Olive oil is the oil of choice because it lowers LDL-cholesterol without lowering HDL-cholesterol. Try using a mild-tasting olive oil in your baked goods. Only your arteries will be able to detect a difference.

You will notice that we recommend grated nutmeg in many recipes. Buy whole nutmegs at your grocery store and simply grate one when you need nutmeg in a recipe. The advantage is that each time you grate one it is fresh and thus has the taste it is supposed to have.

We recommend unbleached white flour because when a flour is bleached, it loses many of its important nutritional qualities.

APPLESAUCE CAKE

1 cup raisins
1/2 cup water
1 cup chunky applesauce
1/3 cup margarine
1/2 cup sugar
1 egg

1 teaspoon vanilla
1 1/2 cups unbleached white flour
1 teaspoon baking soda
1/2 teaspoon cinnamon
1/8 teaspoon ground cloves
1/2 cup chopped walnuts

Preheat oven to 350°F. Grease a loaf pan with margarine.

In a small saucepan, combine raisins and water. Bring to a boil. Reduce heat, cover, and simmer for 1 minute.

Remove from heat. Stir in applesauce. Cool to lukewarm.

Cream margarine and sugar. Beat in egg and vanilla.

Combine flour, baking soda, cinnamon, and cloves and mix into batter.

Add applesauce mixture and nuts.

Pour into greased loaf pan and bake for 1 hour or until a cake tester comes out clean.

Cool for 10 minutes before removing from pan.

Makes 10 slices
Calories per slice: 250 Total; 89 Fat; 14 Sat-fat

APPLE CAKE

A moist, hearty cake that is easy to make.

3/4 cup brown sugar
1/2 cup olive oil
1 teaspoon vanilla
1 egg
1 egg white
3/4 cup unbleached white flour
1 cup whole-wheat flour

1/2 teaspoon salt
1 teaspoon baking soda
1 1/2 teaspoons cinnamon
1/4 teaspoon grated nutmeg
4 cups Delicious apples, peeled
  and cut into chunks
1/2 cup chopped walnuts

Preheat oven to 350°F. Grease an 8-inch springform pan with margarine and dust with flour.

In an electric mixer, beat together brown sugar and oil.

Add vanilla, egg, and egg white and beat until smooth.

Add flours, salt, baking soda, cinnamon, and nutmeg and beat until smooth.

With a large (wooden) spoon or rubber spatula, mix in apples and walnuts. The batter will be *very* sticky and stiff.

Spoon batter into pan and bake for 50–60 minutes or until a cake tester comes out clean.

Makes 12 slices
Calories per slice: 220 Total; 114 Fat; 13 Sat-fat

BANANA CAKE

This banana cake is out of the ordinary. Rich and full-bodied.

1 cup whole-wheat flour	1/3 cup olive oil
1/2 cup unbleached white flour	1/2 cup brown sugar
1/4 cup wheat germ	3/4 teaspoon vanilla
1 teaspoon cinnamon	1 egg
1/2 teaspoon grated nutmeg	3 bananas, mashed
2 teaspoons baking powder	1/2 cup chopped walnuts
1/4 teaspoon baking soda	5 prunes, chopped
1/4 teaspoon salt	

Preheat oven to 350°F. Grease a loaf pan with margarine.

Mix flours, wheat germ, cinnamon, nutmeg, baking powder, baking soda, and salt and set aside.

In an electric mixer, mix oil and brown sugar. Add vanilla and egg and mix well.

Add bananas and blend until smooth. Mix in flour mixture.

Fold in nuts and prunes.

Pour batter into loaf pan and bake for 45–60 minutes or until a cake tester comes out clean.

Makes 10 slices
Calories per slice: 263 Total; 110 Fat; 12 Sat-fat

LEMON LOAF

Crunchy, lemony goodness.

1 cup walnuts*
½ cup sugar
½ cup margarine
Grated peel of 1 lemon
2 cups unbleached white flour
¼ teaspoon salt

2 teaspoons baking powder
1 teaspoon baking soda
¾ cup buttermilk
¼ cup fresh lemon juice
2 tablespoons fresh lemon juice
3 tablespoons sugar

Preheat oven to 375°F. Grease a loaf pan with margarine.

Chop walnuts with food processor or nut chopper. Set aside.

Cream ½ cup sugar and margarine with mixer.

Add grated lemon peel and mix until smooth.

Mix together flour, salt, baking powder, and baking soda and set aside.

Mix buttermilk and lemon juice and set aside.

Add flour mixture to creamed mixture alternately with buttermilk mixture. *Do not overmix.*

Stir in walnuts.

Pour into loaf pan and bake for 30–45 minutes or until a cake tester comes out clean.

Let cool in pan 10 minutes.

In a small saucepan, combine lemon juice and 3 tablespoons sugar and stir over low heat until sugar dissolves.

Pierce top of cake with a fork or skewer. Spoon lemon-sugar mixture into holes.

Let cool for easy slicing. (A whiff of lemon loaf may cause your impatient family to force you to slice the cake warm!)

Makes 10 slices

Calories per slice:	*Total*	*Fat*	*Sat-fat*
	290	142	21
Without walnuts	215	76	15

---

*Lemon Loaf is delicious even without the walnuts. Eliminate walnuts and reduce total calories to 215, fat calories to 76, sat-fat calories to 15, per slice.

PHILIP WAGENAAR'S RAISIN-GINGER-ORANGE CAKE

This is cake disguised as a quick bread. It is a sweet blending of textures and flavors. We are fortunate that Dr. Wagenaar occasionally takes time off from his biking expeditions around the world to bake.

1¾ cups unbleached white flour
2 teaspoons baking powder
½ teaspoon baking soda
½ teaspoon salt
⅓ cup margarine
¾ cup sugar
1 tablespoon grated orange peel*

1 tablespoon grated lemon peel*
4 egg whites
½ cup nonfat milk
½ teaspoon orange extract
2 tablespoons crystallized ginger**
2 cups raisins

Preheat oven to 350°F and lightly grease a loaf pan.
Combine flour, baking powder, baking soda, and salt. Set aside.
Cream together margarine, sugar, and orange and lemon peels.
Add egg whites, two at a time, beating well after each addition.
Combine milk and orange extract.
Add milk and flour mixtures alternately to batter and beat just to mix.
Stir in ginger and raisins.
Pour batter into loaf pan and bake for 45–60 minutes or until cake tester comes out clean.

Makes 12 slices
Calories per slice: 236 Total; 43 Fat; 9 Sat-fat

---

*A dandy way to grate orange or lemon peel is to chop a few slices of the peel in a mini-chopper. Be sure to wash the fruit thoroughly before you cut the slices.
**Available in the spice section of most supermarkets

PUMPKIN CAKE

1¼ cups unbleached white flour
½ cup rye flour
1 teaspoon baking soda
1 teaspoon baking powder
½ teaspoon salt
1½ teaspoons cinnamon
1 teaspoon cardamom

½ cup raisins
1 cup pumpkin purée
¾ cup brown sugar
6 tablespoons margarine
¼ cup skim milk
1 egg
1 egg white

Preheat oven to 350°F. Grease a loaf pan with margarine and lightly flour.

Combine flours, baking soda, baking powder, salt, cinnamon, cardamom, and raisins. Set aside.

In a large mixing bowl, mix together pumpkin purée, brown sugar, and margarine. Add skim milk, whole egg, and egg white and mix until smooth.

Stir in flour mixture.

Pour batter into loaf pan and bake for 45–60 minutes or until a cake tester comes out clean.

Makes 18 ½-inch slices
Calories per slice: 128 Total; 34 Fat; 7 Sat-fat

THE YORK BLUEBERRY CAKE

½ cup brown sugar
½ cup chopped walnuts
1 teaspoon cinnamon
2 cups unbleached white flour
1 teaspoon baking soda
½ teaspoon salt
2 cups blueberries

½ cup margarine
¾ cup sugar
1 egg
2 egg whites
1 cup nonfat yogurt
1 teaspoon vanilla

Preheat oven to 350°F and grease a 13 × 9-inch baking pan with margarine.

Combine brown sugar, nuts, and cinnamon and set aside.

In a large bowl, combine flour, baking soda, and salt.

Mix ¼ cup of the flour mixture with the blueberries and set aside.

In a large mixing bowl, cream margarine and sugar until fluffy.

Beat in egg and egg whites.

Stir in yogurt and vanilla.

Add remaining flour to batter and beat until smooth.

Stir in floured blueberries.

Spread half of the batter into the baking pan and sprinkle half of the brown sugar mixture over it.

Cover with remaining batter (it will barely cover the entire surface) and top with remaining brown sugar mixture.

Bake for 40–45 minutes until cake tester comes out clean.

Makes 24 squares
Calories per square: 141 Total; 46 Fat; 8 Sat-fat

CARROT CAKE SANS OEUFS

¾ cup sugar
1 cup grated carrot (food processor grates quickly)
1 cup raisins
1 teaspoon cinnamon
1 teaspoon grated nutmeg
1 teaspoon ground cloves

1½ cups water
3 tablespoons margarine
2 cups flour
2 teaspoons baking soda
¼ teaspoon salt
1 cup chopped walnuts

Preheat oven to 325°F. Grease a 13 × 9-inch baking pan with margarine.

In a small saucepan, combine sugar, carrot, raisins, cinnamon, nutmeg, cloves, water, and margarine. Bring to a boil. Reduce heat, and simmer for 5 minutes.

Pour into a mixing bowl and cool to lukewarm.

Add flour, baking soda, and salt. Mix well.

Stir in walnuts.

Pour into pan and bake for 45–60 minutes or until a cake tester comes out clean.

Makes 24 squares
Calories per square: 122 Total; 40 Fat; 5 Sat-fat

GINGER CAKE WITH PEAR SAUCE

Ginger Cake tastes good with or without pear sauce.

⅓ cup margarine	½ teaspoon salt
2 tablespoons maple syrup	1 teaspoon cinnamon
⅓ cup sugar	1½ teaspoons ginger
1 egg	½ teaspoon allspice
1½ cups unbleached white flour	¼ teaspoon grated nutmeg
½ teaspoon baking powder	1 cup buttermilk
½ teaspoon baking soda	

Pear Sauce

2 cups water	3 ripe Anjou or other pears
¼ cup sugar	1 tablespoon sugar

The Ginger Cake

Preheat oven to 350°F. Grease an 8 × 8-inch baking pan with margarine.

Cream margarine, maple syrup, and sugar until smooth.

Mix in egg.

Combine flour, baking powder, baking soda, salt, cinnamon, ginger, allspice, and nutmeg. Add to batter, alternating with buttermilk. Mix until smooth. Pour batter into baking pan and bake for 30 minutes or until a cake tester comes out clean.

Meanwhile, make the pear sauce.

The Pear Sauce

In a large saucepan, combine water and ¼ cup sugar and bring to a simmer.

Poach pears in simmering sugar water for about 10 minutes or until soft.

Drain pears and purée them with 1 tablespoon sugar in a blender until smooth.

Serve over cooled cake.

Makes 9 squares

Calories	Total	Fat	Sat-fat
Per square	183	63	14
with Pear Sauce	194	63	14

PINEAPPLE POUND CAKE

This pound cake will remind you of cakes that are made with a pound of butter and 6 eggs. Nonfat yogurt and margarine make the difference in the saturated fat content of our pound cakes, but not in their taste and appearance.

2½ cups flour
1½ teaspoons baking soda
½ teaspoon salt
1 can (20 oz) pineapple chunks
   in heavy syrup
½ cup margarine

¾ cup sugar
3 egg whites
1 tablespoon grated orange peel
1 teaspoon vanilla
1 cup nonfat yogurt
¼ cup sugar

Preheat oven to 375°F. Grease a 10-inch tube pan with margarine.
Mix flour, baking soda, and salt and set aside.
Drain syrup from can of pineapple, reserving ¼ cup.
Cream margarine and ¾ cup of the sugar.
Add egg whites, orange peel, and vanilla and beat well.
Add flour mixture and yogurt alternately to sugar mixture and mix well.
Pour half the batter into pan. Spread 1 cup (or more) of pineapple evenly over batter. Cover with remaining batter.
Bake for 40 minutes or until a cake tester comes out clean.
Let the cake cool for 5 minutes.
Meanwhile, in a small saucepan, combine ¼ cup sugar with reserved pineapple syrup.
Bring to a boil, reduce heat, and simmer for 3–5 minutes or until syrup thickens slightly.
Remove cake from pan. Pierce it with a fork and spoon pineapple juice mixture into holes and over the top of the cake.

Makes 16 slices
Calories per slice: 177 Total; 47 Fat; 9 Sat-fat

CHEESECAKE!

I never believed you could make a cheesecake low in fat. With this recipe I have become a believer. While not *exactly* the same as real cheesecake, this low-fat version is delicious.

NOTE: Start this cake more than a day in advance because it takes 24 hours to make the yogurt cheese and then you need to chill the cake for a few hours after you bake it.

Yogurt Cheese (page 347), made from 2 32-oz containers vanilla nonfat yogurt

Graham Cracker Crust* (page 400), made with 1 tablespoon or no margarine

Filling

Yogurt Cheese	2 tablespoons cornstarch
½ cup sugar	5 egg whites

The day before you plan to serve the cheesecake, prepare the yogurt cheese. But instead of draining the yogurt overnight, drain it for a full 24 hours to create a cheesecake consistency.

When the yogurt cheese is ready, prepare the Graham Cracker Crust in a 9-inch pie plate.

Preheat oven to 325°F.

Place yogurt cheese in a large bowl. In a small bowl, mix sugar and cornstarch together and then add to yogurt cheese. Blend. Mix in egg whites. Blend well, but do not beat air into the batter.

Pour batter into crust and bake about 60–70 minutes, until center is set. Cool slightly and then refrigerate until chilled. You may top with fruit topping.

Makes 12 slices

Calories per slice:	Total	Fat	Sat-fat
With crust made with 1 tablespoon margarine	120	16	4
With crust made with no fat	112	8	3

---

*If you use a commercial crust, divide total, fat, and sat-fat calories of crust by 12 and add to filling (70 total calories/slice and no fat) to determine amounts per slice.

ORANGE CAKE

1½ cups unbleached white flour   ½ cup sugar
2 teaspoons baking powder   ½ cup orange juice
¼ teaspoon salt   3 egg whites
½ cup margarine   2 tablespoons orange juice

Preheat oven to 350°F. Grease a loaf pan with margarine.

Combine flour, baking powder, and salt. Set aside.

In a large mixing bowl, beat margarine until soft. Gradually add sugar until creamy.

Add flour mixture, alternating with ½ cup orange juice, until batter is smooth.

In another bowl, whip egg whites until stiff but not dry.

Fold egg whites into batter.

Pour batter into loaf pan and bake for 40–50 minutes or until a cake tester comes out clean.

Cool in pan for 10 minutes.

Poke holes in top of cake. Pour 2 tablespoons orange juice into holes.

Makes 10 slices
Calories per slice: 180 Total; 74 Fat; 15 Sat-fat

COCOA ANGEL FOOD CAKE

¾ cup cake flour   1 teaspoon cream of tartar
¼ cup unsweetened cocoa   1 teaspoon vanilla
1¼ cups sugar   ½ teaspoon almond extract
1¼–1½ cups egg whites (about
   10–12)

Preheat oven to 350°F.

Sift together three times: cake flour, cocoa, and ¼ cup of the sugar. Set aside.

Sift remaining 1 cup sugar and set aside.

Whip egg whites until foamy. Add cream of tartar. Continue beating until whites are stiff but not dry.

Fold in sugar a little at a time.

Fold in vanilla and almond extract.

Sift flour-cocoa mixture over batter (¼ at a time) and fold into batter.

Pour batter into an ungreased 10-inch tube pan and bake for 45 minutes or until a cake tester comes out clean.

Invert the tube pan and let cake cool.

Makes 12 slices
Calories per slice: 119 Total; <1 Fat; 0 Sat-fat

MARBLE CAKE

To make a special occasion even more special, bake a marble cake and ice it with Cocoa Frosting (page 394).

3½ cups cake flour
½ teaspoon baking soda
2½ teaspoons baking powder
½ cup buttermilk
½ cup skim milk
1 teaspoon vanilla
½ cup margarine
¾ cup sugar
1 egg yolk

1 tablespoon unsweetened cocoa
1 tablespoon sugar
1 teaspoon cinnamon
⅛ teaspoon ground cloves
⅛ teaspoon baking soda
1 tablespoon margarine
4 egg whites, at room temperature

Preheat oven to 375°F. Grease a 10-inch tube pan with margarine.

Combine cake flour, baking soda, and baking powder and set aside.

Combine buttermilk, skim milk, and vanilla and set aside.

In a large mixing bowl, cream ½ cup margarine and ¾ cup sugar. Mix in egg yolk.

Add half the flour mixture and half the milk mixture and stir until smooth.

Add remaining flour mixture and milk mixture and stir until smooth.

Combine cocoa, cinnamon, cloves, baking soda, and 1 tablespoon sugar.

In a small saucepan, melt 1 tablespoon margarine and blend into cocoa-sugar mixture. Blend 1 cup of batter into cocoa mixture.

Whip egg whites until stiff but not dry.

Fold ⅔ of the egg whites into plain batter and remaining ⅓ egg whites into cocoa batter.

Pour plain batter into tube pan.

Drop spoonfuls of cocoa batter onto plain batter.

With a knife, swirl the cocoa batter through the plain batter.

Bake for 30 minutes or until a cake tester comes out clean.

Makes 12 slices
Calories per slice: 238 Total; 75 Fat; 15 Sat-fat

DIVINE BUTTERMILK POUND CAKE

You will not believe how light and fine-grained this cake is.

1¾ cup cake flour	¾ cup sugar
½ teaspoon baking soda	1 egg + 2 egg whites
1 teaspoon baking powder	½ teaspoon vanilla
¼ teaspoon salt	¼ teaspoon almond extract
½ cup margarine	¾ cup buttermilk

Preheat oven to 375°F and grease an 8-inch springform pan with margarine.

Combine flour, baking soda, baking powder, and salt, and set aside.

In an electric mixer, cream margarine and sugar.

Add egg and egg whites, vanilla, and almond extract, and mix until smooth.

Add flour mixture and buttermilk, and mix until smooth.

Pour into springform pan and bake for 30–40 minutes, or until cake tester comes out clean.

When cool, frost it with our number-one favorite choice, Mocha Frosting (page 395). The following Walnut Glaze also tastes good.

Walnut Glaze

¼ cup brown sugar	½ teaspoon margarine
½ tablespoon cornstarch	1 tablespoon chopped walnuts
¼ cup cold water	

In a small saucepan, mix together brown sugar and cornstarch. Slowly add water, making sure mixture is smooth.

At medium-high temperature, stir for 3–4 minutes, until mixture is thick and begins to boil.

Stir in margarine and walnuts. Spoon over cool cake.

Makes 12 slices

Calories per slice:	Total	Fat	Sat-fat
	175	66	13
With Mocha Frosting	225	81	18
With Walnut Glaze	199	71	14

SPICE CAKE

2⅓ cups cake flour
1½ teaspoons baking powder
½ teaspoon baking soda
1 teaspoon grated nutmeg
1 teaspoon cinnamon
½ teaspoon cloves
½ teaspoon salt

¾ cup margarine
1 cup sugar
1 egg yolk
1 cup less 2 tablespoons
  buttermilk
3 egg whites

Preheat oven to 350°F and grease 10-inch tube pan with margarine.

Mix together flour, baking powder, baking soda, nutmeg, cinnamon, cloves, and salt, and set aside.

In a large mixing bowl, cream margarine and sugar until fluffy.

Mix in 1 egg yolk.

Add dry mixture alternately with buttermilk.

Whip 3 egg whites until stiff but not dry and fold them into batter.

Pour into prepared pan and bake for 45–60 minutes, or until cake tester comes out clean.

Cool and ice with Cocoa Frosting (page 394) or Mocha Frosting (page 395).

Makes 12 slices

Calories per slice:	Total	Fat	Sat-fat
	238	96	19
With frosting	288	118	24

CHOCOLATEY-CHOCOLATE COCOA CAKE

3 tablespoons unsweetened cocoa
4 tablespoons margarine
1 cup boiling water
1 cup sugar
1 teaspoon vanilla

1 egg yolk
1 teaspoon baking soda
½ cup buttermilk
2 cups unbleached white flour
1 teaspoon baking powder
2 egg whites

Cocoa Frosting

3 tablespoons margarine
3 tablespoons unsweetened cocoa

1 teaspoon vanilla
1½ cups confectioners' sugar
1 tablespoon skim milk

Preheat oven to 350°F. Grease a 10-inch tube pan with margarine and dust with flour.

Place cocoa and margarine in a large mixing bowl and add boiling water.

When margarine is melted, stir in sugar and vanilla and beat until smooth.

Stir in egg yolk and beat until smooth.

Stir baking soda into buttermilk. Add to batter and mix well.

Add flour and baking powder and mix well.

Whip egg whites until stiff but not dry and fold into batter.

Pour batter into pan and bake on middle rack of oven for 40–50 minutes or until a cake tester comes out clean.

Cool. Then make cocoa frosting.

The Cocoa Frosting

In a mixing bowl, blend margarine and cocoa.
Add vanilla.
Beat in confectioners' sugar.
Add milk.
If too stiff, add more milk. If too runny, add more sugar.
Frost top and sides of cake.

Makes 10 slices
Calories per slice: 273 Total; 71 Fat; 13 Sat-fat

MOCHA CAKE

A rich, dark chocolate cake with a taste of mocha.

1¾ cups unbleached white flour
⅓ cup unsweetened cocoa
1 teaspoon baking soda
½ teaspoon baking powder
¼ teaspoon salt
1 teaspoon cinnamon
½ cup margarine

¾ cup sugar
1 egg
1 egg white
⅔ cup buttermilk
⅔ cup brewed coffee
1 teaspoon vanilla

Mocha Frosting

2 tablespoons margarine
1 cup confectioners' sugar
2 tablespoons unsweetened cocoa

Dash of salt
1 tablespoon brewed coffee
¼ teaspoon vanilla

Preheat oven to 350°F. Grease an 8 × 8-inch baking pan or an 8-inch springform pan with margarine.

Combine flour, cocoa, baking soda, baking powder, salt, and cinnamon. Set aside.

In a large mixing bowl, cream margarine and sugar.

Add egg and egg white and beat well.

Combine buttermilk, coffee, and vanilla.

Alternately add flour mixture and buttermilk mixture to sugar mixture, beating until smooth. Pour into baking pan and bake for 40 minutes or until a cake tester comes out clean.

Cool. Then make the frosting.

The Mocha Frosting

Cream margarine. Add confectioners' sugar. Beat until smooth.

Add cocoa, salt, coffee, and vanilla. Beat until smooth.

Add more sugar if frosting is too thin.

Add more coffee if frosting is too thick.

Frost top and sides of cake.

Makes 16 squares

Calories per square:	Total	Fat	Sat-fat
	140	50	10
With icing	174	61	13

CINNAMON SUGAR COFFEE CAKE

This coffee cake is moist and delicious.

1½ cups unbleached white flour
1½ teaspoons baking powder
1 teaspoon baking soda
½ teaspoon salt
¼ cup brown sugar
¾ cup sugar
1 teaspoon cinnamon
½ cup margarine
1 egg
1 egg white
1 teaspoon vanilla
1 cup nonfat yogurt

Preheat oven to 350°F. Grease an 8-inch springform pan with margarine.

Combine flour, baking powder, baking soda, and salt together in a bowl. Set aside.

In small bowl combine ¼ cup brown sugar, ¼ cup of the granulated sugar, and cinnamon and set aside.

Cream the remaining ½ cup sugar with margarine until light and fluffy.

Add egg and egg white and vanilla and mix until batter is smooth.

Add flour and yogurt alternately and mix until batter is smooth.

Pour batter into baking pan.

Pour sugar mixture on top of the batter and, with a knife, swirl the sugar into the batter.

Bake for 45–50 minutes or until cake tester comes out clean.

Makes 8 slices
Calories per slice: 299 Total; 98 Fat; 20 Sat-fat

NUTMEG TORTE

This is a very rich cake. It is rather silly-looking because it is so flat, but it tastes delicious.

¾ cup brown sugar
1 cup unbleached white flour
¼ cup margarine
1 cup nonfat yogurt
1 egg

½ teaspoon freshly grated nutmeg
1 teaspoon baking soda
1 walnut half

Grease an 8-inch springform pan with margarine and preheat oven to 350°F.

With pastry blender or your fingers combine sugar, flour, and margarine to make a crumbly mixture.

Press 1¼ cups of the crumbs into the bottom of the pan. Reserve the rest.

Combine yogurt, egg, nutmeg, and baking soda.

Stir yogurt mixture into reserved crumb mixture to make a batter. Pour batter over crumb crust.

Bake for about 40–50 minutes or until cake tester comes out clean.

Place walnut half in the center of the torte.

Makes 8 slices
Calories per slice: 204 Total; 54 Fat; 11 Sat-fat

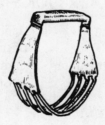

TANTE NANCY'S APPLE CRUMB CAKE

Apple Crumb Cake is luscious. The crust is thick, crunchy, and sweet. The slightly tart apples melt in your mouth.

2–2½ pounds tart apples*
   (about 6–7 large), peeled,
   cored, and sliced
⅓ cup water
¼ cup sugar

2 cups unbleached white flour
¾ cup sugar
1½ teaspoons baking powder
½ cup margarine
1 egg yolk

Preheat oven to 350°F. Grease an 8-inch springform pan with margarine.

In a large pot, cook apple slices with water and ¼ cup sugar until apples are tender but not mushy. Drain and reserve.

In a small bowl, mix flour, ¾ cup sugar, and baking powder.

With a pastry blender, cut in ½ cup margarine.

Cut in egg yolk.

Reserve 1 cup of flour mixture for the topping. Press remainder into bottom and sides of pan.

Spoon drained apples into pan.

Cover with reserved topping.

Bake for about 1 hour or until crust is golden brown.

Makes 12 slices
Calories per slice: 220 Total; 60 Fat; 14 Sat-fat

PIE, TART, OR QUICHE CRUST

1 ice cube
⅓–½ cup cold water
1⅓ cups unbleached white flour
2 tablespoons sugar
Pinch of salt
3 tablespoons tub margarine,
   frozen

½ tablespoon olive oil
(For nonsweet pie dough,
   eliminate sugar and add ¾
   teaspoon salt)

Place ice cube in the cold water. Set aside.

---

*You can use as few as 5 large apples, but more is better. Or substitute 2–2½ pounds peaches or 4 cups blueberries.

Place 1½ cups flour in food processor fitted with steel blade or in a mixing bowl.

Add sugar and salt and mix until well blended.

Cut margarine into ½-inch pieces and add to flour mixture.

Process briefly or use pastry blender until flour mixture resembles coarse meal or oatmeal flakes.

Add oil and ⅓ cup of ice water (without ice cube).

Process 2–3 seconds or blend until dough begins to collect into a ball. *Do not overprocess.*

If dough is too dry, carefully add a few drops more cold water and blend briefly.

Remove ball of dough, lightly flour, and wrap in wax paper. Place in a plastic bag and chill in refrigerator for at least 2 hours. (Dough will keep 2–3 days in refrigerator or for several months in freezer.)

To Bake

Preheat oven to 450°F. Grease an 8- or 9-inch pie or quiche pan with margarine.

On a piece of wax paper, roll dough into an ⅛-inch-thick circle slightly larger than the pie pan.

Turn over the wax paper so the dough is facing downward and lay it over the pan. Peel wax paper off the dough.

Gently push the dough to conform to the shape of the pan.

Trim excess dough, except for about ¼ inch above the rim of the pan. Form a ridge.

Spread margarine on a piece of aluminum foil larger than the pan. Set foil, greased-side down, onto pie dough.

Fill with dried beans or aluminum pie weights to keep the crust from bubbling up.

Bake for 7–8 minutes.

Remove foil and beans. Prick crust with a fork to release air bubbles.

For partially baked pie crust, bake 3–4 minutes more or until crust is just beginning to brown and shrink from the edges.

For fully baked pie crust, bake 7–10 minutes more or until lightly browned.

Calories	Total	Fat	Sat-fat
Sweet pie crust	1051	344	62
Nonsweet pie crust	961	344	62

GRAHAM CRACKER CRUST

Not only do Honey Graham Crackers make a delicious cookie, Honey Graham Cracker crumbs make a delicious pie crust, particularly for lemon meringue or Key lime pie. Commercial graham crackers, graham cracker crumbs, and ready-to-bake graham cracker crusts are often made with lard or hydrogenated vegetable oil. Make your own using the Honey Graham Crackers recipe on page 408.

8 homemade graham crackers crumbled (1¼ cups)	1 teaspoon sugar
	1 tablespoon margarine

Preheat oven to 375°F.
In food processor or blender, finely crush 8 graham crackers.
Combine crumbs and sugar and pour into pie plate.
Melt margarine and mix into crumbs.
Press crumbs into pie plate to make a crust.
Bake 8 minutes, or until lightly browned.

Makes one pie crust
Calories per crust: 600 Total; 186 Fat; 34 Sat-fat

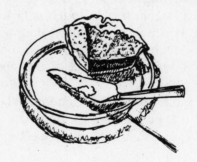

KEY LIME PIE

This pie is as pretty to look at as it is delightful to eat. It never fails to wow guests and please the most discriminating palate. Many Key lime pies call for 3 egg yolks and butter. You will use only 1 egg yolk and margarine to create this divine dessert. You can use lemon juice instead of lime juice and call this Lemon Meringue Pie.

Partially baked sweet pie crust (pages 398–99) or
    Graham Cracker Crust (above)

Filling

¾ cup sugar
¼ cup unbleached white flour
3 tablespoons cornstarch
¼ teaspoon salt

½–⅔ cup fresh lime juice +
   water to equal 2¼ cups
1 egg yolk
1 teaspoon margarine

Meringue

5 egg whites, at room
   temperature

¼ teaspoon cream of tartar
½ cup + 2 tablespoons sugar

The Filling

In a medium saucepan, thoroughly mix sugar, flour, cornstarch, and salt.

Add ¼ cup lime water and blend into a smooth paste.

Add remaining lime water and mix until smooth.

Stir filling over medium heat until it begins to boil and thicken. Remove saucepan from heat.

In a small bowl, combine egg yolk with a small amount of filling and blend until smooth. Mix back into filling in saucepan. (This step is important. If you were to add the egg yolk directly into the hot filling, the egg yolk would curdle.) Stir margarine into the filling and pour into crust. Cool until filling gels.

The Meringue

Preheat oven to 375°F.

Whip egg whites with cream of tartar until stiff but not dry.

Add sugar and continue beating until whites form stiff peaks.

Gently cover lime filling with egg whites, making sure whites cover pie completely.

Bake for 8–10 minutes or until meringue is golden brown.

Cool at room temperature.

Makes 10 slices

Calories per slice:	Total	Fat	Sat-fat
With pastry crust	249	42	9
With Graham Cracker Crust	201	27	6

STRAWBERRY TART

Another pièce de résistance to end any meal on a high note. Make this tart with strawberries, kiwi fruit, peaches, or most any other fruit, even lemons. Try a combination of many fruits on one tart. Tarts are typically filled with crème patissière. Instead of the 6 egg yolks normally used in this French custard, this strawberry tart uses packaged vanilla pudding and pie filling.

Fully baked sweet pie crust
  (pages 398–99)
2 quarts strawberries
1 package vanilla pudding and
  pie filling

1¾ cups skim milk
1 scant tablespoon vanilla
½ cup apricot preserves
1 tablespoon sugar

Wash and hull strawberries.

On a plate the size of your tart pan, make a pleasing arrangement of strawberries.

Make vanilla pudding according to package instructions but use 1¾ cups skim milk and 1 scant tablespoon of vanilla instead of the ingredients listed on the box.

Spread pudding evenly over the bottom of the pie crust.

Immediately arrange fruit on crust.

Combine apricot jam and sugar and heat until syrup is thick and forms a ball at the end of your spoon.

Paint fruit with glaze. Refrigerate tart.

Makes 10 slices
Calories per slice: 194 Total; 35 Fat; 6 Sat-fat

STRAWBERRY-RHUBARB PIE

The combination of rhubarb and strawberries gives this pie a wonderful blending of sweet and sour.

Partially baked sweet pie crust
  (pages 398–99)
3 stalks rhubarb
2 pints strawberries, washed
  and hulled

1½ teaspoons margarine
¾–1 cup sugar
2⅔ tablespoons quick-cooking
  tapioca
½ teaspoon margarine

Prepare partially baked sweet pastry for pie bottom crust, but use 1¾ cups flour.

Refrigerate extra pastry.

Preheat oven to 400°F.

Slice rhubarb into ¼-inch pieces. Cut strawberries into quarters.

Gently sauté rhubarb in 1½ teaspoons of the margarine until slightly softened (about 5 minutes).

Combine rhubarb, strawberries, sugar, and tapioca, and set aside for 15 minutes.

Fill crust with fruit mixture.

Dot with the remaining ½ teaspoon margarine.

Roll out remaining pastry and cut into strips. Cover pie with lattice top. Bake for 25–40 minutes or until crust is browned.

Makes 10 slices
Calories per slice: 219 Total; 40 Fat; 7 Sat-fat

APPLE PANDOWDY

1¼ cups unbleached white flour	½ cup brown sugar
1 tablespoon sugar	1 tablespoon flour
¼ teaspoon salt	1 teaspoon cinnamon
3 tablespoons margarine	3 tablespoons molasses
1 tablespoon olive oil	7 cups tart apples (about 7),
3 tablespoons + 1 teaspoon	peeled and sliced
skim milk	½ cup chopped walnuts

Preheat oven to 400°F. Grease a 2-quart shallow baking pan with margarine.

In a small bowl, combine flour, sugar, and salt.

Cut in margarine with a pastry blender until margarine is the size of small peas.

Add oil and 3 tablespoons of skim milk. Mix until dough forms a ball. If too dry, add 1 teaspoon of milk.

Wrap dough in wax paper, place in a plastic bag, and refrigerate for 30 minutes.

In a large bowl, combine brown sugar, flour, and cinnamon.

Mix in molasses. Mixture will be sticky.

Mix in apples and walnuts. Molasses mixture will clump. Don't worry.

Pour into pan. Spread molasses mixture over apples as evenly as possible.

Roll out pastry into a rectangle and place over apples.

Bake for 30–40 minutes or until crust is golden brown.

Makes 10 pieces
Calories per piece: 243 Total; 74 Fat; 11 Sat-fat

DEEP-DISH PEAR PIE

This pie is absolutely scrumptious! Your fortunate guests will never suspect that nonfat yogurt (no saturated fat) was substituted for the traditional sour cream (270 sat-fat calories per cup).

Partially baked sweet pie crust (pages 398–99)

Filling

2 tablespoons unbleached white flour
½ cup sugar
⅛ teaspoon salt
1 cup nonfat yogurt
1 egg

¼ teaspoon grated nutmeg
1 teaspoon vanilla
5 cups peeled pears (or tart apples), cut into bite-size pieces

Topping

3 tablespoons sugar
3 tablespoons unbleached white flour

½ teaspoon cinnamon
4 teaspoons margarine

Preheat oven to 400°F.

In a large bowl, combine flour, sugar, and salt. Mix in nonfat yogurt. Blend in egg. Add nutmeg and vanilla. Fold in pears.

Pour pear mixture into pie crust and bake at 400°F for 15 minutes. Lower heat to 350°F and continue baking for 25 minutes more.

Mix together topping ingredients.

Remove pie from oven and sprinkle topping over filling.

Raise heat to 375°F and bake until topping is brown.

Makes 12 slices
Calories per slice: 215 Total; 43 Fat; 8 Sat-fat

Q COCOA BROWNIES

1/3 cup margarine	1 egg white
1/2 cup sugar	1/3 cup unsweetened cocoa
1/4 cup light corn syrup	1/2 cup flour
2 teaspoons vanilla	1/2 teaspoon salt
1 egg	1/2 cup chopped walnuts

Preheat oven to 350°F. Grease an 8 × 8-inch baking pan with margarine.

In a large bowl, cream margarine and sugar.

Add corn syrup, vanilla, egg, and egg white and mix until well blended.

Combine cocoa, flour, and salt and slowly add to batter.

Fold in nuts and pour batter into baking pan.

Bake for 25–30 minutes or until a cake tester comes out clean.

Makes 16 squares
Calories per brownie: 115 Total; 54 Fat; 9 Sat-fat

Q CINNAMON SWEET CAKES

A family favorite that can be made on the spur of the moment.

1/4 cup olive oil	3/4 cup whole-wheat flour
1 egg	3/4 cup unbleached white flour
1/2 cup skim milk	2 teaspoons baking powder
1/2 cup sugar	1/2 teaspoon salt

Topping

1/2 cup brown sugar	1 tablespoon margarine
1/2 cup coarsely chopped walnuts	1 teaspoon cinnamon
1 tablespoon unbleached white flour	

Preheat oven to 375°F. Grease an 8 × 8-inch baking pan with margarine.

In a large mixing bowl, beat together oil, egg, and skim milk.

Add sugar, whole-wheat flour, white flour, baking powder, and salt and beat until smooth.

Spoon batter into baking pan. (Batter will be thick.)

To make the topping, combine brown sugar, walnuts, flour, and cinnamon in a small bowl.

Melt margarine and stir into mixture.

Sprinkle topping over batter.

Bake for about 25 minutes or until a cake tester comes out clean.

Makes 16 squares
Calories per square: 148 Total; 61 Fat; 8 Sat-fat

GLAZED CINNAMON BUNS

1 tablespoon active dry yeast
3 tablespoons sugar
½ cup warm water
1½ cups whole-wheat flour
1½ + cups unbleached white
   flour
1 teaspoon salt
1 teaspoon cinnamon
1½ tablespoons olive oil

½ cup nonfat skim milk
1 egg white
⅓ cup firmly packed brown
   sugar
2 teaspoons cinnamon
½ cup raisins
1 cup confectioners' sugar
1–3 tablespoons nonfat
   skim milk

Place yeast, sugar, and water in a large bowl or the bowl of a food processor. Let proof until foamy.

Add 1½ cups of whole-wheat flour, 1½ cups of white flour, salt, oil, 1 teaspoon cinnamon, milk, and egg white and mix or process. Keep adding white flour until dough becomes fairly stiff.

Knead dough for 10 minutes or process for 15 seconds or until dough is smooth and elastic, adding more flour if necessary.

Place dough in bowl you have greased with a drop or two of olive oil, cover with a dish towel, and let rise in a warm place for 1 hour or until doubled in bulk.

When the dough has doubled in size, place it on a lightly floured surface.

Grease a 12-cup muffin tin with margarine. Set aside.

While the dough rests, combine brown sugar, 2 teaspoons cinnamon, and raisins and set aside.

Roll dough into a 9 × 12-inch rectangle.

Sprinkle cinnamon mixture evenly over the dough.

Starting with the long side of the rectangle, roll the dough *tightly* into a jelly roll. Cut it crosswise into 12 even pieces.

Place each piece, cut side up, into a muffin cup. Cover with a towel and let rise 45 minutes.

Preheat oven to 400°F. Bake buns for 15–20 minutes or until nicely browned. Transfer them to a cooling rack.

Place confectioners' sugar in bowl of an electric mixer. Add 1 tablespoon of milk and mix on low speed until smooth. Add more milk very slowly if mixture is too thick.

Spoon glaze over tops of buns.

Makes 12 buns
Calories per bun: 120 Total; 18 Fat; 3 Sat-fat

[Q]   **MANDELBROT**

These cookies are addictive. Thank you, Esther Krashes!

⅔ cup sugar   1½ cups unbleached white flour
¼ cup olive oil   1 teaspoon baking powder
3 egg whites   ½ cup coarsely ground almonds
1 egg   1 teaspoon orange extract

Preheat oven to 350°F.

Lightly grease a cookie sheet with margarine or olive oil.

In a large mixing bowl, cream sugar and olive oil.

Mix in egg whites and egg.

Add flour and baking powder and mix until smooth.

Stir in almonds and orange extract.

Pour onto cookie sheet. Spread into rectangle (8 × 8 inches), about ½ inch thick.

Bake for 20 minutes or until lightly browned.

Remove cookie sheet from oven.

Cut dough into strips about 3 inches wide and then score (do not cut through) into bars about ¾ inch wide.

Turn strips over and bake 10 more minutes or until crisp.

Break into bars.

Makes 4 dozen bars
Calories per bar: 46 Total; 18 Fat; 2 Sat-fat

☒ HONEY GRAHAM CRACKERS

1 cup whole-wheat flour	2 tablespoons margarine
½ cup unbleached white flour	2 tablespoons light brown sugar
½ teaspoon baking powder	2 tablespoons honey
¼ teaspoon baking soda	½ teaspoon vanilla
Pinch of salt	2 tablespoons skim milk

Preheat oven to 350°F and grease a cookie sheet with margarine.

Combine flours, baking powder, baking soda, and salt, and set aside.

Cream margarine, sugar, and honey in an electric mixer.

Mix in vanilla.

Add flour mixture and milk.

Gather dough together (add a drop of milk if too dry) and knead into a ball.

Roll dough onto cookie sheet into a rectangle, ⅛ inch thick.

If dough is too sticky, sprinkle it with flour.

Without moving dough, cut into 3-inch squares.

Lightly score a line through the center of each square and pierce each side several times with a fork.

Bake 10–15 minutes, until edges brown. Remove crackers and cool on a wire rack.

Crackers will become crisp as they cool.

Makes 18 crackers
Calories per cracker: 58 Total; 12 Fat; 2 Sat-fat

☒ SUGAR COOKIES

These cookies are habit forming. They contain only 3 sat-fat calories each, but the 11 total fat calories per cookie can quickly add up.

3 tablespoons margarine	1 tablespoon skim milk
⅔ cup + ⅓ cup sugar	1¾ cups + ⅓ cup unbleached
1 egg	white flour
2 teaspoons vanilla	½ teaspoon baking soda

Preheat oven to 350°F. Grease a cookie sheet with margarine.

In a large mixing bowl, cream the 3 tablespoons margarine and ⅔ cup of the sugar.

Mix in egg, vanilla, and skim milk.

Add 1¾ cups flour and baking soda and mix until smooth.

Pour the remaining sugar on a small plate. Pour the remaining flour on another small plate. Dip your fingers in the flour, pick up a small amount of dough, and roll the dough into a small ball in your hand.

Roll the ball in the sugar. Place the ball on the cookie sheet and gently flatten it with your hand. Continue with the rest of the dough.

Bake for 10–15 minutes or until golden brown.

Makes 32 cookies
Calories per cookie: 65 Total; 11 Fat; 2 Sat-fat

APPLE-NUT COOKIES

⅓ cup margarine
½ cup brown sugar
1 egg
1 cup unbleached white flour
½ cup whole-wheat flour
½ teaspoon baking soda
1 teaspoon baking powder
½ teaspoon salt

1 teaspoon cinnamon
¼ teaspoon grated nutmeg
3 tablespoons milk
¼ cup raisins
½ cup chopped walnuts
  (optional)
2½ cups peeled, diced cooking
  apples

Preheat oven to 400°F. Lightly grease a cookie sheet with margarine.

In a large mixing bowl, cream margarine and brown sugar.

Add egg and beat until batter is smooth.

Combine white flour, whole-wheat flour, baking soda, baking powder, salt, cinnamon, and nutmeg.

Mix into batter alternately with milk.

Stir in raisins and nuts. Fold in apples.

Drop batter by teaspoonfuls onto cookie sheet and bake for 10–12 minutes or until golden brown.

Makes 3 dozen cookies

Calories per cookie:	*Total*	*Fat*	*Sat-fat*
	62	25	4
Without walnuts	51	16	3

OATMEAL COOKIES

¼ cup olive oil	2 cups rolled oats
⅓ cup brown sugar	⅓ cup unbleached white flour
2 tablespoons sugar	⅓ cup whole-wheat flour
1 egg white	¼ teaspoon salt
¾ teaspoon vanilla	½ teaspoon baking soda
3 tablespoons water	1 teaspoon cinnamon

Preheat oven to 350°F. Grease a cookie sheet with margarine.
Cream oil and sugars.
Mix in egg white, vanilla, and water.
Add oats, white flour, whole-wheat flour, salt, baking soda, and cinnamon and mix until blended. Do not overmix or you will lose the texture of the oats.
Drop batter by teaspoonfuls onto cookie sheet and bake for 10–15 minutes.

Makes 2 dozen cookies
Calories per cookie: 65 Total; 25 Fat; 3 Sat-fat

MERINGUE SHELLS WITH FRESH STRAWBERRIES AND WARM RASPBERRY SAUCE

Here's a delectable dessert that has no saturated fat or total fat. It is extremely simple to prepare and, later, to assemble. Make sure to budget in 1 to 2 hours baking time for the meringue.

Meringue Shells

4 egg whites at room temperature	¾ cup sugar
⅛ teaspoon salt	½ teaspoon vanilla
⅛ teaspoon cream of tartar	¼ teaspoon almond extract

Filling

1 pint strawberries, washed, hulled, and halved (actually any berry or cut-up fruit will do)

Sauce

1 package (10 oz) frozen raspberries	1 teaspoon cornstarch
	½ teaspoon lemon juice

The Meringue

Preheat oven to 275°F. Completely cover your baking sheet with a piece of brown paper. Set aside.

In a very clean mixing bowl, whip egg whites until foamy. Continue whipping as you add salt and cream of tartar. When egg whites form soft peaks, slowly add sugar while continuing to beat until whites are glossy and stiff. Mix in vanilla and almond extract.

On the brown paper, use a spoon or spatula to spread the meringue into 6 shells, 4–5 inches across with a raised edge about 1 inch high. You may also use a pastry tube to squeeze out concentric circles to form a base and sides. The shells should be deep enough to hold the fruit.

Bake for 2 hours. Turn off heat and let meringues sit in closed oven for 2 hours or overnight. Gently remove meringues, as they crack easily.

The Filling

Fill the shell cavity with a mound of strawberries.

The Raspberry Sauce

Thaw raspberries or, if you forgot to plan ahead, place pouch containing raspberries into a bowl of warm water for about 2 minutes to thaw. When partially thawed, purée the raspberries in a blender.

Place cornstarch in a small saucepan. Add 1 tablespoon of purée and mix with cornstarch until smooth. Stir in remaining purée and add lemon juice. Bring to a boil and simmer for 1 minute.

Spoon several tablespoons of the warm sauce over the strawberries. You may also refrigerate the sauce and serve it cold.

6 servings
Calories per serving: 130 Total; 0 Fat; 0 Sat-fat

Q

PEARS HÉLÈNE

Pears Hélène made with cocoa and margarine are wonderful, just like their counterpart made with chocolate and butter.

The chocolate sauce is a good all-purpose dessert sauce. You can store it in the refrigerator for weeks.

Pears

4 ripe pears	¼ cup sugar
2 cups water	1 tablespoon fresh lemon juice

Chocolate Sauce

3 tablespoons sugar	2 tablespoons water
2 tablespoons unsweetened cocoa	1 tablespoon light corn syrup
1 tablespoon cornstarch	1 tablespoon margarine
	½ teaspoon vanilla

The Pears

Peel pears, cut them in half, core them, and cut off the stems.

In a pot large enough to hold pears, combine water, sugar, and lemon juice and bring to a boil.

Spoon pears into liquid, reduce heat, and simmer, covered, for 5 minutes. Pears should be tender, not mushy.

Drain poached pears and chill.

The Chocolate Sauce

In a small saucepan, combine sugar, cocoa, and cornstarch.

Mix in water and corn syrup and blend well.

Cook over medium heat until mixture comes to a boil.

Remove from heat and stir for about 1 minute.

Add margarine and vanilla and continue to stir until sauce is well blended.

On each plate, place 2 pear halves, cut-side up, and pour warm sauce over them.

4 servings
Calories per serving: 205 Total; 23 Fat; 5 Sat-fat

THREE

FOOD TABLES

CONTENTS

INTRODUCTION TO THE FOOD TABLES

The Food Tables in this new edition of *Eater's Choice* contain both saturated fat calories and total fat calories. Total fat is the sum of saturated fat, monounsaturated fat, and polyunsaturated fat. Each has a different effect on heart health, but all are equally fattening. Knowing both the saturated and total fat calories in a food will help you make more informed choices.

People who are keeping track of saturated fat to lower their blood cholesterol should know how much total fat a food contains. For example, if you are only considering saturated fat you might blithely consume a Wendy's baked potato with broccoli and cheese because it has only 18 sat-fat calories. However, if you had looked at the total fat calories for this "healthy" potato you would see that it contains 126 fat calories. This is a heaping amount of fat — almost half the Fat Budget for a woman wanting to weigh 120 pounds, or about one-third the Fat Budget of a man wanting to weigh 150.

Those who are reducing total fat may also be interested in the amount of saturated fat in foods to help them make healthier choices. For instance, both olive oil, the most heart-healthy of all the fats, and butter, a highly heart-risky food, are 100 percent fat and fattening. However, a tablespoon of olive oil, which has 119 total fat calories, has only 16 sat-fat calories. A tablespoon of butter has 100 fat calories and 65 sat-fat calories. By using the Food Tables, you can quickly see that butter is a poorer choice because it is very saturated.

Because products are constantly changing, always look at nutrition labels for the most up-to-date nutrition information. If you don't know where to look for a food in the Food Tables, turn to the Food Tables Index, immediately following the Food Tables. (This is different from the general index at the end of the book.)

The abbreviation "NA" means the sat-fat calories are "not available."

We would like to thank the Center for Science in the Public Interest for permission to use their nutrition analyses of Italian restaurant foods, Mexican restaurant foods, and popcorn.

Foods are often measured in grams instead of ounces. To put amounts into perspective, remember that 1 ounce = approximately 28 grams.

BEVERAGES

FOOD	AMOUNT	CALORIES TOTAL	FAT	SAT-FAT
Alcoholic				
Beer	12 fl oz	150	0	**0**
Lite beer	12 fl oz	100	0	**0**
Gin, rum, vodka, whiskey				
80–90 proof	1.5 fl oz	95–110	0	**0**
Other				
brandy Alexander	3 fl oz	254	52	**32**
Irish coffee	8 fl oz	210	99	**60**
piña colada	6 fl oz	392	103	**85**
eggnog	8 fl oz	342	171	**102**
Wine				
dessert	3.5 fl oz	140	0	**0**
table	3.5 fl oz	75	0	**0**
Carbonated				
Club soda	12 fl oz	0	0	**0**
Cola	12 fl oz	160	0	**0**
Ginger ale	12 fl oz	125	0	**0**
Lemon-lime	12 fl oz	150	0	**0**
Orange, grape	12 fl oz	180	0	**0**

BEVERAGES

FOOD	AMOUNT	CALORIES		
		TOTAL	FAT	SAT-FAT
Cocoa				
Hershey's				
made with whole milk	6 fl oz	135	58	**34**
made with 2% milk	6 fl oz	113	35	**20**
made with skim milk	6 fl oz	87	5	**0**
Swiss Miss with water	1 pkt (28 g)	110	10	**0**
Coffee				
Nescafé cappuccino	1 pkt (27 g)	110	20	**5**
International Coffees				
Cafe Amaretto	6 fl oz prep.	50	27	**NA**
Cafe Français	6 fl oz prep.	60	27	**NA**
Cafe Vienna	6 fl oz prep.	60	18	**NA**
Italian cappuccino	6 fl oz prep.	50	18	**NA**

Coffee Bar Coffees

If whipped cream is added to your coffee, add 60 total calories and 45 fat calories.

Coffee Beanery				
Cafe Mocha				
with whole milk	8 fl oz	94	45	**NA**
with 2% milk	8 fl oz	76	27	**NA**
with skim milk	8 fl oz	54	0	**NA**
Cappuccino				
with whole milk	12 fl oz	296	81	**NA**
with 2% milk	12 fl oz	267	54	**NA**
with skim milk	12 fl oz	232	9	**NA**
Espresso	2.4 fl oz	0	0	**NA**
Latte				
with whipped cream and				
grated chocolate	16 fl oz	350	180	**NA**
with whole milk	16 fl oz	263	126	**NA**
with 2% milk	16 fl oz	211	72	**NA**
with skim milk	16 fl oz	151	9	**NA**
Gloria Jean's (made with 2% milk)				
Cafe Mocha	8 fl oz	222	36	**NA**
grande	16 fl oz	312	63	**NA**
iced	12 fl oz	282	54	**NA**
Espresso	2.7 fl oz	0	0	**NA**
Latte	8 fl oz	76	27	**NA**
grande	16 fl oz	166	54	**NA**

BEVERAGES

FOOD	AMOUNT	CALORIES TOTAL	FAT	SAT-FAT
Starbucks				
Cafe Mocha				
short				
with whole milk	8 fl oz	195	135	NA
with 2% milk	8 fl oz	175	117	NA
with skim milk	8 fl oz	156	99	NA
grande				
with whole milk	16 fl oz	409	279	NA
with 2% milk	16 fl oz	365	243	NA
with skim milk	16 fl oz	324	189	NA
iced	12 fl oz	271	171	NA
Cappuccino	8 fl oz	99	45	NA
grande	16 fl oz	249	117	NA
Espresso	2.7 fl oz	0	0	NA
Latte				
short				
with whole milk	8 fl oz	114	54	NA
with 2% milk	8 fl oz	90	36	NA
with skim milk	8 fl oz	68	9	NA
grande				
with whole milk	16 fl oz	247	117	NA
with 2% milk	16 fl oz	195	72	NA
with skim milk	16 fl oz	146	18	NA
Fruit Drinks				
Noncarbonated				
canned	6 fl oz	85–100	0	0
frozen	6 fl oz	80	0	0
Hot Chocolate	8 fl oz	232	122	72
with whipped cream	¼ cup	334	221	133
Instant Breakfast Shakes				
Carnation				
Creamy Milk Chocolate	1 pkt (37 g)	130	10	5
Creamy Milk Chocolate, sugar-free	1 pkt (21 g)	70	10	5
Tea	8 fl oz	0	0	0

Dairy drinks (milk, milk shakes, etc.): *see* **DAIRY AND EGGS** and **FAST FOODS**.
Fruit juices: *see* **FRUITS AND FRUIT JUICES**.

DAIRY AND EGGS

FOOD	AMOUNT	CALORIES		
		TOTAL	FAT	SAT-FAT
Butter				
Regular	1 pat	36	36	23
	1 tbsp	100	100	65
	1 stick (½ cup)	813	813	515
Whipped	1 tbsp	67	67	38
	1 stick (½ cup)	542	542	344

Margarine and other butter substitutes: *see* **FATS AND OILS.**

FOOD	AMOUNT	CALORIES		
		TOTAL	FAT	SAT-FAT
Cheese				
American	1 oz	106	80	50
Blue	1 oz	100	73	48
Bonbel (Laughing Cow)	1 oz	70	50	36
Brie	1 oz	90	70	27
Camembert	1 oz	90	70	27
Cheddar	1 oz	114	85	54
shredded	¼ cup	110	80	54
Colby	1 oz	112	82	54
Cottage cheese				
4%	½ cup	110	43	23
2% fat	½ cup	102	20	14
1% fat	½ cup	90	10	7
dry curd	½ cup	80	9	4
Cream cheese				
regular	1 tbsp	52	48	26
with salmon or strawberries	2 tbsp	100	80	54
soft	2 tbsp	100	90	63
whipped	1 tbsp	37	34	19
Edam	1 oz	101	71	45
Feta	1 oz	75	54	38
with basil and tomato	1 oz	80	60	36
Farmer				
Friendship	1 oz	40	27	18
May-Bud	1 oz	90	63	41
Gouda	1 oz	101	70	45
Gruyère	1 oz	117	83	48
Limburger	1 oz	93	69	43
Monterey	1 oz	106	77	45
Mozzarella				
whole milk	1 oz	80	50	36
shredded	1 oz	90	65	42
part skim	1 oz	72	45	27

DAIRY AND EGGS

FOOD	AMOUNT	CALORIES		
		TOTAL	FAT	SAT-FAT
Muenster	1 oz	104	77	49
Neufchâtel	1 oz	74	60	38
Parmesan	1 tbsp	23	14	9
	1 oz	129	77	49
Port du Salut	1 oz	100	72	43
Provolone	1 oz	100	68	44
Ricotta				
whole milk	½ cup	216	145	93
part skim	½ cup	171	88	55
Romano	1 oz	110	70	49
Roquefort	1 oz	105	78	49
String	1 oz	80	50	36
Swiss	1 oz	107	70	45
Tilsit	1 oz	96	66	43

Cheese, Fat-free

FOOD	AMOUNT	TOTAL	FAT	SAT-FAT
All brands	1 slice (21 g)	25–30	0	0
Cream cheese	2 tbsp	30	0	0
Mozzarella, shredded	¼ cup (28 g)	45	0	0

Cheese, Reduced-Calorie or Lite

FOOD	AMOUNT	TOTAL	FAT	SAT-FAT
Alouette Lite Herbs & Garlic	2 tbsp	60	35	27
Bonbel Light Wedge				
(Laughing Cow)	1 piece (28 g)	50	30	18
Cheddar, shredded				
⅓ Less Fat Kraft	¼ cup	90	50	36
Sargento	¼ cup	70	40	18
Cream cheese				
Philadelphia ⅓ Less Fat	2 tbsp	70	60	36
Monterey Jack				
Dorman's	1 slice	120	60	41
Kraft	28 g	80	45	27
Mozzarella	¼ cup	60	30	18
Ricotta	¼ cup	75	35	18
Rondelé Soft Spreadable Lite	2 tbsp	60	35	23
String (Poly-O)	1 piece (28 g)	80	50	36
Weight Watchers, all	1 slice (21 g)	50	20	0

Cheese Spreads

FOOD	AMOUNT	TOTAL	FAT	SAT-FAT
Alouette				
Garlic and Spices	2 tbsp	70	60	41
Spinach	2 tbsp	60	50	32
Boursin	2 tbsp	120	110	45

DAIRY AND EGGS

FOOD	AMOUNT	CALORIES		
		TOTAL	FAT	SAT-FAT
Cheez Whiz (Kraft)	2 tbsp	100	70	45
Rondelé Soft Spreadable				
Black Pepper & Garden				
Vegetable	2 tbsp	90	80	54
Garlic & Herbs	2 tbsp	100	80	54
Cream				
Half-and-half	1 tbsp	20	15	10
Light, coffee or table	1 tbsp	29	26	16
	1 cup	469	417	260
Nondairy				
Frozen				
Rich's Coffee Rich	1 tbsp	25	15	0
Powdered				
Coffee Mate	1 tbsp	30	15	14
flavored	1⅓ tbsp	60	25	23
Refrigerated				
Farm Rich				
fat-free	1 tbsp	10	0	0
light	1 tbsp	10	5	0
original	1 tbsp	20	15	0
Sour cream	2 tbsp	60	50	36
	1 cup	493	434	270
fat-free	2 tbsp	20	0	0
light	2 tbsp	35	25	14
Whipping cream				
heavy, fluid	1 cup	821	792	493
Whipped	½ cup	205	198	123
light, fluid	1 cup	699	665	416
nondairy (Cool Whip)	2 tbsp	25	15	14
	½ cup	200	120	108
Pressurized topping				
whipped light	2 tbsp	30	20	14
Reddi Wip	2 tbsp	20	15	9
Milk				
1% fat	1 cup	104	23	14
2% fat	1 cup	121	42	27
Buttermilk	1 cup	99	0–36	0–12
Chocolate				
2% milk	1 cup	179	45	28
whole milk	1 cup	208	76	47

DAIRY AND EGGS

FOOD	AMOUNT	CALORIES TOTAL	FAT	SAT-FAT
Condensed, sweetened	1 tbsp	62	15	9
Evaporated				
skim	1 cup	200	5	2
	1 tbsp	13	0	0
whole	1 cup	340	172	104
	1 tbsp	21	11	7
Nonfat				
dry	¼ cup	109	2	1
instant	to make 1 qt	326	6	4
Skim	1 cup	86	4	0–3
Whole	1 cup	150	73	45
dry	¼ cup	159	77	48

Yogurt
Custard-style
FOOD	AMOUNT	TOTAL	FAT	SAT-FAT
Whitney's Original 100%				
Natural, all flavors	6 oz	190	45	27
Yoplait, all flavors	6 oz	170	25	14

French-style
FOOD	AMOUNT	TOTAL	FAT	SAT-FAT
La Yogurt				
All flavors but Piña				
Colada	6 oz	180	25	14
Piña colada	6 oz	180	30	14

Low-fat
FOOD	AMOUNT	TOTAL	FAT	SAT-FAT
Astro vanilla				
with apple crisp granola				
topping	6 oz	230	35	23
with chocolate fudge				
crunch	6 oz	230	45	23
with oat bran raisin				
granola topping	6 oz	230	40	23
Breyers	8 oz	250	25	14
Colombo	8 oz	120	40	23
Dannon, all flavors	8 oz	210	30	18
Fruit on the Bottom, all				
flavors	8 oz	240	25	14
Premium	8 oz	150	35	23
Lucerne, Pre-Stirred, all				
flavors	8 oz	250	25	14
Whitney's Supreme, all				
flavors	6 oz	200	20	9
Yoplait Original, all flavors	6 oz	170	15	9
Yoplait Trix	6 oz	180	25	14

DAIRY AND EGGS

FOOD	AMOUNT	CALORIES		
		TOTAL	FAT	SAT-FAT
Nonfat				
Colombo				
fruit flavors	8 oz	190	0	0
other flavors	8 oz	160	0	0
Colombo Light 100, all				
flavors	8 oz	100	0	0
Dannon	8 oz	110	0	0
Blended, all flavors	6 oz	150–160	0	0
Lucerne Light, all flavors	6 oz	90	0	0
Lucerne, Pre-Stirred, all				
flavors	8 oz	180	0	0
Weight Watchers Ultimate				
90, all flavors	8 oz	90	0	0
Yoplait Light, all flavors	6 oz	90	0	0
Egg, chicken				
Whole, large	1 egg	79	50	15
White	1 white	16	0	0
Yolk	1 yolk	63	50	15
Egg substitute				
Egg Beaters™ (Fleischmann's)	¼ cup	30	0	0
Healthy Choice Egg Product	¼ cup	25	<5	0
Scramblers (Morningstar				
Farms)	¼ cup	35	0	0
Simply Eggs	½ cup	80	20	9
	3 tbsp	35	10	0

FAST FOODS

FOOD	AMOUNT	CALORIES		
		TOTAL	FAT	SAT-FAT
Arby's				
Bacon platter	1	593	297	83
Baked potato				
Broccoli and Cheddar	1	417	162	63
Deluxe	1	621	328	163
Mushroom and Cheese	1	515	240	52

FAST FOODS

| FOOD | AMOUNT | CALORIES | | |
		TOTAL	FAT	SAT-FAT
Biscuit				
Bacon	1	318	162	39
Ham	1	323	150	36
Plain	1	280	135	30
Sausage	1	460	288	85
Blueberry Muffin	1	240	63	9
Croissant				
Bacon and Egg	1	430	270	139
Butter	1	260	140	94
Ham and Swiss	1	345	186	109
Mushroom and Swiss	1	495	340	137
Sausage and Egg	1	520	353	167
Cheesecake	1 serving	305	205	65
Chicken Breast Sandwich	1	445	203	27
Chicken Club Sandwich	1	505	243	63
Chicken Cordon Bleu				
Sandwich	1	520	243	48
Chocolate Chip Cookie	1	130	36	18
Cinnamon Nut Danish	1	360	99	9
Egg Platter	1	460	216	65
Fish Fillet Sandwich	1	526	243	63
Fries				
Cheddar Fries	1 sm order	399	197	81
Curly Fries	1 sm order	337	169	67
French Fries	1 sm order	246	119	27
Grilled Chicken Barbecue				
Sandwich	1	385	118	32
Grilled Chicken Deluxe				
Sandwich	1	430	180	32
Ham n' Cheese Sandwich	1	353	128	46
Ham Platter	1	518	234	72
Horsey Sauce	1 oz	120	54	18
Italian Sub	1	671	349	115
Light Sandwiches				
Roast Beef Deluxe	1	294	90	32
Roast Chicken Deluxe	1	276	63	15
Roast Turkey Deluxe	1	260	54	14
Polar Swirl				
Butterfinger	1	457	163	76
Heath	1	543	196	47
Oreo	1	482	177	94
Peanut Butter Cup	1	517	216	73

FAST FOODS

FOOD	AMOUNT	CALORIES		
		TOTAL	FAT	SAT-FAT
Polar Swirl (*cont.*)				
Snickers	1	510	170	60
Potato Cakes	1 serving	201	108	20
Roast Beef Sandwich				
Arby Q	1	389	137	50
Bac'n Cheddar Deluxe	1	512	284	78
Beef 'n Cheddar	1	508	239	69
French Dip	1	368	139	50
French Dip 'n Swiss	1	429	171	79
Giant	1	544	237	99
Junior	1	233	97	37
Philly Beef 'n Swiss	1	467	228	87
Regular	1	383	164	63
Super	1	552	255	68
Roast Beef Sub	1	623	288	104
Salads (without dressing)				
Chef	1	205	86	35
Chicken	1	204	65	30
Garden	1	117	47	24
Salad dressings				
Blue Cheese	1 packet	295	281	52
Buttermilk Ranch	1 packet	349	347	50
Honey French	1 packet	322	242	36
Italian, light	1 packet	23	10	1
Thousand Island	1 packet	298	263	39
Sausage platter	1	640	370	120
Shakes				
Chocolate	10.6 fl oz	450	105	25
Jamocha	10.8 fl oz	368	95	23
Vanilla	8.8 fl oz	330	100	36
Soup				
Boston Clam Chowder	1 cup	193	90	40
Cream of Broccoli	1 cup	166	65	34
Potato with Bacon	1 cup	184	79	39
Wisconsin Cheese	1 cup	281	162	81
Toastix	1 serving	420	225	41
Tuna Sub	1	663	333	74
Turnover				
Apple	1	310	165	63
Blueberry	1	320	180	57
Cherry	1	280	160	48
Turkey Sub	1	486	171	48

FAST FOODS

| FOOD | AMOUNT | CALORIES | | |
		TOTAL	FAT	SAT-FAT
Arthur Treacher's				
Chicken, fried	1 serving	369	198	**36**
Chicken Sandwich	1	413	171	**27**
Chips (french fries)	1 serving	276	117	**18**
Chowder	1 serving	112	45	**18**
Cole Slaw	1 serving	123	72	**9**
Fish, broiled	5 oz	245	126	**NA**
Fish, fried	2 pieces	355	180	**27**
Krunch Pup (batter-fried hot dog)	1	203	135	**36**
Lemon Luv (fried pie)	1 serving	276	126	**18**
Shrimp, fried	1 serving	381	216	**27**
Burger King				
Apple Pie	1	311	126	**36**
BK Broiler Chicken Sandwich, no mayo	1	267	72	**18**
BK Broiler Sauce	1	37	36	**9**
Blueberry Mini Muffins	1 serving	292	126	**27**
Breakfast Buddy with sausage, egg, and cheese	1	255	144	**54**
Burger Buddies	1 pair	349	153	**63**
Cheeseburger	1	317	135	**63**
Deluxe	1	390	207	**72**
Double	1	483	243	**117**
Bacon	1	510	279	**126**
Bacon Deluxe	1	584	342	**144**
Chef Salad	1	178	81	**36**
Chicken Sandwich	1	685	360	**81**
Chicken Tenders	6 pieces	236	117	**27**
Chunky Chicken Salad	1	142	36	**9**
Croissan'wich				
Bacon, Egg, and Cheese	1	355	216	**72**
Ham, Egg, and Cheese	1	351	198	**63**
Sausage, Egg, and Cheese	1	534	360	**126**
French Fries, regular	1 serving	372	180	**45**
French Toast Sticks	1 serving	538	288	**72**
Garden Salad	1	95	45	**27**
Hamburger	1	275	99	**36**
Deluxe	1	344	171	**54**
Hash Browns	1 serving	215	108	**27**
Ocean Catch Fish Fillet Sandwich	1	479	297	**72**

FAST FOODS

FOOD	AMOUNT	CALORIES		
		TOTAL	FAT	SAT-FAT
Onion Rings, regular	1 serving	339	171	45
Pies				
Cherry	1	360	117	36
Lemon	1	290	72	27
Ranch Dipping Sauce	1	171	162	27
Scrambled Egg Platter (eggs,				
croissant, hash browns)	1 serving	549	306	81
with bacon	1 serving	610	351	99
with sausage	1 serving	768	477	135
Shakes				
Chocolate	10 fl oz	326	90	54
Vanilla	10 fl oz	334	90	54
Specialty Sandwiches				
Chicken	1	688	360	72
Ham and Cheese	1	471	216	81
Whaler Sandwich	1	488	243	54
with cheese	1	530	270	72
Whopper	1	614	324	108
with cheese	1	709	396	144
Double Whopper	1	844	477	171
with cheese	1	935	549	216
Whopper Jr.	1	322	153	54
with cheese	1	364	180	72
Carl's Jr.				
Breakfast Burrito	1	430	234	108
Carl's Catch Fish Sandwich	1	560	270	36
Charbroiler Sandwich				
BBQ Chicken	1	310	54	18
Chicken Club	1	570	261	72
Cheeseburger				
Western Bacon	1	730	351	180
Double	1	1030	567	288
Cheesecake	1 piece	310	153	72
Chicken Strips	6 pieces	260	171	45
Chocolate Cake	1 piece	300	99	27
Chocolate Chip Cookie	1	330	153	63
Cinnamon Rolls	1 serving	460	162	9
CrissCut Fries, regular	1 serving	330	198	27
Danish	1	520	144	36
French Fries, regular	1 serving	420	180	45
French Toast Dips	1 serving	490	234	54
Fudge Moussecake	1 piece	400	207	99

FAST FOODS

FOOD	AMOUNT	CALORIES		
		TOTAL	FAT	SAT-FAT
"Great Stuff" Potato				
Bacon and Cheese	1	730	387	135
Broccoli and Cheese	1	590	279	99
Cheese	1	690	324	135
Sour Cream and Chive	1	470	171	63
Hamburger	1	320	126	45
Carl's Original	1	460	180	81
Famous Star	1	610	342	117
Super Star	1	820	477	216
Hash Brown Nuggets	1 serving	270	153	36
Hot Cakes with Margarine	1 serving	510	216	45
Muffin				
Blueberry	1	340	81	9
Bran	1	310	63	<9
Onion Rings	1 serving	520	234	54
Roast Beef Club Sandwich	1	620	306	99
Roast Beef Deluxe Sandwich	1	540	234	90
Santa Fe Chicken Sandwich	1	540	117	27
Teriyaki Chicken Sandwich	1	330	54	18
Turkey Club Sandwich	1	530	207	54
Shakes, regular	1	350	63	36
Sunrise sandwich	1	300	117	54
Zucchini	1 serving	390	207	54
Chick-Fil-A				
Chargrilled Chicken				
Garden salad	1	126	19	NA
Sandwich	1	258	43	NA
Deluxe	1	266	44	NA
Chicken Nuggets	8	287	135	NA
Chicken Salad Plate	1	291	168	NA
Chicken Salad Sandwich	1	449	238	NA
Chick-n-Q Sandwich	1	206	61	NA
Fudge Brownie with Nuts	1	369	172	NA
Grilled 'n Lites	2 skewers	97	18	NA
Icedream	1 reg cone	134	44	NA
Lemon Pie	1 slice	329	46	NA
Original Chicken Sandwich	1	360	76	NA
Church's Fried Chicken				
Catfish, fried	3 pieces	201	108	NA
Chicken, fried				
breast	1 serving	278	153	NA

FAST FOODS

FOOD	AMOUNT	CALORIES		
		TOTAL	FAT	SAT-FAT
Chicken, fried (cont.)				
leg	1 serving	147	81	NA
thigh	1 serving	305	198	NA
wing	1 serving	303	180	NA
Chicken Breast Fillet				
Sandwich	1	608	306	NA
Chicken Nuggets				
regular	6 pieces	330	171	NA
spicy	6 pieces	312	153	NA
Coleslaw	1 serving	83	63	NA
Corn on the Cob, buttered	9 oz	165	27	NA
Dinner Roll	1	83	18	NA
Fish Fillet Sandwich	1	430	162	NA
French Fries, regular	3 oz	256	117	NA
Hush Puppies	2	156	54	NA
Pie				
Apple	1 serving	300	171	NA
Pecan	1 serving	367	180	NA
Dairy Queen				
Banana Split	1	510	99	72
BBQ Beef Sandwich	1	225	36	9
Buster Bar	1	460	261	81
Chicken Fillet Sandwich,				
breaded	1	430	180	36
with cheese	1	480	225	63
Chicken Fillet Sandwich,				
grilled	1	300	72	18
Chocolate cone				
large	1	350	99	72
regular	1	230	63	45
Chocolate cone, dipped				
large	1	510	216	140
regular	1	340	144	90
small	1	190	81	54
Dilly Bar	1	210	117	54
Double Delight	1 serving	490	180	NA
DQ Frozen Cake	1 slice	380	162	72
DQ Sandwich	1	140	36	24
Fish Fillet Sandwich	1	370	144	27
with cheese	1	420	189	54
Float	1	410	63	41

FAST FOODS

| FOOD | AMOUNT | CALORIES | | |
		TOTAL	FAT	SAT-FAT
Freeze	1	500	108	72
French fries	1 regular	300	126	27
	1 large	390	162	36
Garden Salad, no dressing	1	200	117	63
Hamburger	1	310	117	54
with cheese	1	365	162	81
DQ Homestyle Ultimate				
Burger	1	700	423	189
Double	1	460	225	108
with cheese	1	570	306	162
Single	1	360	144	54
with cheese	1	410	180	81
Heath Blizzard	1 regular	820	324	153
Heath Breeze	1 regular	680	189	54
Hot Dog	1	280	144	54
with cheese	1	330	189	81
with chili	1	320	180	63
Super Hot Dog	1	520	243	100
with cheese	1	580	306	142
with chili	1	570	288	112
quarter pound	1	590	342	144
Hot Fudge Brownie Delight	1	710	261	126
Malt				
Chocolate				
large	20 fl oz	1060	225	NA
regular	14 fl oz	760	162	NA
small	10 fl oz	520	117	NA
Vanilla	1 regular	610	126	72
Mr. Misty Float	1	390	63	41
Mr. Misty Freeze	1	500	108	70
Mr. Misty Kiss	1	70	0	0
Mr. Misty				
large	1	340	0	0
regular	1	250	0	0
small	1	190	0	0
Nutty Double Fudge	1	580	198	90
Onion Rings	1 regular	240	108	27
Parfait	1 serving	430	72	47
Peanut Buster	1 serving	710	288	90
QC Chocolate Big Scoop	1	310	126	90

FAST FOODS

FOOD	AMOUNT	CALORIES		
		TOTAL	FAT	SAT-FAT
Shake				
Chocolate				
large	20 fl oz	990	234	**128**
regular	14 fl oz	710	171	**111**
small	10 fl oz	490	117	**64**
Vanilla	1 regular	520	126	**72**
Soft ice cream, without cone	4 oz	180	54	**36**
Soft ice cream cone				
large	1	340	90	**63**
regular	1	240	63	**45**
small	1	140	36	**27**
Strawberry Blizzard	1 regular	570	144	**99**
Strawberry Breeze	1 regular	420	9	**<9**
Strawberry Shortcake	1 serving	540	99	**NA**
Strawberry Waffle Cone				
Sundae	1	350	108	**45**
Sundae				
Chocolate				
large	8.4 fl oz	440	90	**58**
regular	6 fl oz	310	72	**45**
small	3.5 fl oz	190	36	**23**
Vanilla cone	1 regular	230	65	**45**
Yogurt Cup	1 regular	170	<9	**<9**
Yogurt Strawberry Sundae	1 regular	200	<9	**<9**
Denny's				
Baked Potato	1	180	0	**NA**
Biscuit	1	217	63	**NA**
BLT Sandwich	1	492	306	**NA**
Blueberry Muffin	1	309	126	**NA**
Catfish	1 entree	576	432	**NA**
Chicken Strips	4 oz	240	90	**NA**
Chili	8 oz	238	135	**NA**
Cinnamon Roll	1	450	126	**NA**
Club Sandwich	1	590	180	**NA**
Coleslaw	1 cup	119	86	**NA**
Country Gravy	1 oz	140	72	**NA**
Eggs Benedict	1	658	320	**NA**
French Fries	1 order	303	142	**NA**
French Toast	2 slices	729	504	**NA**
Fried Chicken	1 entree	463	266	**NA**
Fried Shrimp	1 entree	230	135	**NA**

FAST FOODS

| FOOD | AMOUNT | CALORIES | | |
		TOTAL	FAT	SAT-FAT
Grilled Cheese Sandwich	1	454	261	NA
Grilled Chicken	1 entree	192	36	NA
Grilled Chicken Sandwich	1	439	108	NA
Guacamole	1 oz	60	55	NA
Hamburger				
Bacon Swiss	1	819	468	NA
Denny	1	629	340	NA
San Fran	1	872	432	NA
Works	1	944	549	NA
Hash Browns	4 oz	164	18	NA
Liver with Bacon and Onions	1 entree	334	130	NA
Mozzarella Sticks	1	88	60	NA
Omelet				
Denver	1	567	243	NA
Ultimate	1	577	369	NA
Onion Rings	3 rings	258	135	NA
Pancakes	2	272	36	NA
Patty Melt	1	761	423	NA
Rice Pilaf	⅓ cup	89	21	NA
Sausage	1 link	113	90	NA
Soup				
Cheese	1 bowl	309	198	NA
Chicken Noodle	1 bowl	105	30	NA
Clam Chowder	1 bowl	235	126	NA
Potato	1 bowl	141	120	NA
Split Pea	1 bowl	231	45	NA
Stir-fry	1 entree	328	99	NA
Stuffing	½ cup	180	81	NA
Super Bird	1	625	216	NA
Salad				
Chef	1	492	180	NA
Chicken, no shell	1	207	36	NA
Taco, no shell	1	514	180	NA
Tuna	1	340	162	NA
Steak				
Fried Chicken, no gravy	1 entree	252	131	NA
Hamburger	1 entree	669	484	NA
New York	1 entree	582	324	NA
Top Sirloin	1 entree	223	57	NA
Tortilla Shell, fried	1	439	270	NA
Turkey, no gravy	1 entree	505	130	NA

FAST FOODS

FOOD	AMOUNT	CALORIES		
		TOTAL	FAT	SAT-FAT
Veggie Cheese	1	350	180	NA
Waffle	1	261	94	NA

Domino's Pizza
12" Pizza

FOOD	AMOUNT	TOTAL	FAT	SAT-FAT
Cheese	2 slices	360	90	45
Deluxe	2 slices	540	207	95
Extravaganza	2 slices	510	216	104
Pepperoni	2 slices	410	135	68
with extra cheese	2 slices	460	176	86
Pepperoni Feast	2 slices	460	171	81
Pepperoni, Sausage, Mushroom	2 slices	460	180	81
Sausage	2 slices	430	149	68
Vegi Feast	2 slices	390	117	59

Dunkin' Donuts
Cookie

FOOD	AMOUNT	TOTAL	FAT	SAT-FAT
Chocolate Chunk	1	200	90	NA
with nuts	1	210	99	NA
Oatmeal Pecan Raisin	1	200	81	NA
Croissant	1	310	171	NA
Almond	1	420	243	NA
Chocolate	1	440	261	NA
Donut				
Apple-filled with Cinnamon Sugar	1	250	99	NA
Bavarian with Chocolate Frosting	1	240	99	NA
Blueberry-filled	1	210	72	NA
Glazed French Cruller	1	140	72	NA
Jelly-filled	1	220	81	NA
Lemon-filled	1	260	108	NA
Glazed Coffee Roll	1	280	108	NA
Rings				
Cake	1	270	153	NA
Chocolate-frosted Yeast	1	200	90	NA
Glazed				
Buttermilk	1	290	126	NA
Chocolate	1	324	189	NA
Whole-Wheat	1	330	162	NA
Yeast	1	200	81	NA

FAST FOODS

FOOD	AMOUNT	CALORIES		
		TOTAL	FAT	SAT-FAT
Muffin				
Apple 'n Spice	1	300	72	NA
Banana Nut	1	310	90	NA
Blueberry	1	280	72	NA
Bran with Raisins	1	310	81	NA
Corn	1	340	108	NA
Cranberry Nut	1	290	81	NA
Oat Bran	1	330	99	NA
Hardee's				
Apple Turnover	1	270	108	36
Big Cookie Treat	1	250	117	36
Big Country Breakfast				
Bacon	1	660	360	90
Country Ham	1	670	342	81
Ham	1	620	297	63
Sausage	1	849	630	144
Big Twin	1	450	225	99
Bagel				
Bacon	1	280	81	34
Bacon and Egg	1	330	108	41
Bacon, Egg, and Cheese	1	375	144	68
Egg	1	250	54	24
Egg and Cheese	1	295	90	NA
Plain	1	200	27	5
Sausage	1	350	144	59
Sausage and Egg	1	400	171	68
Sausage, Egg, and Cheese	1	445	207	86
Biscuit	1	257	112	29
Bacon	1	360	189	36
Bacon and Egg	1	410	216	45
Bacon, Egg, and Cheese	1	460	252	72
Canadian Rise 'n Shine	1	482	250	72
Cheese	1	304	142	NA
Chicken	1	430	198	36
Cinnamon 'n Raisin	1	320	153	45
Country Ham	1	350	162	27
Country Ham and Egg	1	400	198	36
Ham	1	320	144	18
Ham and Egg	1	370	171	36
Ham, Egg, and Cheese	1	420	207	54
'N Gravy	1	440	216	54

FAST FOODS

FOOD	AMOUNT	CALORIES		
		TOTAL	FAT	SAT-FAT
Biscuit (*cont.*)				
Rise 'n Shine	1	320	162	27
Sausage	1	440	255	63
Sausage and Egg	1	503	280	72
Steak	1	500	261	63
Steak and Egg	1	550	288	72
Western Omelet	1	400	243	72
Breadstick	1	150	36	0
Cheeseburger	1	300	134	54
Bacon	1	610	351	144
Quarter-pound	1	500	261	126
Chicken Fillet Sandwich	1	370	117	18
Coleslaw	4 oz	240	180	27
Combo Sub	1	380	54	27
Cool Twist Sundae (hot fudge)	1	320	90	45
Crispy Curls	1 order	300	144	27
Fisherman's Fillet Sandwich	1	469	190	45
French Fries	1 large	360	153	27
	1 regular	230	100	18
Fried Chicken				
Breast	1	340	171	63
Chicken Stix	6 pieces	210	81	18
Leg	1	152	72	27
Thigh	1	370	234	81
Wing	1	205	117	45
Frisco Breakfast Sandwich	1	430	180	63
Frisco Chicken Sandwich	1	680	369	90
Frisco Club Sandwich	1	670	378	108
Grilled Chicken Breast Sandwich	1	310	81	9
Hamburger	1	260	90	36
Big Deluxe	1	503	270	108
Frisco Burger	1	730	423	153
Ham Sub	1	370	63	36
Hash Rounds	1 serving	249	126	27
Hot Dog	1	290	144	36
Hot Ham 'n Cheese Sandwich	1	330	108	45
Mushroom 'n Swiss Burger Sandwich	1	509	243	117
Muffin				
Blueberry	1	400	153	36
Oatbran Raisin	1	410	144	27

FAST FOODS

FOOD	AMOUNT	CALORIES		
		TOTAL	FAT	SAT-FAT
Pancakes	1 order	280	18	9
with 2 strips of bacon	1 order	350	81	27
with a sausage patty	1 order	430	144	54
Roast Beef Sandwich				
Big	1	380	162	72
Regular	1	280	99	36
Roast Beef Sub	1	370	45	27
Salad				
Chef	1	215	117	72
Green	1	184	108	63
Grilled Chicken, no dressing	1	120	36	9
Potato	1 small	260	171	27
Shrimp 'n Pasta	1 serving	362	261	NA
Shakes				
Chocolate	1	390	90	54
Peach	1	530	99	63
Strawberry	1	390	72	45
Vanilla	1	370	81	54
Turkey Club Sandwich	1	390	144	36
Turkey Sub	1	390	63	36
Jack in the Box				
Apple Turnover	1	354	171	NA
Breakfast Jack	1	307	117	46
Cheeseburger	1	315	126	51
Bacon	1	705	405	135
Double	1	467	243	111
Ultimate	1	942	621	238
Cheesecake	1 slice	309	162	85
Chicken and Mushroom Sandwich	1	438	162	45
Chicken Fajita Pita	1	292	72	27
Chicken Strips	4 pieces	285	117	28
Chicken Supreme Sandwich	1	641	351	90
Chicken Wings	6 pieces	846	396	96
Country-Fried Steak Sandwich	1	450	225	63
Crescent				
Sausage	1	584	387	140
Supreme	1	547	360	119
Curly Fries	1 serving	358	180	42
Double Fudge Cake	1 piece	288	81	20
Egg Rolls	3	437	216	61

FAST FOODS

FOOD	AMOUNT	CALORIES		
		TOTAL	FAT	SAT-FAT
Fish Supreme Sandwich	1	510	243	55
French Fries	1 regular	351	153	36
Grilled Chicken Fillet				
Sandwich	1	431	171	42
Hamburger	1	276	108	37
Grilled Sourdough	1	712	450	143
Ham and Swiss	1	638	351	NA
Mushroom	1	477	243	NA
Swiss and Bacon	1	643	387	NA
Hash browns	1 order	156	99	23
Jumbo Jack	1	584	306	99
with cheese	1	677	360	126
Mini Chimichangas	4 pieces	571	252	77
Moby Jack	1	444	225	NA
Old-Fashioned Patty Melt	1	713	414	133
Onion Rings	1 serving	382	207	50
Pancake Platter	1	612	198	77
Salad				
Chef	1	325	162	76
Pasta Seafood	1 serving	394	198	NA
Taco	1	503	279	121
Scrambled Egg				
Platter	1	560	288	78
Pocket	1	431	189	68
Shakes				
Chocolate	1	330	63	39
Strawberry	1	320	63	39
Vanilla	1	320	54	32
Sirloin Steak Sandwich	1	517	207	45
Sourdough Breakfast				
Sandwich	1	381	180	64
Supreme Nachos	1 serving	718	360	NA
Taco				
regular	1 serving	191	99	34
super	1 serving	288	153	53
Toasted Raviolis	7 pieces	537	252	72
Tortilla Chips	1 serving	139	54	NA
KFC (Kentucky Fried Chicken)				
Buttermilk Biscuit	1	235	108	29
Chicken Little Sandwich	1	169	90	18
Coleslaw	1 serving	114	54	9

FAST FOODS

FOOD	AMOUNT	CALORIES		
		TOTAL	FAT	SAT-FAT
Colonel's Chicken Sandwich	1	482	243	**51**
Corn on the Cob	1 serving	176	27	**9**
Kentucky Fried Chicken				
Extra Tasty Crispy Chicken				
breast	1	344	189	**45**
drumstick	1	205	126	**27**
thigh	1	415	280	**72**
wing	1	230	153	**36**
Hot and Spicy Chicken				
breast	1	382	225	**54**
drumstick	1	207	126	**27**
thigh	1	412	270	**72**
wing	1	244	162	**36**
Hot	6	471	297	**72**
Original Recipe Chicken				
breast	1	276	126	**36**
drumstick	1	150	81	**18**
thigh	1	290	189	**45**
wing	1	181	108	**27**
Kentucky Fried Chicken Dinner				
Original Recipe				
wing and breast	1 dinner	604	289	**NA**
drumstick and thigh	1 dinner	643	317	**NA**
wing and thigh	1 dinner	661	340	**NA**
Extra Crispy				
wing and breast	1 dinner	755	383	**NA**
drumstick and thigh	1 dinner	765	483	**NA**
wing and thigh	1 dinner	902	434	**NA**
Kentucky Fries	1 serving	244	108	**27**
Kentucky Nuggets	6 pieces	280	162	**38**
Long John Silver's				
Baked Chicken	1 order	130	36	**11**
Dinner	1 order	550	135	**29**
Baked Fish	1 order	150	9	**NA**
Dinner	1 order	570	108	**19**
Baked Shrimp	1 order	120	45	**NA**
Batter-Dipped Chicken Sandwich	1	280	72	**19**
Batter-Dipped Fish Sandwich	1	340	117	**29**
Batter-Fried Fish	1 piece	180	100	**18**

FAST FOODS

FOOD	AMOUNT	TOTAL	FAT	SAT-FAT
		CALORIES		
Batter-Fried Shrimp	1 piece	47	27	6
Dinner	1 serving	711	405	NA
Breaded Clams	1 order	526	279	46
Breaded Oysters	1 piece	60	27	NA
Breaded Shrimp	1 order	388	207	21
Platter	1 order	962	513	NA
Chicken Nuggets Dinner	6 pieces	699	405	NA
Chicken Plank	1 piece	120	54	14
Chicken Planks	2 pieces	240	108	29
with fries	2 pieces	490	234	51
with fries	3 pieces	885	459	86
for kids	2 pieces	560	261	57
Chocolate Chip Cookie	1	230	81	51
Chowder				
Clam	1 serving			
	(6.6 oz)	128	45	16
Seafood	1 cup	140	54	18
Clam Dinner	1 order	990	522	99
Coleslaw	½ cup	140	54	9
Combination entrees, with				
fries, slaw, 2 hush puppies				
1 fish and 2 chicken	1 order	950	441	99
2 fish and 8 shrimp	1 order	1140	585	127
2 fish, 5 shrimp, and				
1 chicken	1 order	1160	585	128
2 fish, 4 shrimp, and 3 oz				
clams	1 order	1240	630	137
Corn Cobbette	1 piece	140	72	23
Fish and Chicken				
with fries	1 piece each	550	288	61
for kids	1 piece each	620	306	67
Fish and Fryes				
2 pieces of fish	1 order	651	324	72
3 pieces of fish	1 order	853	432	91
Fish Dinner, fried, 3 pieces	1 order	1180	630	NA
Fish Sandwich, Homestyle	1 order	510	198	44
Fryes	1 order	247	135	23
Hush Puppies	1	70	18	4
Oatmeal Raisin Cookie	1	160	90	18
Ocean Chef Salad	1 order	110	9	4
Oyster Dinner	1 order	789	405	NA

FAST FOODS

| FOOD | AMOUNT | CALORIES | | |
		TOTAL	FAT	SAT-FAT
Pie				
Apple	1 piece	320	117	**41**
Cherry	1 piece	360	117	**40**
Lemon	1 piece	340	81	**27**
Pumpkin	1 piece	251	99	**NA**
Scallop Dinner	1 order	747	405	**NA**
Saltines	2	25	9	**NA**
Seafood Gumbo	1 cup	120	72	**19**
Seafood Platter	1 order	976	522	**NA**
Seafood Salad	1 order	380	279	**46**
Tartar Sauce	1	50	45	**9**
Walnut Brownie	1	440	198	**49**
McDonald's				
Apple Pie	1	260	135	**43**
Big Mac	1	570	315	**104**
Biscuit with Biscuit Spread	1	330	164	**68**
Bacon, Egg, and Cheese	1	483	284	**83**
Sausage	1	467	278	**105**
Sausage and Egg	1	585	360	**131**
Cheeseburger	1	318	144	**60**
Chef Salad	1	170	81	**36**
Chicken McNuggets	6 pieces	323	182	**46**
Cookies				
Chocolaty Chip	1 box	342	144	**74**
McDonaldland	1 box	308	99	**38**
Danish				
Apple	1	390	162	**31**
Cinnamon Raisin	1	440	189	**38**
Iced Cheese	1	390	198	**54**
Raspberry	1	410	144	**28**
Egg McMuffin	1 order	340	142	**53**
English Muffin with Butter	1 order	186	45	**21**
Filet-O-Fish	1 order	435	231	**50**
Fries				
small	1 order	220	108	**23**
medium	1 order	320	153	**32**
large	1 order	400	198	**45**
Hamburger	1	263	99	**40**
Hash Brown Potatoes	1 order	144	81	**26**
Hotcakes with Syrup and Butter	1 order	500	90	**34**

FAST FOODS

FOOD	AMOUNT	CALORIES		
		TOTAL	FAT	SAT-FAT
McChicken	1	490	257	**49**
McD.L.T.	1 order	680	396	**133**
McLean Deluxe	1	320	90	**36**
with cheese	1	370	126	**45**
Quarter Pounder	1	427	212	**82**
with cheese	1	525	284	**115**
Sausage	1	210	171	**45**
Sausage McMuffin	1	427	237	**91**
with egg	1	517	296	**115**
Scrambled Eggs	1 serving	180	117	**46**
Shake				
Chocolate	1	383	81	**37**
Strawberry	10.2 fl oz	362	81	**37**
Soft Serve and Cone	1 serving	189	45	**20**
Sundae				
Caramel	1	361	90	**31**
Hot fudge	1 order	357	99	**49**
Strawberry	1 serving	320	81	**29**
Pizza Hut				
Hand-Tossed Pizza, medium				
Cheese	2 slices	518	180	**122**
Pepperoni	2 slices	500	207	**116**
Super Supreme	2 slices	556	225	**117**
Supreme	2 slices	540	234	**124**
Pan Pizza, medium				
Cheese	2 slices	492	162	**81**
Pepperoni	2 slices	540	198	**83**
Super Supreme	2 slices	563	234	**108**
Supreme	2 slices	589	270	**124**
Personal Pan Pizza				
Pepperoni	1 pizza	675	261	**113**
Supreme	1 pizza	647	252	**101**
Thin 'n Crispy pizza, medium				
Cheese	2 slices	398	153	**94**
Pepperoni	2 slices	413	180	**95**
Super Supreme	2 slices	463	189	**94**
Supreme	2 slices	459	198	**99**
Red Lobster				
Alaskan Snow Crab Legs	1 order	200	99	**54**
Bay Platter	1	680	243	**81**
Bayou-style Seafood Gumbo	6 oz	180	45	**9**

FAST FOODS

FOOD	AMOUNT	CALORIES		
		TOTAL	FAT	SAT-FAT
Broiled Flounder Fillets	1 order	150	54	27
Broiled Rock Lobster	1 order	250	45	18
Fish Fillet Sandwich	1	230	85	<9
Grilled Chicken Breast	1	170	54	18
Grilled Chicken and Shrimp	1 order	490	180	54
Grilled Chicken Sandwich	1	340	90	36
Grilled Shrimp Skewers	1 order	290	81	36
Ice Cream	1 order	260	126	81
Live Maine Lobster	1 order	200	45	18
Seafood Lover's Platter	1	650	243	108
Sherbet	1 order	180	27	18
Shrimp				
Cocktail	1	90	18	4
in the Shell	6 oz	130	18	<9
Scampi	1 order	310	207	126
Today's Fresh Catch (for lunch portions, halve the calories and fat calories)				
Atlantic Cod	1 dinner	300	108	54
Atlantic Salmon	1 dinner	460	306	108
Catfish	1 dinner	440	270	108
Coho Salmon	1 dinner	480	252	90
Grouper	1 dinner	300	108	54
Haddock	1 dinner	320	108	54
King Salmon	1 dinner	580	360	72
Mahi Mahi	1 dinner	320	108	54
Ocean Perch	1 dinner	360	162	90
Orange Roughy	1 dinner	440	270	54
Rainbow Trout	1 dinner	440	252	72
Red Rockfish	1 dinner	280	108	54
Sea Bass	1 dinner	360	144	72
Snapper	1 dinner	320	108	54
Sole	1 dinner	320	108	54
Swordfish	1 dinner	300	162	108
Walleye Pike	1 dinner	340	108	54
Yellow Lake Perch	1 dinner	340	108	54
Roy Rogers				
Bacon Bits	1 tsp	24	9	NA
Baked Potato, Hot-Topped				
Bacon 'n Cheese	1	397	198	NA
Broccoli 'n Cheese	1	376	162	NA
Plain	1	211	0	NA
Sour Cream 'n Chives	1	408	189	NA

FAST FOODS

| FOOD | AMOUNT | CALORIES | | |
		TOTAL	FAT	SAT-FAT
Baked Potato (*cont.*)				
Taco Beef 'n Cheese	1	463	198	NA
with margarine	1	274	63	NA
Biscuit	1	231	108	NA
Breakfast Crescent Sandwich	1	401	243	NA
Bacon	1	431	270	NA
Ham	1	557	378	NA
Sausage	1	449	261	NA
Brownie	1	264	99	NA
Cheddar Cheese	¼ cup	112	81	NA
Cheeseburger	1	563	333	NA
Bacon	1	581	351	NA
Chicken				
breast	1	324	171	NA
breast and wing	1	466	261	NA
leg	1	117	63	NA
thigh	1	282	180	NA
thigh and leg	1	399	234	NA
wing	1	142	90	NA
Chinese Noodles	¼ cup	55	27	NA
Coleslaw	1 order	110	63	NA
Crescent Roll	1	287	162	NA
Danish				
Apple	1	249	108	NA
Cheese	1	271	108	NA
Cherry	1	271	126	NA
Egg and Biscuit Platter	1	394	243	NA
Bacon	1	435	270	NA
Ham	1	442	261	NA
Sausage	1	550	369	NA
French Fries				
large	1 order	357	162	NA
regular	1 order	268	126	NA
Hamburger	1	456	252	NA
RR Bar Burger	1	611	351	NA
Hot Chocolate	1	123	18	NA
Macaroni	1 order	186	99	NA
Pancake Platter (with syrup				
and butter)	1	452	135	NA
Bacon	1	493	162	NA
Ham	1	506	153	NA
Sausage	1	608	270	NA

FAST FOODS

FOOD	AMOUNT	CALORIES		
		TOTAL	FAT	SAT-FAT
Potato Salad	1	107	54	NA
Roast Beef Sandwich	1	317	90	NA
with cheese	1	424	171	NA
large	1	360	108	NA
with cheese	1	467	189	NA
Shake				
Chocolate	1	358	90	NA
Strawberry	1	315	90	NA
Vanilla	1	306	99	NA
Strawberry Shortcake	1 piece	447	171	NA
Sundae				
Caramel	1	293	72	NA
Strawberry	1	216	63	NA
Taco Bell				
Burritos				
Bean	1	447	126	18
Beef	1	493	189	72
Chicken	1	334	108	NA
Combo	1	407	144	45
Supreme	1	503	198	NA
Chilito	1	383	162	72
Cinnamon Twists	1 order	171	72	27
Guacamole	2 tbsp	34	18	0
MexiMelt				
Beef	1	266	135	72
Chicken	1	257	135	NA
Nacho Cheese Sauce	2 tbsp	103	72	27
Nachos	1 order	346	162	54
BellGrande	1 order	649	315	108
Supreme	1 order	367	243	45
Pintos 'n Cheese	1 order	190	81	36
Salsa	1 serving	18	0	0
Soft Taco	1	225	108	NA
Chicken	1	213	90	36
Supreme	1	272	144	72
Taco	1	183	99	45
Supreme	1	230	135	72
Taco Salad	1	905	549	171
without shell	1	680	279	126
Taco Sauce	1 serving	3	0	0
Tostada	1	243	99	36

FAST FOODS

FOOD	AMOUNT	CALORIES		
		TOTAL	FAT	SAT-FAT
Wendy's				
Baked Potato, plain	1	250	0	**0**
Bacon and Cheese	1	510	153	**36**
Broccoli and Cheese	1	450	126	**18**
Cheese	1	550	216	**72**
Chili and Cheese	1	600	225	**81**
Sour Cream and Chives	1	500	207	**84**
Big Classic Sandwich	1	570	297	**54**
Breaded Chicken	1 fillet	220	90	**18**
Sandwich	1	450	180	**36**
Chicken Club Sandwich	1	520	225	**54**
Cheeseburger				
Double	1	590	297	**128**
Jr. Cheeseburger	1	320	117	**45**
Bacon	1	440	225	**72**
Deluxe	1	390	180	**63**
Kid's Meal	1	310	117	**45**
Chicken Nuggets	6	280	180	**40**
Chili				
large	1	290	81	**36**
small	1	190	54	**18**
Chocolate Chip Cookie	1	275	117	**38**
Chow Mein Noodles	¼ cup	74	36	**5**
Cole Slaw	½ cup	90	72	**18**
Country-Fried Steak Sandwich	1	460	234	**63**
Fish Sandwich	1	460	225	**42**
French Fries				
large	1 order	450	198	**45**
small	1 order	240	108	**23**
Frosty Dairy Dessert				
large	1	578	153	**76**
small	1	340	90	**45**
Fruit-Flavored Drink	12 fl oz	110	0	**0**
Grilled Chicken	1 fillet	100	27	**9**
Sandwich	1	290	63	**9**
Hamburger	1	350	135	**54**
with Everything	1	440	207	**63**
Double Hamburger	1	520	243	**96**
Jr. Hamburger	1	270	81	**27**
Kid's Meal	1 serving	270	81	**27**
Hot Chocolate	6 fl oz	100	27	**9**

FAST FOODS

FOOD	AMOUNT	CALORIES		
		TOTAL	FAT	SAT-FAT
Mexican Fiesta Superbar				
Cheese Sauce	4 tbsp	40	36	9
Picante Sauce	2 tbsp	10	0	0
Refried Beans	4 tbsp	70	18	8
Spanish Rice	4 tbsp	60	9	2
Taco Chips	8	160	54	9
Taco Sauce	2 tbsp	12	0	0
Taco Shells	1	50	27	6
Tortilla	1	100	27	4
Pasta Superbar				
Alfredo Sauce	4 tbsp	30	9	7
Fettuccine	½ cup	120	36	9
Garlic Toast	1 piece	70	27	9
Macaroni and Cheese	½ cup	130	54	27
Pasta Medley	4 tbsp	60	18	3
Rotini	4 tbsp	90	18	3
Spaghetti Meat Sauce	4 tbsp	45	9	6
Spaghetti Sauce	4 tbsp	30	0	0
Salad				
Caesar Side Salad	1	160	54	9
Chicken (salad bar)	¼ cup	120	72	14
Deluxe Garden, without dressing	1	110	45	9
Grilled Chicken, without dressing	1	200	72	9
Side, without dressing	1	60	27	<9
Taco, without dressing	1	640	270	108
Sunflower Seeds and Raisins	2 tbsp	140	90	67
Turkey Ham	¼ cup	35	18	4

FATS AND OILS

FOOD	AMOUNT	CALORIES		
		TOTAL	FAT	SAT-FAT
Animal Fats				
Beef tallow	1 tbsp	116	116	58
Butter				
regular	1 pat	36	36	23
	1 tbsp	100	100	65
	1 stick	813	813	515

FATS AND OILS

FOOD	AMOUNT	CALORIES TOTAL	FAT	SAT-FAT
Butter (*cont.*)				
whipped	1 tsp	23	23	**12**
	1 tbsp	67	67	**38**
Chicken fat	1 tbsp	115	115	**34**
Duck fat	1 tbsp	115	115	**39**
Goose fat	1 tbsp	115	115	**32**
Lard (pork)	1 tbsp	116	116	**45**
Mutton tallow	1 tbsp	116	116	**55**
Turkey fat	1 tbsp	115	115	**34**
Butter Substitutes				
Butter Buds Sprinkles	1 tsp (2 g)	8	0	**0**
Molly McButter	1 tsp (2 g)	5	0	**0**
Margarines				
Stick				
Fleischmann's	1 tbsp (14 g)	90	90	**18**
lower fat	1 tbsp (14 g)	40	40	**0**
Imperial	1 tbsp (14 g)	90	90	**18**
Land O Lakes				
Country Morning Blend	1 tbsp (14 g)	100	100	**36**
light	1 tbsp (14 g)	50	50	**27**
Spread with Sweet Cream	1 tbsp (14 g)	90	90	**18**
Move Over Butter	1 tbsp (14 g)	90	90	**18**
Promise	1 tbsp (14 g)	90	90	**18**
Shedd's Spread Country Crock				
Churn-Style	1 tbsp (14 g)	80	80	**18**
Spreadable Stick	1 tbsp (14 g)	80	80	**14**
Tub				
Fleischmann's	1 tbsp (14 g)	90	90	**18**
I Can't Believe It's Not Butter,				
light	1 tbsp (14 g)	70	70	**14**
Land O Lakes Spread with				
Sweet Cream	1 tbsp (14 g)	80	80	**14**
Move Over Butter	1 tbsp (10 g)	60	60	**14**
Parkay				
soft	1 tbsp (14 g)	100	100	**18**
spread	1 tbsp (14 g)	60	60	**14**
Promise	1 tbsp (14 g)	90	90	**14**
ultra	1 tbsp (14 g)	35	35	**0**
ultra-fat-free	1 tbsp (14 g)	5	5	**0**

FATS AND OILS

| FOOD | AMOUNT | CALORIES | | |
		TOTAL	FAT	SAT-FAT
Shedd's Spread Country Crock	1 tbsp (14 g)	60	60	14
Churn-Style	1 tbsp (14 g)	60	60	14
Smart Beat, super light	1 tbsp (14 g)	20	20	0

Oils

FOOD	AMOUNT	TOTAL	FAT	SAT-FAT
Canola	1 tbsp	120	120	9
Cocoa butter	1 tbsp	120	120	73
Coconut	1 tbsp	120	120	106
Corn	1 tbsp	120	120	15
Cottonseed	1 tbsp	120	120	32
Olive	1 tbsp	119	119	16
Palm	1 tbsp	120	120	60
Palm kernel	1 tbsp	120	120	100
Peanut	1 tbsp	119	119	21
Safflower	1 tbsp	120	120	11
Sesame	1 tbsp	120	120	17
Soybean	1 tbsp	120	120	18
Sunflower	1 tbsp	120	120	13
Walnut	1 tbsp	120	120	11

Salad Dressings and Spreads

FOOD	AMOUNT	TOTAL	FAT	SAT-FAT
Bacon and Tomato (Kraft)	2 tbsp	140	130	23
Balsamic and Basil Vinaigrette				
(Ken's)	2 tbsp	110	110	14
Blue Cheese				
chunky (Wish-Bone)	2 tbsp	150	140	27
Free (Kraft)	2 tbsp	45	0	0
regular (Kraft)	2 tbsp	90	70	36
Caesar				
Gourmet (Good Seasons)	2 tbsp prep.	150	140	23
light (Ken's)	2 tbsp	70	60	5
regular (Ken's)	2 tbsp	140	120	18
Caesar Ranch (Kraft)	2 tbsp	140	130	23
Catalina				
Free (Kraft)	2 tbsp	45	0	0
regular (Kraft)	2 tbsp	140	100	18
Coleslaw Dressing				
Hidden Valley Ranch	2 tbsp	150	140	27
Kraft	2 tbsp	150	110	18
Cucumber and Chive, fat-free				
(Ken's)	2 tbsp	30	0	0
Cucumber Ranch (Kraft)	2 tbsp	60	45	9

FATS AND OILS

FOOD	AMOUNT	CALORIES		
		TOTAL	FAT	SAT-FAT
French (Kraft)	2 tbsp	120	100	18
Free (Kraft)	2 tbsp	50	0	0
Garlic and Herb (Good Seasons)	2 tbsp prep.	140	140	20
Honey Dijon				
fat-free (Ken's)	2 tbsp	40	0	0
light (Hidden Valley)	2 tbsp	35	0	0
regular (Kraft)	2 tbsp	140	120	18
Italian				
Free (Kraft)	2 tbsp	10	0	0
light (Wish-Bone)	2 tbsp	15	5	0
regular (Good Seasons)	2 tbsp prep.	140	140	20
regular (Kraft)	2 tbsp	120	110	18
zesty (Good Seasons)	2 tbsp prep.	140	140	20
zesty (Kraft)	2 tbsp	110	100	14
Mayonnaise				
Hellman's				
light	1 tbsp (15 g)	50	45	9
regular	1 tbsp (15 g)	100	100	14
Kraft				
Free	1 tbsp (15 g)	10	0	0
light	1 tbsp (15 g)	50	45	9
regular	1 tbsp	100	100	18
Mayonnaise substitute				
Miracle Whip (Kraft)	1 tbsp	70	60	9
light	1 tbsp	40	30	9
Nacho Cheese Ranch (Hidden Valley)	2 tbsp	130	120	18
Oriental Sesame (Good Seasons)	2 tbsp prep.	150	140	23
Parmesan, creamy low-fat (Hidden Valley Ranch)	2 tbsp	30	0	0
Parmesan Pepper, light (Ken's)	2 tbsp	80	60	14
Peppercorn Free (Kraft)	2 tbsp	50	0	0
Pizza Ranch (Hidden Valley)	2 tbsp	140	130	18
Ranch				
Free (Kraft)	2 tbsp	50	0	0
light (Hidden Valley)	2 tbsp	80	60	9
original (Hidden Valley)	2 tbsp	140	130	18
regular (Kraft)	2 tbsp	170	170	27
super creamy (Hidden Valley Ranch)	2 tbsp	140	130	NA

FATS AND OILS

FOOD	AMOUNT	CALORIES		
		TOTAL	FAT	SAT-FAT
Raspberry Walnut, light				
(Ken's)	2 tbsp	80	50	0
Russian	2 tbsp	166	160	29
Salsa Zesty Garden (Kraft)	2 tbsp	70	60	9
Sun-Dried Tomato Vinaigrette,				
free (Ken's)	2 tbsp	15	0	0
Taco Ranch (Hidden Valley				
Ranch)	2 tbsp	130	120	18
Thousand Island				
Free (Kraft)	2 tbsp	45	0	0
regular (Kraft)	2 tbsp	110	90	14
Shortening				
Crisco	1 tbsp	110	110	27

FISH AND SHELLFISH

Unless otherwise noted, fish is baked, steamed, or broiled with *no added fat.* If fish is baked in butter or margarine and you are keeping track of total fat, for each teaspoon of butter or margarine you use, add 33 total calories to the total calories listed for each fish and 33 fat calories to the fat calories listed for each fish. If you are keeping track of saturated fat, for each teaspoon of butter you use, add 33 total calories to the total calories listed for each fish and 22 sat-fat calories to the sat-fat calories listed for each fish. For margarine, add 33 total calories to the total calories listed for each fish and 18 sat-fat calories to the sat-fat calories listed for each fish. *See also* **FROZEN, MICROWAVE, AND REFRIGERATED FOODS** and **FAST FOODS.**

*Remember that most of the following calorie figures are for **only 1 ounce** of seafood!*

FOOD	AMOUNT	CALORIES		
		TOTAL	FAT	SAT-FAT
Abalone				
raw	1 oz	30	2	0
cooked, fried	1 oz	54	17	4
Anchovy				
raw	1 oz	37	12	3
canned in oil, drained	1 oz	60	25	6
	5 anchovies (20 g)	42	17	4

FISH AND SHELLFISH

FOOD	AMOUNT	CALORIES		
		TOTAL	FAT	SAT-FAT
Bass				
freshwater, raw	1 oz	32	9	2
	1 fillet (79 g)	90	26	6
striped, raw	1 oz	27	6	1
	1 fillet (159 g)	154	33	7
Bluefish				
raw	1 oz	35	11	2
	1 fillet (150 g)	186	57	12
Burbot, raw	1 oz	25	2	0
	1 fillet (116 g)	104	8	2
Butterfish, raw	1 oz	41	20	NA
	1 fillet (32 g)	47	23	NA
Carp				
raw	1 oz	36	14	3
	1 fillet (218 g)	276	110	21
cooked, dry heat	1 oz	46	18	4
	1 fillet (170 g)	276	110	21
Catfish, channel				
breaded and fried	1 oz	65	34	8
	1 fillet (87 g)	199	104	26
raw	1 oz	33	11	3
	1 fillet (79 g)	92	30	7
Caviar, black and red	1 tbsp	40	26	15
	1 oz	71	45	27
Cisco (lake herring)				
raw	1 oz	28	5	1
	1 fillet (79 g)	78	14	3
smoked	1 oz	50	30	4
Clams				
raw, cherrystones or littlenecks	9 large or 20 small (180 g)	133	16	1
	1 oz	22	3	0
breaded and fried	1 oz	57	28	7
	20 small clams (188 g)	379	189	45
canned, drained solids	1 oz	42	5	0
	½ cup	118	14	1
cooked, moist heat	1 oz	42	5	0
	20 small clams (90 g)	133	16	2
fritters	1 fritter	124	54	NA

FISH AND SHELLFISH

| FOOD | AMOUNT | CALORIES | | |
		TOTAL	FAT	SAT-FAT
Cod, Atlantic				
raw	1 oz	23	2	0
	1 fillet (231 g)	190	14	3
baked	1 oz	30	2	0
	1 fillet (180 g)	189	14	3
canned	1 oz	30	2	1
dried and salted	1 oz	81	6	0
Cod, Pacific, raw	1 oz	23	2	0
	1 fillet (116 g)	95	7	1
Crab				
Alaska king, steamed	1 oz	27	4	0
	1 leg (172 g)	129	18	2
Alaska king, imitation, made from surimi	1 oz	29	3	NA
Blue				
raw	1 oz	25	3	0
	1 crab (21 g)	18	2	0
cooked, moist heat	1 oz	27	4	1
canned	1 oz	28	3	0
	½ cup	67	7	2
Crab cakes	1 cake	93	41	8
	1 oz	44	19	4
Chesapeake Bay Deluxe Crab Cakes, frozen	1 oz	65	41	NA
Dungeness, raw	1 oz	24	2	0
Nutri Sea Crab Sticks	1 oz	29	3	NA
Nutri Sea King Crab	1 oz	31	3	NA
Sea Legs, Crabmeat Salad Style	1 oz	27	3	NA
Crayfish				
raw	1 oz	25	3	0
	8 crayfish (27 g)	24	2	0
steamed	1 oz	32	3	0
Croaker, Atlantic				
raw	1 oz	30	8	3
	1 fillet (79 g)	83	22	8
breaded and fried	1 oz	63	32	9
	1 fillet (87 g)	192	99	27
Cusk, raw	1 oz	25	2	NA
Cuttlefish, raw	1 oz	22	2	

FISH AND SHELLFISH

FOOD	AMOUNT	CALORIES		
		TOTAL	FAT	SAT-FAT
Dolphinfish, raw	1 oz	24	2	0
	1 fillet (204 g)	174	13	3
Drum, freshwater, raw	1 oz	34	13	3
	1 fillet (198 g)	236	88	20
Eel				
raw	1 oz	52	30	6
baked	1 oz	67	38	8
	1 fillet (159 g)	375	214	43
Flatfish (flounder or sole)				
raw	1 oz	26	3	1
	1 fillet (163 g)	149	17	4
baked or steamed	1 oz	33	4	1
	1 fillet (127 g)	148	17	4
Gefilte fish	1 piece	35	7	2
	1 oz	24	4	1
Grouper				
raw	1 oz	26	3	1
	1 fillet (259 g)	238	24	5
baked or steamed	1 oz	33	3	1
	1 fillet (202 g)	238	24	5
Haddock				
raw	1 oz	25	2	0
	1 fillet (193 g)	168	12	2
baked or steamed	1 oz	32	2	0
	1 fillet (150 g)	168	12	2
smoked	1 oz	33	2	0
Halibut, Atlantic and Pacific				
baked or steamed	1 oz	40	7	1
	½ fillet (159 g)	223	42	6
Herring, Atlantic				
raw	1 oz	45	23	5
	1 fillet (184 g)	291	150	34
baked or steamed	1 oz	57	30	7
canned	1 oz	59	35	7
in tomato sauce	1 herring (37 g)	97	52	10
pickled	1 oz	65	39	6
	1 herring	112	68	9
	1 piece (15 g)	33	21	3
smoked, kippered	1 oz	60	33	7
	1 fillet (40 g)	87	45	10
Herring, Pacific, raw	1 oz	55	35	8

FISH AND SHELLFISH

FOOD	AMOUNT	CALORIES		
		TOTAL	FAT	SAT-FAT
Lobster, northern				
raw	1 oz	26	2	0
	1 lobster (150 g)	136	12	NA
cooked, moist heat	1 oz	28	2	0
	1 cup	142	8	1
Newburg (with butter, eggs, sherry, cream)	1 cup	485	239	160
salad (with mayonnaise)	½ cup or 4 oz	286	149	NA
Lox (smoked salmon)	1 oz	33	11	2
Mackerel, Atlantic				
raw	1 oz	58	35	8
	1 fillet (112 g)	229	140	33
baked or steamed	1 oz	74	45	11
	1 fillet (88 g)	231	141	33
Mackerel, Jack, canned	1 cup	296	108	30
Mackerel, king, raw	1 oz	30	9	1
	½ fillet (198 g)	207	36	6
Mackerel, Pacific and Jack, raw	1 oz	44	20	6
	1 fillet (225 g)	353	160	46
Mackerel, Spanish				
raw	1 oz	39	16	5
	1 fillet (187 g)	260	106	31
baked or steamed	1 oz	45	16	5
	1 fillet (146 g)	230	83	24
Milkfish, raw	1 oz	42	17	NA
Monkfish, raw	1 oz	21	4	NA
Mullet, striped				
raw	1 oz	33	10	3
	1 fillet (119 g)	139	41	12
baked	1 oz	42	12	4
	1 fillet (93 g)	139	41	12
Mussels, blue				
raw	1 oz	24	6	1
	1 cup	129	30	6
Ocean perch, Atlantic				
raw	1 oz	27	4	1
	1 fillet (64 g)	60	9	1
baked	1 oz	34	5	1
	1 fillet (50 g)	60	9	1

FISH AND SHELLFISH

FOOD	AMOUNT	CALORIES		
		TOTAL	FAT	SAT-FAT
Ocean perch, Atlantic *(cont.)*				
breaded and fried	1 fillet	185	99	NA
Octopus, raw	1 oz	23	3	1
Oyster, eastern				
raw	6 medium (84 g)	58	19	5
	1 cup	170	55	14
breaded and fried	1 oz	56	32	8
	6 medium (88 g)	173	100	25
canned	1 oz	19	6	2
	½ cup	85	28	7
steamed	1 oz	39	13	3
	6 medium (42 g)	58	19	5
stew (2 parts milk, 1 part oyster)	1 cup	233	139	80
Oyster, Pacific, raw	1 oz	23	6	1
	1 medium (50 g)	41	10	2
Pike, northern				
raw	1 oz	25	2	0
	½ fillet (198 g)	175	12	2
baked	1 oz	32	2	0
	½ fillet (155 g)	176	12	2
Pike, walleye, raw	1 oz	26	3	1
	1 fillet (159 g)	147	17	4
Pollock, Atlantic, raw	1 oz	26	2	0
	½ fillet (193 g)	177	17	2
Pollock, walleye				
raw	1 oz	23	2	0
	1 fillet (77 g)	62	6	1
baked	1 oz	32	3	1
	1 fillet (60 g)	68	6	1
Pompano, Florida				
raw	1 oz	47	24	9
	1 fillet (112 g)	184	95	35
baked	1 oz	60	31	11
	1 fillet (88 g)	185	96	36
Pout, ocean, raw	1 oz	22	2	1
	½ fillet (176 g)	40	14	5

FISH AND SHELLFISH

| FOOD | AMOUNT | CALORIES | | |
		TOTAL	FAT	SAT-FAT
Rockfish, Pacific				
raw	1 oz	27	4	1
	1 fillet (191 g)	180	27	6
baked	1 oz	34	5	1
	1 fillet (149 g)	180	27	6
Roughy, orange, raw	1 oz	36	18	0
Sablefish				
raw	1 oz	55	39	8
	½ fillet (193 g)	377	266	56
smoked	1 oz	72	51	10
Salmon, Atlantic, raw	1 oz	40	16	3
Salmon, chinook				
raw	1 oz	51	27	6
smoked	1 oz	33	11	2
Salmon, chum				
raw	1 oz	34	10	2
canned	1 oz	40	14	4
Salmon, coho				
raw	1 oz	41	15	3
Salmon, pink				
raw	1 oz	33	9	1
canned	1 oz	39	15	4
Salmon, sockeye				
raw	1 oz	48	22	4
canned, drained	1 oz	40	14	4
Salmon, smoked (lox)	1 oz	33	11	2
Sardines, Atlantic, canned in				
oil, drained	1 oz	59	29	3
	2 sardines (24 g)	50	25	3
	1 can (3¼ oz)	192	95	13
Sardines, Pacific, canned in				
tomato sauce, drained	1 oz	51	31	8
	1 sardine (38 g)	68	41	11
Scallops				
raw	1 oz	25	2	0
	2 large or 5 small (30 g)	26	2	0
breaded, fried	1 oz	61	28	6
	2 large (31 g)	67	31	7
steamed	1 oz	32	4	1

FISH AND SHELLFISH

FOOD	AMOUNT	CALORIES		
		TOTAL	FAT	SAT-FAT
Scup, raw	1 oz	30	7	NA
	1 fillet (64 g)	67	16	NA
Sea bass				
raw	1 oz	27	5	1
	1 fillet (129 g)	125	23	6
baked	1 oz	35	7	2
	1 fillet (101 g)	125	23	6
Sea trout, raw	1 oz	29	9	3
	1 fillet (238 g)	248	77	22
Shad				
raw	1 oz	56	35	NA
	1 fillet (184 g)	362	228	NA
baked	1 oz	57	29	NA
Shark				
raw	1 oz	37	11	2
batter-dipped and fried	1 oz	65	35	8
Sheepshead				
raw	1 oz	31	6	2
	1 fillet (238 g)	257	52	13
baked	1 oz	36	4	1
	1 fillet (186 g)	234	27	6
Shrimp				
raw	1 oz	30	4	1
	4 large (28 g)	30	4	1
breaded, fried	1 oz	69	31	5
	4 large (30 g)	73	33	6
canned	1 oz	34	5	1
	½ cup	77	11	2
cocktail (Sau-Sea)	½ cup	90	0	0
steamed	1 oz	28	3	1
	4 large (22 g)	22	2	1
Smelt, rainbow				
raw	1 oz	28	6	1
baked	1 oz	35	8	2
Snapper				
raw	1 oz	28	3	1
	1 fillet (218 g)	217	26	6
baked	1 oz	36	4	1
	1 fillet (170 g)	217	26	6
Sole (see Flatfish)				

FISH AND SHELLFISH

FOOD	AMOUNT	CALORIES		
		TOTAL	FAT	SAT-FAT
Spiny lobster, raw	1 oz	32	4	1
	1 lobster (209 g)	233	28	4
Spot, raw	1 oz	35	12	4
	1 fillet (64 g)	79	28	8
Squid				
raw	1 oz	26	4	1
fried	1 oz	50	19	5
Sturgeon				
raw	1 oz	30	10	2
baked	1 oz	38	13	3
smoked	1 oz	48	11	3
Sucker, white, raw	1 oz	26	6	1
	1 fillet (159 g)	147	33	6
Sunfish, pumpkinseed, raw	1 oz	25	2	0
	1 fillet (48 g)	43	3	0
Surimi	1 oz	28	2	0
Swordfish				
raw	1 oz	34	10	3
baked	1 oz	44	13	4
Tilefish				
raw	1 oz	27	6	1
	½ fillet (193 g)	184	40	8
baked	1 oz	42	12	2
	½ fillet (150 g)	220	63	12
Trout, rainbow				
raw	1 oz	33	9	2
	1 fillet (79 g)	93	24	5
baked	1 oz	43	11	2
	1 fillet (62 g)	94	24	5
Tuna				
raw	1 oz	41	12	3
baked	1 oz	52	16	4
canned, drained				
solid white in water	1 oz	37	6	2
chunk light in oil	1 oz	56	21	4
Tuna salad	½ cup	190	85	14
Turbot, European, raw	1 oz	27	8	NA
	½ fillet (204 g)	194	54	NA
Whelk				
raw	1 oz	39	1	0
steamed	1 oz	78	2	0

FISH AND SHELLFISH

FOOD	AMOUNT	CALORIES		
		TOTAL	FAT	SAT-FAT
Whitefish				
raw	1 oz	38	15	2
	1 fillet (198 g)	266	104	16
smoked	1 oz	30	2	1
Whiting				
raw	1 oz	26	3	1
	1 fillet (92 g)	83	11	2
baked	1 oz	33	4	1
	1 fillet (72 g)	83	11	2
Wolffish, Atlantic, raw	1 oz	27	6	1
	½ fillet (153 g)	147	33	5
Yellowtail, raw	1 oz	41	13	NA
	½ fillet (187 g)	273	88	NA

FROZEN, MICROWAVE, AND REFRIGERATED FOODS

FOOD	AMOUNT	CALORIES		
		TOTAL	FAT	SAT-FAT
Breakfast Foods				
Blintzes				
Ratner's				
Cheese	1 (71 g)	100	5	5
Cherry	1 (71 g)	110	5	5
Potato	1 (71 g)	120	30	18
Breakfast Burritos				
Great Starts				
Bacon (Swanson)	1 pkg (99 g)	250	100	36
Breakfast Sandwich				
Great Starts (Swanson)				
Egg, Canadian Bacon, and Cheese on a Muffin	1 pkg (116 g)	290	140	54
Pancakes with Sausage	1 pkg (170 g)	490	230	99
Sausage, Egg, and Cheese on a Biscuit	1 pkg (156 g)	490	270	108
Scrambled Eggs and Bacon with Home-Fried Potatoes	1 pkg (149 g)	290	170	81

FROZEN, MICROWAVE, AND REFRIGERATED FOODS

FOOD	AMOUNT	CALORIES		
		TOTAL	FAT	SAT-FAT
Breakfast Sandwich				
Great Starts (Swanson) (*cont.*)				
Scrambled Eggs and Sausage with Hashed Brown Potatoes	1 pkg (177 g)	360	230	**90**
Morningstar Farms				
Breakfast Links	2 (45 g)	90	50	**9**
Breakfast Patties	1 (38 g)	90	50	**14**
Grillers	1 (64 g)	140	65	**9**
Weight Watchers				
English Muffin Sandwich	1 (113 g)	220	60	**18**
Croissants				
Original (Sara Lee)	1 (43 g)	170	70	**27**
Eggs				
Great Starts (Swanson)				
Scrambled Eggs and Bacon	1 pkg (149 g)	290	170	**81**
Scrambled Eggs and Home-Fried Potatoes	1 pkg (120 g)	200	110	**72**
Scrambled Eggs and Sausage	1 pkg (177 g)	360	230	**90**
French Toast, Frozen				
Aunt Jemima, all types	2 (118 g)	240	50	**0**
Breakfast Blast Mini Sticks (Swanson)	1 pkg (120)	310	130	**36**
Downyflake				
Cinnamon Swirl	2 (113 g)	270	50	**14**
Plain	2 (113 g)	260	60	**14**
Great Starts (Swanson)				
Cinnamon Swirl French Toast with Sausage	1 pkg (156 g)	440	250	**108**
French Toast Sticks	1 pkg (120 g)	320	90	**45**
French Toast with Sausage	1 pkg (156 g)	410	230	**81**
Muffins				
Blueberry (Sara Lee)	1 (64 g)	220	100	**18**
Pancakes, Frozen				
Aunt Jemima				
Buttermilk Pancake Batter	½ cup batter	260	25	**9**
Low-fat	3 (97 g)	130	15	**0**

FROZEN, MICROWAVE, AND REFRIGERATED FOODS

FOOD	AMOUNT	CALORIES		
		TOTAL	FAT	SAT-FAT
Great Starts (Swanson)				
Silver Dollar	1 pkg (106 g)	340	160	**81**
with sausage	1 pkg (170 g)	490	230	**99**
Hungry Jack				
Blueberry	3 (116 g)	230	30	**5**
Buttermilk	3 (116 g)	240	35	**9**
Toaster Strudel				
Pillsbury, all flavors	1 (54 g)	180	60	**14**
Waffles, Frozen				
Aunt Jemima				
Blueberry	2 (71 g)	190	60	**14**
Buttermilk	2 (71 g)	170	50	**14**
Low-fat	2 (74 g)	160	10	**0**
Oatmeal	2 (84 g)	200	70	**14**
Original	2 (71 g)	180	60	**14**
Belgian Chef Belgian				
Waffles	2 (70 g)	140	25	**5**
Breakfast Blast 5 Waffle				
Sticks	1 pkg (78 g)	330	150	**63**
Downyflake				
Homestyle and Buttermilk	2 (68 g)	170	35	**0**
Eggo				
Blueberry, Buttermilk, or				
Homestyle	2 (78 g)	220	70	**14**
Common Sense Oat Bran	2 (78 g)	200	60	**14**
Fat-free	2 (58 g)	140	0	**0**
Minis, plain or blueberry	2 (85 g)	240	70	**14**
Special K	2 (58 g)	140	0	**0**
Nutri-Grain Eggo				
Multi-bran or Whole-grain	2 (78 g)	180	50	**9**
Dishes or Dinners				
Amy's				
Black Bean, Vegetable				
Enchilada	1 (135 g)	130	40	**<9**
Burrito, nondairy	1 (236 g)	250	45	**23**
Cheese Enchilada	1 (135 g)	210	80	**0**
Mexican Tamale Pie	1 (227 g)	220	27	**0**
Shepherd's Pie	1 (227 g)	160	35	**0**
Vegetable Lasagna	1 (269 g)	300	90	**36**

FROZEN, MICROWAVE, AND REFRIGERATED FOODS

FOOD	AMOUNT	CALORIES		
		TOTAL	FAT	SAT-FAT
Banquet				
Beef Pot Pie	1 (198 g)	330	140	63
Chicken Breast Patties	1 (70 g)	200	110	23
Chicken Breast Tenders	3 (85 g)	210	90	18
Chicken Nugget Meal	1 (191 g)	410	190	45
Chicken Nuggets	9 (84 g)	240	130	27
Chicken Patties	1 (70 g)	200	110	23
Chicken Pot Pie	1 (198 g)	350	160	63
Country Fried Chicken	3 oz (84 g)	270	160	45
Fried Chicken	3 oz (84 g)	270	160	45
Fried Chicken Meal	1 (255 g)	470	240	81
Mozzarella Cheese Nuggets	3 pieces (36 g)	110	50	23
Salisbury Steak Meal	1 (269 g)	310	150	63
Skinless Fried Chicken	3 oz (84 g)	210	120	27
Southern Chicken Chunks	19 nuggets (84 g)	230	140	27
Southern Fried Chicken	3 oz (84 g)	270	160	45
Spicy 'n Hot Fried Chicken	3 oz (84 g)	260	160	45
Turkey and Gravy	1 meal (262 g)	270	90	27
Turkey Pot Pie	1 (198 g)	370	180	72
Vegetable-Cheese Pot Pie	1 (198 g)	390	160	72
Banquet Extra Helping				
Southern Fried Chicken	1 meal (496 g)	750	330	81
Turkey and Gravy	1 meal (532 g)	560	180	45
Budget Gourmet				
Beef Cantonese	1 entree	280	70	27
Cheese Manicotti with Meat Sauce	1 entree	440	230	108
Cheese Tortellini	1 pkg	190	70	18
Chicken and Egg Noodles	1 entree	410	210	108
Chicken Marsala	1 entree	270	60	36
Chicken with Fettucini	1 entree	380	170	90
Escalloped Noodles and Turkey	1 entree	440	180	90
Fettucini Alfredo	1 entree	480	210	117
Italian Sausage Lasagna	1 entree	400	180	90
Linguini with Bay Shrimp and Clams Marinara	1 entree	300	100	54
Oriental Rice with Vegetables	1 pkg	220	110	45

FROZEN, MICROWAVE, AND REFRIGERATED FOODS

FOOD	AMOUNT	CALORIES		
		TOTAL	FAT	SAT-FAT
Pepper Steak with Rice	1 entree	290	70	27
Rice Pilaf with Green Beans	1 pkg	230	110	27
Roast Sirloin Supreme	1 entree	300	110	63
Sirloin Cheddar Melt	1 entree	370	190	90
Sirloin Tips	1 entree	260	130	54
Swedish Meatballs	1 entree	550	300	144
Szechuan Vegetables and Chicken	1 entree	300	80	14
Three-Cheese Lasagna	1 entree	370	140	90
Wide Ribbon Pasta with Ricotta and Chunky Tomato Sauce	1 entree	420	200	72
Ziti in Marinara Sauce	1 pkg	220	90	36
Budget Gourmet Light & Healthy				
Chicken Oriental and Vegetable	1 entree	300	60	18
Chinese-Style Vegetables and Chicken	1 entree	290	80	14
Glazed Turkey	1 entree	250	35	18
Italian Style Vegetables and Chicken	1 entree	280	60	18
Lasagna with Meat Sauce	1 entree	250	60	27
Linguini with Scallops and Clams	1 entree	300	90	54
Macaroni and Cheese	1 entree	350	70	45
Mandarin Chicken	1 entree	250	40	9
Orange-Glazed Chicken Breast	1 entree	270	25	9
Oriental Beef	1 entree	290	80	45
Penne Pasta with Chunky Tomato Sauce and Italian Sausage	1 entree	330	70	23
Roast Chicken Breast with Herb Gravy	1 dinner	240	60	18
Sirloin of Beef in Herb Sauce	1 entree	280	80	36
Spaghetti with Chunky Tomato and Meat Sauce	1 entree	320	70	23
Special Recipe Sirloin of Beef	1 dinner	330	70	27

FROZEN, MICROWAVE, AND REFRIGERATED FOODS

FOOD	AMOUNT	CALORIES		
		TOTAL	FAT	SAT-FAT
Budget Gourmet Light & Healthy (*cont.*)				
Stuffed Turkey Breast	1 dinner	260	50	18
Yankee Pot Roast	1 dinner	270	60	23
Celentano				
Cheese Ravioli	6 (182 g)	400	80	45
Manicotti with Sauce	1 (202 g)	320	140	63
Dinty Moore				
Beef Stew (canned)	1 cup	230	120	63
Beef Stew	1 cup	190	90	36
Chicken Stew	1 cup	180	70	18
Chicken and Dumplings	1 cup	190	50	14
Corned Beef Hash	1 cup	350	200	81
Don Miguel				
Bean and Cheese Burrito	1 (198 g)	420	120	54
Bean and Cheese Chimichanga	1 (198 g)	470	160	54
Beef and Cheese Burrito	1 (198 g)	390	100	36
Chicken and Cheese Burrito	1 (198 g)	410	130	36
Chicken Burrito	1 (198 g)	360	70	18
Gorton's				
Batter-Dipped Fish Portions	1 portion (70 g)	160	90	18
Crispy Fish Fillets in Batter	2 fillets (108 g)	280	170	45
Crispy Flounder	2 fillets (108 g)	290	190	36
Crispy Haddock	2 fillets (108 g)	270	170	36
Crunchy Breaded Fish Fillets	2 fillets (108 g)	270	150	45
Crunchy Breaded Fish Sticks	6 sticks (104 g)	250	140	36
Healthy Choice				
Beef and Peppers Cantonese	1 meal	270	50	23
Beef Broccoli Beijing	1 meal	330	30	9
Beef Burrito Ranchero	1 meal	300	70	23
Beef Macaroni	1 meal	200	10	5
Beef Pepper Steak Oriental	1 meal	250	35	14
Beef Tips	1 meal	260	50	18
Breast of Chicken	1 meal	280	25	9
Breast of Turkey	1 meal	280	25	9
Cacciatore Chicken	1 meal	260	25	5
Chicken Bangkok	1 meal	270	30	5

FROZEN, MICROWAVE, AND REFRIGERATED FOODS

FOOD	AMOUNT	CALORIES		
		TOTAL	FAT	SAT-FAT
Chicken Cantonese	1 meal	210	5	0
Chicken con Queso Burrito	1 meal	280	60	23
Chicken Dijon	1 meal	280	35	14
Chicken Fettuccine Alfredo	1 meal	250	30	9
Chicken Parmigiana	1 meal	300	15	5
Chicken Teriyaki	1 meal	270	20	5
Chicken and Vegetables Marsala	1 meal	220	10	0
Country Glazed Chicken	1 meal	200	15	5
Country Herb Chicken	1 meal	270	35	14
Country Inn Roast Turkey	1 meal	250	30	9
Country Roast Turkey	1 meal	220	35	9
Fettuccine Alfredo	1 meal	240	45	18
Fiesta Chicken Fajitas	1 meal	260	35	9
Garden Potato Casserole	1 meal	200	35	14
Ginger Chicken Hunan	1 meal	350	20	5
Honey Mustard Chicken	1 meal	260	20	0
Lemon Pepper Fish	1 meal	290	45	9
Macaroni and Cheese	1 meal	290	45	18
Mandarin Chicken	1 meal	280	20	0
Meat Loaf	1 meal	320	80	36
Mesquite Beef	1 meal	310	40	14
Mesquite Chicken BBQ	1 meal	320	20	5
Pasta Shells Marinara	1 meal	360	25	14
Salisbury Steak	1 meal	320	60	27
Sesame Chicken Shanghai	1 meal	310	45	9
Shrimp and Vegetables Maria	1 meal	260	15	5
Southwestern Glazed Chicken	1 meal	300	30	9
Spaghetti Bolognese	1 meal	260	25	9
Sweet and Sour Chicken	1 meal	310	45	9
Three-Cheese Manicotti	1 meal	310	80	45
Vegetable Pasta Italiano	1 meal	220	10	0
Yankee Pot Roast	1 meal	280	50	18
Hormel				
Chili, no beans	1 cup	360	230	90
Macaroni and Cheese	1 cup	270	100	54
Noodles and Chicken	1 cup	250	100	27
Kid Cuisine				
Chicken Nuggets	1 meal	440	150	41

FROZEN, MICROWAVE, AND REFRIGERATED FOODS

FOOD	AMOUNT	CALORIES		
		TOTAL	FAT	SAT-FAT
Kids Fun Feast (Swanson)				
Frazzlin' Fried Chicken	1 pkg	660	320	117
Frenzied Fish Sticks	1 pkg	360	130	45
Kid's Kitchen (Hormel)				
Beans and Weiners	1 cup	310	110	45
Beefy Mac	1 cup	190	50	23
Kosherific				
Fish Fillets	2 (109 g)	280	140	27
Lean Cuisine				
Angel Hair Pasta	1 pkg	210	35	9
Beef Pot Roast	1 pkg	210	60	14
Cheese Cannelloni	1 pkg	270	70	32
Cheese Ravioli	1 pkg	250	70	27
Chicken Chow Mein	1 pkg	210	45	9
Chicken Enchilada Suiza	1 pkg	290	40	18
Chicken Fettucini	1 pkg	270	60	23
Chicken à l'Orange	1 pkg	260	20	5
Chicken Parmesan	1 pkg	220	40	14
Chicken in Peanut Sauce	1 pkg	280	60	9
Chicken and Vegetables	1 pkg	240	45	9
Classic Cheese Lasagna	1 pkg	290	60	27
Deluxe Cheddar Potato	1 pkg	270	90	32
Fettucini Alfredo	1 pkg	270	60	27
Fettucini Primavera	1 pkg	260	70	23
Fiesta Chicken	1 pkg	240	40	9
Glazed Chicken	1 pkg	240	60	9
Honey Mustard Chicken	1 pkg	250	40	9
Lasagna with Meat	1 pkg	270	50	23
Macaroni and Beef	1 pkg	280	70	18
Meatloaf	1 pkg	270	90	36
Oriental Beef	1 pkg	250	70	27
Rigatoni	1 pkg	180	35	14
Spaghetti with Meat Sauce	1 pkg	290	60	14
Swedish Meatballs	1 pkg	290	80	27
Three-Bean Chili	1 pkg	210	60	18
Turkey	1 pkg	230	50	14
Zucchini Lasagna	1 pkg	240	35	14

FROZEN, MICROWAVE, AND REFRIGERATED FOODS

FOOD	AMOUNT	CALORIES		
		TOTAL	FAT	SAT-FAT
Lean Cuisine Lunch				
Express				
Broccoli and Cheddar				
Cheese Sauce over				
Baked Potato	1 pkg	250	80	**36**
Cheese Lasagna Casserole	1 pkg	270	60	**23**
Chicken Fettucini	1 pkg	250	60	**23**
Macaroni and Cheese	1 pkg	240	60	**27**
Mandarin Chicken	1 pkg	270	50	**9**
Teriyaki Stir-Fry	1 pkg	260	45	**9**
Mama Lucia				
Italian-Style Meatballs	3 (84 g)	270	190	**81**
Matlaw's				
Stuffed Clams	1 clam (71 g)	120	50	**5**
Michelina's				
Creamed Sauce, Beef	1 pkg	360	180	**54**
Egg Noodles, Gravy,				
Swedish Meatballs	1 pkg	340	130	**36**
Fettuccine Alfredo	1 pkg	390	130	**45**
Lasagna with Meat Sauce	1 pkg	290	90	**36**
Macaroni and Cheese	1 pkg	370	130	**54**
Noodles Stroganoff	1 pkg	310	150	**45**
Penne Pollo	1 pkg	330	130	**45**
Risotto Parmesano	1 pkg	360	180	**54**
Spaghetti Bolognese	1 pkg	270	70	**27**
Spaghetti Marinara	1 pkg	250	20	**9**
Morton				
Macaroni and Cheese	1 cup	230	35	**18**
Mrs. Budd's				
White Meat Chicken Pie				
Fancy Vegetables	1 cup	310	140	**45**
Original Recipe	1 cup	330	150	**45**
Mrs. Paul's				
Breaded Fish Fillets	1 (113 g)	170	25	**14**
Deviled Crabs	1 cake (80 g)	180	80	**27**
Healthy Treasures	1 fillet (113 g)	170	25	**14**
Nancy's French Baked				
Quiche				
Broccoli Cheddar	1 (170 g)	490	290	**144**
Classic French	1 (170 g)	520	330	**162**
Florentine	1 (170 g)	480	290	**144**

FROZEN, MICROWAVE, AND REFRIGERATED FOODS

FOOD	AMOUNT	CALORIES		
		TOTAL	FAT	SAT-FAT
Patio Burritos				
Beef and Bean	1	280	60	**27**
Beef and Bean Green Chili	1	260	40	**14**
Beef and Bean with Red				
Chili Peppers	1	270	60	**18**
Chicken	1	260	35	**14**
Perdue				
BBQ Chicken	1 breast (154 g)	220	70	**23**
	2 drumsticks			
	(84 g)	110	35	**9**
	2 thighs (84 g)	180	110	**32**
Breaded Chicken Breast				
Nuggets	5 (84 g)	200	110	**27**
Breaded Chicken Breast				
Tenders	3 oz (84 g)	160	60	**23**
Ratner's				
Potato Pancakes (Latkes)	1 (43 g)	110	60	**27**
Rymel Menu Maker				
Beef, teriyaki	196 g	240	90	**36**
Chicken breasts, boneless				
without skin				
Breaded	1 (100 g)	130	10	**0**
Lemon Herb and Teriyaki	1 (100 g)	110	10	**0**
Teriyaki	1 (100 g)	110	10	**0**
Sea Pak				
Breaded Butterfly Shrimp	8 (112 g)	150	10	**0**
Clam Strips	1 pkg	410	200	**36**
Fantail Style Shrimp 'n				
Butter Batter	6 pieces	190	80	**18**
Jumbo Butterfly Shrimp	4 (84 g)	200	80	**9**
Popcorn Shrimp	15 (84 g)	210	110	**18**
Shrimp Fajitas	3 (340 g)	370	60	**0**
Shrimp Oriental Stir-Fry	½ pkg (269 g)	190	25	**0**
Shrimp Poppers	20 pieces (83 g)	210	110	**18**
Shrimp Primavera	½ pkg (284 g)	280	70	**5**
Tuna Steak	1 (170 g)	210	50	**0**
Spare the Rib				
Pork, no bones	5 oz	380	260	**72**
Stouffer's				
Baked Chicken Breast	1 pkg	270	110	**27**
Beef Pot Roast	1 pkg	270	90	**27**

FROZEN, MICROWAVE, AND REFRIGERATED FOODS

		CALORIES		
FOOD	AMOUNT	TOTAL	FAT	SAT-FAT
Cheese Tortellini in Alfredo Sauce	1 pkg	550	300	**162**
Chicken Breast Parmigiana	1 pkg	320	100	**18**
Chicken à la King	1 pkg	320	90	**27**
Chicken Monterey	1 pkg	410	180	**81**
Chicken Pie	1 pkg	520	300	**72**
Chili with Beans	1 pkg	270	90	**36**
Creamed Chicken	1 pkg	280	180	**63**
Creamed Chipped Beef	½ cup	160	100	**27**
Escalloped Chicken and Noodles	1 pkg	440	260	**54**
Fettucini Alfredo	1 pkg	480	260	**153**
Fish Filet	1 pkg	430	190	**45**
Four-Cheese Lasagna	1 pkg	410	170	**90**
Fried Chicken Breast	1 pkg	330	150	**36**
Green Pepper Steak	1 pkg	330	80	**27**
Lasagna with Meat and Sauce	1 pkg	360	120	**45**
Lasagna with Tomato Sauce and Italian Sausage	1 pkg	370	160	**63**
Macaroni and Beef	1 pkg	340	110	**45**
Macaroni and Cheese	1 cup	330	150	**54**
Meatloaf	1 pkg	390	210	**72**
Noodles Romanoff	1 pkg	490	230	**54**
Roast Turkey Breast	1 pkg	280	100	**27**
Salisbury Steak	1 pkg	370	170	**54**
Spaghetti with Meatballs	1 pkg	420	130	**36**
Spinach Soufflé	½ cup	150	90	**18**
Stuffed Peppers	1 pepper	180	70	**9**
Swedish Meatballs	1 pkg	440	200	**72**
Tuna Noodle Casserole	1 pkg	330	130	**18**
Turkey Tetrazzini	1 pkg	360	170	**27**
Veal Parmigiana	1 pkg	420	170	**36**
Vegetable Lasagna	1 pkg	370	170	**45**
Welsh Rarebit	¼ cup	120	80	**36**
Stouffer's Lunch Express				
Cheese Ravioli	1 pkg	310	100	**36**
Chicken Alfredo	1 pkg	360	150	**54**
Chicken Chow Mein	1 pkg	260	35	**9**
Fettucini Alfredo	1 pkg	460	240	**135**
Fettucini Primavera	1 pkg	420	220	**108**

FROZEN, MICROWAVE, AND REFRIGERATED FOODS

FOOD	AMOUNT	CALORIES		
		TOTAL	FAT	SAT-FAT
Stouffer's Lunch Express				
(*cont.*)				
Lasagna	1 pkg	350	100	**45**
Macaroni and Cheese	1 pkg	360	170	**45**
Rigatoni	1 pkg	340	100	**23**
Spaghetti with Meat Sauce	1 pkg	280	70	**27**
Swanson Dinners				
Chicken Pot Pie	1 pie	390	200	**81**
Fish 'n' Chips	1 pkg	500	210	**135**
Fried Chicken				
Dark portions	1 pkg	560	250	**99**
White portions	1 pkg	550	230	**99**
Salisbury Steak	1 pkg	610	310	**153**
Sirloin Beef Tips	1 pkg	450	140	**54**
Turkey (Mostly White Meat)	1 pkg	310	70	**18**
Turkey Pot Pie	1 pie	390	190	**81**
Veal Parmigiana	1 pkg	400	160	**72**
Yankee Pot Roast	1 pkg	270	60	**36**
Swanson Hungry Man				
Beef Pot Pie	1 pkg	620	260	**126**
Chicken Pot Pie	1 pkg	620	320	**126**
Fried Chicken (Mostly				
White Meat)	1 pkg	810	360	**126**
Sirloin Beef Tips	1 pkg	450	140	**54**
Turkey	1 pkg	490	120	**54**
Tyson				
Blackened Chicken	1 meal	270	45	**9**
Chicken Marsala	1 meal	180	35	**9**
Chicken Mesquite	1 meal	310	70	**27**
Chicken Picatta	1 meal	190	25	**9**
Chicken Supreme	1 meal	260	180	**18**
Grilled Chicken	1 meal	220	25	**9**
Grilled Italian-Style Chicken	1 meal	210	35	**9**
Honey Roasted Chicken	1 meal	220	35	**9**
Roasted Chicken	1 meal	240	25	**9**
Van de Kamp's				
Breaded Butterfly Shrimp	7 (112 g)	280	120	**23**
Breaded Fish Portions	3 portions (128 g)	330	190	**27**
Breaded Popcorn Shrimp	20 (112 g)	270	110	**18**
Breaded Shrimp	7 (112 g)	240	90	**14**

FROZEN, MICROWAVE, AND REFRIGERATED FOODS

FOOD	AMOUNT	CALORIES		
		TOTAL	FAT	SAT-FAT
Weight Watchers				
Broccoli and Cheese Baked Potato	10 oz	230	60	18
Cheese Manicotti	1 meal	260	70	23
Cheese Tortellini	1 cup	290	35	18
Chicken Enchiladas Suiza	1 meal	230	60	14
Chicken Fettucini	1 meal	280	80	27
Fettucini Alfredo	1 cup	220	50	23
Garden Lasagna	1¼ cups	230	45	9
Grilled Chicken Suiza	1 entree	240	50	18
Grilled Salisbury Steak	1 entree	250	80	27
Italian Cheese Lasagna	1 meal	300	70	27
Lasagna with Meat Sauce	1 meal	270	50	18
Macaroni and Cheese	1¼ cups	260	50	18
Nacho Grande Chicken Enchiladas	1 pkg	290	70	23
Penne Pasta with Sun-dried Tomatoes	1 pkg	290	80	23
Spaghetti with Meat Sauce	1¼ cups	240	60	14
Stuffed Turkey Breast	1 entree	240	70	23
Swedish Meatballs	1 entree	280	70	27
Tex-Mex Chicken	1 entree	260	35	14
Three-Cheese Rotini	1¼ cups	270	80	27
Tuna Noodle Casserole	1¼ cups	240	60	23
Vegetable Primavera Baked Potato	1¼ cups	220	60	27
Weight Watchers Smart Ones				
Chicken Marsala	1 entree	110	5	0
Honey Mustard Chicken	1 pkg	140	10	5
Lasagna Florentine	1 pkg	190	10	5
Ravioli Florentine	1 pkg	170	10	0
Yu Sing				
Chicken Fried Rice	1 meal	250	45	18
Chicken Lo Mein	1 meal	230	40	18
Szechwan Shrimp with Rice	1 meal	210	35	9
Szechwan Vegetable with Rice	1 meal	220	25	9

FROZEN, MICROWAVE, AND REFRIGERATED FOODS

FOOD	AMOUNT	CALORIES		
		TOTAL	FAT	SAT-FAT
Egg Rolls				
Chung's				
Pork	2 (168 g)	400	180	45
Shrimp	2 (168 g)	360	130	23
Vegetable	2 (168 g)	380	140	23
White Meat Chicken	2 (168 g)	340	100	14
Lo-An				
Beef Steak Teriyaki	1 (78 g)	140	35	9
Chicken and Shrimp	1 (78 g)	140	35	9
Lobster	1 (78 g)	150	35	9
Shrimp	1 (78 g)	150	45	9
White Meat Chicken	1 (78 g)	140	35	9
Matlaw's				
Egg Roll Bites	2 pieces (28 g)	45	5	0
Pizzas				
Celeste				
Pizza Deluxe	¼ pizza (158 g)	350	160	54
Pizza-for-One				
Cheese	1 (184 g)	540	230	117
Four-Cheese				
Original	1 (198 g)	540	270	108
Zesty	1 (198 g)	530	240	117
Pepperoni	1 (191 g)	520	240	90
Suprema	1 (255 g)	580	280	90
Vegetable	1 (213 g)	480	210	72
Fox De Luxe				
Cheese	1 (198 g)	460	100	45
Hamburger	1 (198 g)	470	130	36
Pepperoni	1 (198 g)	530	180	54
Sausage	1 (198 g)	480	150	36
Sausage and Pepperoni	1 (198 g)	490	160	45
Healthy Choice French Bread Pizza				
Cheese	1 (158 g)	310	35	18
Pepperoni	1 (170 g)	360	80	36
Supreme	1 (180 g)	340	50	18
Heinz Mini Bagel Pizzas				
Cheese, Sausage, Pepperoni	4 (88 g)	200	70	23
Extra Cheese	4 (88 g)	190	60	18

FROZEN, MICROWAVE, AND REFRIGERATED FOODS

		CALORIES		
FOOD	**AMOUNT**	**TOTAL**	**FAT**	**SAT-FAT**
Jeno's				
Cheese	½ pizza (106 g)	250	100	**32**
Combination Sausage and				
Pepperoni	½ pizza (111 g)	290	140	**36**
Pepperoni	½ pizza (108 g)	280	140	**32**
Lean Cuisine French Bread				
Pizza				
Pepperoni	1 (148 g)	330	70	**27**
Macabee				
Cheese Bagel Pizza	1 (57 g)	150	45	**23**
McCain Ellio's				
Cheese	1 slice (75 g)	160	45	**18**
	⅓ pizza (151 g)	340	100	**36**
Healthy Slices	2 slices (168 g)	320	45	**18**
Stouffer's French Bread				
Pizza				
Cheese	1 (147 g)	350	120	**45**
Deluxe	1 (175 g)	440	200	**72**
Pepperoni	1 (159 g)	420	180	**72**
Sausage and Pepperoni	1 (177 g)	490	220	**63**
White	1 (144 g)	350	120	**72**
Totino's Party Pizza				
Cheese	½ pizza (139 g)	320	130	**45**
Combination	½ pizza (152 g)	380	180	**45**
Pepperoni	½ pizza (145 g)	380	190	**45**
Weight Watchers				
Deluxe Combo	1 (199 g)	330	70	**36**
Sandwiches				
Banquet Hot Sandwich				
Toppers				
Chicken à la King	1 bag	100	40	**14**
Creamed Chipped Beef	1 bag	100	35	**14**
Gravy and Salisbury Steak	1 bag	220	140	**63**
Gravy and Sliced Beef	1 bag	70	20	**9**
Gravy and Sliced Turkey	1 bag	90	35	**14**
Sloppy Joe	1 bag	140	60	**27**
Hormel Quick Meal				
Sandwich				
Bacon Cheeseburger	1 (142 g)	440	200	**90**
Barbecue Beef	1 (122 g)	360	140	**54**

FROZEN, MICROWAVE, AND REFRIGERATED FOODS

FOOD	AMOUNT	CALORIES		
		TOTAL	FAT	SAT-FAT
Hormel Quick Meal				
Sandwich (*cont.*)				
Cheeseburger	1 (136 g)	400	180	81
Grilled Chicken	1 (133 g)	300	80	27
Hot Pockets				
Pepperoni Pizza	1 (128 g)	350	150	72
Jimmie Dean				
Bacon, Egg, and Cheese				
on a Biscuit	1 (102 g)	300	150	54
Miniburgers with Cheese	2 (91 g)	270	120	81
Sausage, Egg, and Cheese				
on a Biscuit	1 (128 g)	390	240	90
Steak Biscuits	2 (94 g)	280	90	36
Ken & Roberts				
Veggie Burger	1 (71 g)	130	10	0
Morningstar Farms				
Garden Vege patties	1 (67 g)	110	35	5
Quaker Maid				
All-Beef Sandwich Steak	1 steak (56 g)	170	130	54
Philly Cheese Steak	1 (170 g)	400	80	36
Weight Watchers On-the-				
Go! Sandwiches				
Chicken, Broccoli, and				
Cheddar	1 sandwich	250	50	23
English Muffin with Ham				
and Cheese	1 sandwich	220	60	18
Grilled Chicken	1 sandwich	270	50	23
Honey Dijon Turkey Pretzel	1 sandwich	230	35	14
Reuben	1 sandwich	250	50	18
White Castle				
Cheeseburger	2 sandwiches	310	160	81
Hamburger	2 sandwiches	270	130	54
Vegetables				
Corn Soufflé (Stouffer's)	½ cup	170	60	18
Onions				
Onion Ringers (Ore Ida)	6 rings (88 g)	240	130	23
Onion Rings (Ore Ida)	4 pieces (86 g)	220	110	32
Potatoes				
Act II Microwave French				
Fries	1 box	240	110	23

FROZEN, MICROWAVE, AND REFRIGERATED FOODS

| FOOD | AMOUNT | CALORIES | | |
		TOTAL	FAT	SAT-FAT
Potatoes (*cont.*)				
Budget Gourmet				
Cheddared Potatoes	1 pkg	260	150	**81**
Cheddared Potatoes and				
Broccoli	1 pkg	170	80	**54**
McCain				
Crinkle-Cut French Fried				
Potatoes	3 oz	120	30	**0**
Spiral Fries	30 pieces (85 g)	160	70	**14**
Steak Fries	10 pieces (84 g)	110	30	**9**
Ultimate Crinkle Cut	12 pieces (85 g)	170	60	**9**
Ore Ida				
Country-Style Hash				
Browns	1 cup	60	0	**0**
Crispers	17 fries (84 g)	220	110	**18**
Dinner Fries	8 fries (84 g)	110	30	**9**
Fast Fries	23 fries (84 g)	140	50	**18**
Golden Crinkles	16 fries (84 g)	120	35	**9**
Golden Patties Shredded				
Potatoes	1 patty (71 g)	140	70	**14**
Golden Twirls	28 fries (84 g)	160	60	**9**
Hash Browns	¾ cup	70	0	**0**
Hot Tots	9 pieces (84 g)	150	60	**14**
Mashed Potatoes, butter				
flavor	½ cup	80	20	**5**
Onion Tater Tots	9 taters (84 g)	150	60	**14**
Potatoes O'Brien	¾ cup	60	0	**0**
Potato Wedges with skins	9 wedges (84 g)	110	25	**9**
Shoestrings	38 fries (84 g)	150	50	**9**
Shredded Potatoes	1 patty (71 g)	140	70	**14**
Shredded Potato Patties	2 patties (99 g)	190	110	**18**
Tater Tots	9 taters (84 g)	160	70	**14**
Toaster Hash Browns	2 patties (99 g)	190	110	**18**
Topped Baked Potatoes,				
Broccoli, and Cheese	½ potato (159 g)	150	35	**14**
Twice-Baked Potatoes				
Cheddar Cheese	1 potato (140 g)	200	80	**27**
Sour Cream and Chives	1 potato (140 g)	180	60	**36**
Zesties	12 fries (84 g)	160	80	**14**

FROZEN, MICROWAVE, AND REFRIGERATED FOODS

FOOD	AMOUNT	CALORIES		
		TOTAL	FAT	SAT-FAT
Potatoes (cont.)				
Stouffer's				
Potatoes au Gratin	½ cup	130	60	**23**
Spinach and Cheese				
Spanakopita (Apollo)	5 triangles	390	200	**72**
Spinach Soufflé (Stouffer's)	½ cup	150	90	**18**

FRUITS AND FRUIT JUICES

FOOD	AMOUNT	CALORIES		
		TOTAL	FAT	SAT-FAT
Apple				
fresh	1 (3 per lb)	81	0	**0**
cooked, boiled				
canned, sweetened	½ cup slices	68	0	**0**
Apple juice	1 cup	116	0	**0**
Applesauce				
unsweetened	½ cup	53	0	**0**
sweetened	½ cup	97	0	**0**
Apricot	3 (12 per lb)	51	0	**0**
dried, uncooked	10 halves	83	0	**0**
	1 cup halves	310	0	**0**
dried, cooked	1 cup halves	211	0	**0**
Avocado, fresh				
California	1	306	270	**41**
Florida	1	339	243	**48**
Banana, fresh	1	105	5	**2**
Blackberries, fresh	½ cup	37	0	**0**
Blueberries, fresh	1 cup	82	0	**0**
Boysenberries, canned,				
heavy syrup	½ cup	113	0	**0**
Cantaloupe, fresh	½ fruit	94	0	**0**
	1 cup cubes	57	0	**0**
Cherries, sour, fresh	1 cup with pits	51	0	**0**
canned, light syrup	½ cup	94	0	**0**
canned, heavy syrup	½ cup	116	0	**0**
Cherries, sweet, fresh	10	49	0	**0**
	1 cup	104	0	**0**
canned, light syrup	½ cup	85	0	**0**
canned, heavy syrup	½ cup	107	0	**0**

FRUITS AND FRUIT JUICES

FOOD	AMOUNT	CALORIES		
		TOTAL	FAT	SAT-FAT
Cranberries, fresh	1 cup whole	46	0	0
Cranberry juice cocktail	1 cup	147	0	0
Cranberry sauce	½ cup	209	0	0
Dates, pitted	5–6 dates	120	0	0
	1 cup chopped	489	7	3
Figs, fresh	1 medium	37	0	0
	1 large	47	0	0
dried, uncooked	2	150	0	0
	1 cup	508	21	4
dried, cooked	1 cup	279	11	2
Fruit cocktail, canned				
juice pack	1 cup	113	0	0
light syrup pack	1 cup	110	0	0
heavy syrup pack	1 cup	186	0	0
Grapefruit, fresh	½ fruit	38	0	0
	1 cup sections	74	0	0
Grapefruit juice				
fresh	4 oz	47	0	0
canned, unsweetened	4 oz	47	0	0
canned, sweetened	4 oz	57	0	0
Grapes, fresh	10	15	0	0
	1 cup	58	0	0
Grape juice, canned or bottled	1 cup	155	0	0
Guava, fresh	1	45	0	0
Honeydew melon, fresh	1/10	46	0	0
	1 cup cubes	60	0	0
Kiwi, fresh	1 medium	46	0	0
	1 large	55	0	0
Kumquat, fresh	1	12	0	0
Lemon, fresh	1 medium	17	0	0
	1 large	25	0	0
Lemon juice	1 tbsp	4	0	0
	1 cup	60	0	0
Lime, fresh	1	20	0	0
Lime juice	1 tbsp	4	0	0
	1 cup	66	0	0
Mango, fresh	1	135	0	0
	1 cup slices	108	0	0
Mixed fruit, dried	11 oz	712	13	0
Mulberries, fresh	10	7	0	0
	1 cup	61	0	0

FRUITS AND FRUIT JUICES

FOOD	AMOUNT	CALORIES		
		TOTAL	FAT	SAT-FAT
Nectarine, fresh	1	67	0	0
	1 cup slices	68	0	0
Orange, fresh	1	60	0	0
Orange juice	1 cup	111	0	0
Papaya, fresh	1	117	0	0
	1 cup cubes	54	0	0
Peaches, fresh	1 (4 per lb)	37	0	0
canned in juice	1 cup halves	109	0	0
canned in light syrup	1 cup halves	136	0	0
canned in heavy syrup	1 cup halves	190	0	0
dried, uncooked	10 halves	311	9	1
	1 cup halves	383	11	1
dried, cooked	1 cup halves	198	6	1
Pears, fresh	1	98	0	0
canned in juice	1 cup halves	123	0	0
canned in light syrup	1 cup halves	144	0	0
canned in heavy syrup	1 cup halves	188	0	0
dried, uncooked	10 halves	459	10	1
	1 cup halves	472	10	1
dried, cooked	1 cup halves	325	7	0
Pineapple, fresh	1 slice (¾" thick)	42	0	0
	1 cup diced	77	0	0
canned in juice	1 cup chunks	150	0	0
canned in light syrup	1 cup	131	0	0
canned in heavy syrup	1 cup	199	0	0
Pineapple juice	1 cup	139	0	0
Plantain, fresh	1	218	6	NA
cooked	1 cup slices	179	3	NA
Plums, fresh	1	36	0	0
	1 cup slices	91	0	0
Prunes				
canned in heavy syrup	5	90	0	0
	1 cup	245	0	0
dried, uncooked	10	201	0	0
	1 cup	385	7	0
dried, cooked	1 cup	227	4	0
Prune juice	1 cup	181	0	0
Raisins, seedless	1 cup packed	494	7	0
Raspberries, fresh	1 cup	61	0	0
Rhubarb, fresh	1 cup diced	26	0	0

FRUITS AND FRUIT JUICES

FOOD	AMOUNT	CALORIES		
		TOTAL	FAT	SAT-FAT
Strawberries, fresh	1 cup	45	0	0
canned in heavy syrup	1 cup	234	0	0
Tangerine, fresh	1	37	0	0
	1 cup sections	86	0	0
Watermelon, fresh	1 cup diced	50	0	0

GRAINS AND PASTA

FOOD	AMOUNT	CALORIES		
		TOTAL	FAT	SAT-FAT
Bread				
Bagels				
Freshly baked, grocery				
Blueberry	1 (114 g)	310	10	5
Bran	1 (114 g)	310	15	5
Cinnamon Raisin	1 (114 g)	320	10	5
Combination	1 (114 g)	310	10	5
Garlic	1 (114 g)	300	10	0
Honey Wheat	1 (114 g)	310	15	5
Oat Bran	1 (114 g)	310	15	5
Onion	1 (114 g)	300	10	0
Plain	1 (114 g)	300	10	5
Poppy Seed	1 (114 g)	310	20	5
Pumpernickel	1 (114 g)	300	15	5
Raisin Bran	1 (114 g)	300	15	5
Rye	1 (114 g)	310	15	5
Sesame Seed	1 (114 g)	310	20	5
Water	1 (74 g)	210	5	0
Frozen				
Lender's				
Bagelettes	1 (25 g)	70	5	0
Big n'Crusty				
Cinnamon Raisin	1 (85 g)	240	20	0
Plain or Onion	1 (85 g)	220	15	0
Blueberry or Cinnamon				
Raisin	1 (71 g)	200	15	0
Egg, Onion, or Plain	1 (57 g)	160	10–15	0
Soft	1 (71 g)	210	30	5

GRAINS AND PASTA

| FOOD | AMOUNT | CALORIES | | |
		TOTAL	FAT	SAT-FAT
Bagels				
Frozen (*cont.*)				
Sara Lee				
Cinnamon and Raisin	1 (80 g)	220	5	0
Oat Bran or Poppy Seed	1 (80 g)	210	10	0
Plain	1 (80 g)	210	0	0
Bialy	1 (110 g)	270	15	0
Biscuits (*see also* **FAST FOODS**)				
Pillsbury Ready-to-Bake				
Big Country				
Butter Tastin'	1 (34 g)	100	35	9
Country	3 (64 g)	150	20	0
1869 Brand Buttermilk	1 (31 g)	100	45	14
Grands!				
Butter Tastin'	1 (61 g)	200	90	9
Buttermilk	1 (61 g)	200	90	27
Cinnamon Raisin	1 (61 g)	200	70	18
Flaky	1 (61 g)	190	80	18
Southern-Style	1 (61 g)	200	90	23
Hungry Jack				
Biscuits	2 (57 g)	170	60	14
Butter Tastin' or				
Buttermilk	2 (57 g)	170	70	14
Tender Layer Buttermilk	3 (64 g)	160	40	9
Bran'nola	1 slice (38 g)	90	20	0
Country Oat	1 slice (38 g)	90	25	5
Bread Crumbs				
Cracker Meal (OTC)	¼ cup	110	0	0
Progresso Bread Crumbs				
Italian-Style	¼ cup	110	15	0
Plain	¼ cup	100	15	0
Shake 'n Bake				
Barbecue Chicken Glaze	⅛ packet (12 g)	45	10	0
Honey Mustard Chicken				
Glaze	¼ packet (25 g)	100	20	9
Pork Original Recipe	⅛ packet (11 g)	40	0	0
Tangy Honey Glaze	¼ packet (25 g)	90	15	5
Bread Mixes				
Bread Machine				
Dromedary				
Country White	½ inch (50 g)	140	10	5

GRAINS AND PASTA

FOOD	AMOUNT	CALORIES		
		TOTAL	FAT	SAT-FAT
Bread Mixes				
Bread Machine				
Dromedary (cont.)				
Italian Herb	½ inch (50 g)	140	20	**14**
Sourdough	½ inch (50 g)	140	15	**9**
Stoneground Wheat	½ inch (50 g)	140	15	**9**
Pillsbury				
Cracked Wheat	¹⁄₁₂ pkg (36 g)	130	20	**0**
Crusty White	¹⁄₁₂ pkg (36 g)	130	15	**0**
Hot Roll Mix (Pillsbury)	1 pan roll (28 g)	100	10	**0**
Quick Mix (Pillsbury)				
Apple Cinnamon	¹⁄₁₂ loaf			
	(37 g mix)	140	10	**0**
Banana	¹⁄₁₂ loaf			
	(33 g mix)	120	10	**0**
Bread Sticks				
Cheese (Angonoa's)	6 (28 g)	120	20	**5**
Italian	5 (28 g)	120	20	**5**
Italian (Angonoa's)	6 (28 g)	130	40	**5**
Mini Sesame Royale				
(Angonoa's)	24 (28 g)	130	35	**5**
Sesame	5 (28 g)	120	20	**5**
Sesame Royale	6 (28 g)	130	40	**5**
Soft (Bread du Jour)	1 (53 g)	130	10	**0**
Soft (Pillsbury)	1 (39 g)	110	25	**5**
Soft, Cheese	1 (28 g)	80	20	**9**
Bread Stuffing				
Arnold				
Sage and Onion	2 cups (67 g)	240	30	**5**
Seasoned	2 cups (67 g)	250	30	**5**
Kellogg's				
Croutettes Stuffing Mix	1 cup prep.			
	(100 g)	240	120	**18**
Nabisco				
Cracker Meal	¼ cup (26 g)	100	0	**0**
Pepperidge Farm				
Corn Bread Stuffing	¾ cup (43 g)	170	20	**0**
Country Garden Herb				
Stuffing	½ cup (34 g)	150	10	**9**
Country-Style Stuffing	¾ cup (37 g)	140	15	**0**
Herb-Seasoned Stuffing	¾ cup (43 g)	170	15	**0**
Ritz Stuffing Mix	⅔ cup (38 g)	200	80	**18**

GRAINS AND PASTA

FOOD	AMOUNT	CALORIES		
		TOTAL	FAT	SAT-FAT
Challah	1" slice (50 g)	160	35	9
Cocktail bread				
Rye or Pumpernickel	3 slices (31 g)	80	10	0
Cracked wheat (Pepperidge				
Farm)	1 slice (25 g)	70	10	0
Croissant				
Butter (Vie-de-France)	1 (56 g)	230	110	72
Croutons (Pepperidge Farm)	2 tbsp (7 g)	30	10	0
English muffin	1 (57 g)	120	10	0
Bran'nola (Arnold)	1 (66 g)	130	15	0
Raisin	1 (61 g)	140	10	0
Raisin (Sun Maid)	1 (68 g)	160	10	0
Flat Bread (JJ Flats)	1 piece (14 g)	50	10	0
French bread	2" slice	130	0	0
French loaf (Bread du Jour)	3" slice (56 g)	130	10	0
Crusty French loaf				
(Pillsbury)	⅕ loaf (62 g)	150	10	0
French toast (*see also* **FROZEN, MICROWAVE, AND REFRIGERATED**				
FOODS)				
French toast	1 slice	140	70	40
Garlic bread	3½" slice (56 g)	190	80	14
with cheese	3½" slice (56 g)	180	60	14
Italian bread	1¼" slice (46 g)	130	10	0
Pepperidge Farm	⅛th loaf (50 g)	130	15	9
Italian Bread Shell (Boboli)	⅕ shell (57 g)	150	30	9
Italian Olive Bread	2 slices (50 g)	150	30	5
Muffins				
Almond Poppy Seed	2 mini (55 g)	180	50	9
Apple Walnut	1 (127 g)	400	100	18
Banana Walnut (Hostess)	5 mini (57 g)	260	140	18
Blueberry	1 (127 g)	400	140	32
Entenmann's	1 (57 g)	120	0	0
Hostess	5 mini (57 g)	240	120	18
Bran	1 (127 g)	390	90	23
Cinnamon Apple (Hostess)	5 mini (57 g)	260	140	23
Corn	1 (127 g)	400	110	18
	2 mini (55 g)	210	70	18
Corn Muffin Toasties	2 (65 g)	240	80	14
Oat Bran	1 (127 g)	390	90	23
Strawberry	1 (127 g)	400	110	23

GRAINS AND PASTA

FOOD	AMOUNT	CALORIES		
		TOTAL	FAT	SAT-FAT
Muffin Mixes				
Betty Crocker				
Wild blueberry	1 muffin (40 g)	170	50	<5
Gold Medal				
Golden Corn	1 muffin (31 g)	170	50	<5
Pillsbury				
Apple Cinnamon	1 muffin (38 g)	140	35	9
Banana Nut	1 muffin (37 g)	150	45	9
Twice the Blueberries	1 muffin (39 g)	140	35	9
Wild Blueberry	1 muffin (40 g)	170	50	9
Multi-Grain	1″ slice (50 g)	160	20	5
Oatmeal (Pepperidge Farm)	1 slice (25 g)	60	10	0
Soft (Pepperidge Farm)	1 slice (25 g)	60	5	0
Pita				
White	1 (6″ diam)	150	10	0
Whole-wheat	1 (6″ diam)	180	10	0
Pumpernickel	1 slice (32 g)	80	10	0
Raisin (Pepperidge Farm)	1 slice (28 g)	80	10	0
Rolls				
Cinnamon (Pillsbury)	1 (40 g)	140	45	14
Club (Pepperidge Farm)	1 (47 g)	120	10	5
Cornbread Twists (Pillsbury)	1 (41 g)	130	50	14
Dinner				
Arnold	2 (38 g)	110	25	5
Country-Style (Pepperidge Farm)	3 (57 g)	150	30	9
Crescent (Pillsbury)	2 (57 g)	200	100	23
Parker House (Pepperidge Farm)	3 (53 g)	150	40	14
Party (Pepperidge Farm)	5 (53 g)	170	40	14
Egg Twist	1 (47 g)	180	35	14
French (Pepperidge Farm)	½ (71 g)	180	20	5
Seven-Grain (Pepperidge Farm)	1 (38 g)	80	20	0
Hamburger	1 (43 g)	130	20	9
Potato (Martins)	1 (39 g)	110	20	0
Hard	1 (57 g)	160	10	5
Hoagie with Sesame Seeds (Pepperidge Farm)	1 (69 g)	200	40	23
Hot dog	1 (39 g)	110	20	5
Italian (Bread du Jour)	1 (35 g)	80	5	0

GRAINS AND PASTA

FOOD	AMOUNT	CALORIES TOTAL	FAT	SAT-FAT
Rolls (*cont.*)				
Mix (Pillsbury)	1 pan roll			
	(28 g mix)	120	25	0
Oat Bran	1 (52 g)	140	20	5
Pumpernickel	1 (57 g)	160	20	0
Sub (La Parisienne)	⅗ 8″ roll (50 g)	130	0	0
Wheat	1 (57 g)	190	25	5
White	1 (6″ diam)	150	10	0
Whole-wheat	1 (6″ diam)	180	10	0
Rye				
Jewish	1 slice (32 g)	80	10	0
Seeded	1 slice (22 g)	55	8	3
Onion	1 slice (32 g)	80	10	0
Sunflower Seed	1 slice (50 g)	120	7	0
Seven-Grain (Dimplemeier)	1 slice (50 g)	120	18	0
Sicilian	¼ loaf (57 g)	150	15	0
Sourdough	1″ slice (50 g)	130	10	0
Boule (La Parisienne)	1 slice (57 g)	120	10	0
Tortillas				
Corn	1 (28 g)	60	0	0
Flour	1 (35 g)	110	25	0
Wheat Bread, Very Thin				
(Pepperidge Farm)	1 slice (15 g)	37	5	2
White	1 slice (25–27 g)	65–80	8–15	0
Light white	1 slice (22 g)	40	3	0
Whole-wheat				
Pepperidge Farm	1 slice (25 g)	60	10	0
Soft	1 slice (25 g)	60	5	0
Stroehmann	1 slice (36 g)	80	15	0
Wonder	1 slice (34 g)	80	15	0

Breakfast Cereals, Cold

If you are keeping track of total fat, add 73 fat calories per cup of whole milk, 42 per cup of 2% milk, 23 per cup of 1% milk, 4 per cup of skim milk. If you are keeping track of saturated fat, add 45 sat-fat calories per cup of whole milk, 27 per cup of 2% milk, 14 per cup of 1% milk, 0–3 per cup of skim milk.

All-Bran, original	½ cup	80	10	0
All-Bran, Extra Fiber	½ cup	50	10	0
Alpha-Bits	1 cup	130	5	0
Apple Cinnamon Squares	¾ cup	180	10	0

GRAINS AND PASTA

FOOD	AMOUNT	CALORIES		
		TOTAL	FAT	SAT-FAT
Apple Raisin Crisp	1 cup	180	0	0
Apple Jacks	1 cup	110	0	0
Banana Nut Crunch	1 cup	250	50	9
Banana Nut Granola	½ cup	250	80	36
Basic 4	1 cup	210	30	0
Blueberry Morning	1¼ cups	230	30	5
Bran'nola	½ cup	200	25	5
Cap'n Crunch	¾ cup	110	15	0
Deep-Sea Crunch	1 cup	130	20	5
Peanut Butter Crunch	¾ cup	120	25	9
Cheerios	1 cup	110	15	0
Apple Cinnamon	¾ cup	120	25	0
Honey Nut Cheerios	1 cup	120	15	0
Multi-Grain Cheerios	1 cup	110	10	<5
Cinnamon Toast Crunch	¾ cup	130	30	5
Clusters	1 cup	220	40	5
Cocoa Krispies	¾ cup	110	0	0
Cocoa Pebbles	¾ cup	120	10	9
Cocoa Puffs	1 cup	120	10	0
Common Sense Oatbran	¾ cup	110	10	0
Complete Bran Flakes	1 cup	100	5	0
Cookie Crisp Chocolate Chip	1 cup	120	10	0
Corn Chex	1¼ cups	110	0	0
Corn Flakes	1 cup	110	0	0
Corn Pops	1 cup	110	0	0
Count Chocula	1 cup	120	10	0
Cracklin' Oat Bran	¾ cup	230	70	27
Crispix	1 cup	110	0	0
Crispy Wheats'n Raisins	1 cup	190	10	0
Double Chex	1¼ cups	120	0	0
Fiber One	½ cup	60	10	0
Froot Loops	1 cup	120	10	5
Frosted Bran	¾ cup	100	0	0
Frosted Flakes	¾ cup	120	0	0
Frosted Mini-Wheats	1 cup	190	10	0
Frosted Wheat Bites	1 cup	180	0	0
Fruit and Fibre Peaches, Raisins, and Almonds	1 cup	210	25	5
Fruity Pebbles	¾ cup	110	10	5
Golden Crisp	¾ cup	110	0	0
Golden Grahams	¾ cup	120	10	0

GRAINS AND PASTA

FOOD	AMOUNT	CALORIES		
		TOTAL	FAT	SAT-FAT
Graham Chex	1 cup	210	15	0
Granola, low-fat (Kellogg's)				
with raisins	⅔ cup	200	30	0
without raisins	½ cup	210	30	0
Grape Nuts	½ cup	200	0	0
Grape Nuts Flakes	¾ cup	100	10	0
Healthy Choice				
Multi-Grains Flakes	1 cup	110	0	0
Multi-Grains Raisins,				
Crunchy Oat				
Clusters, and Almonds	1¼ cups	200	20	0
Multi-Grains Squares	1¼ cups	190	10	0
Hidden Treasures	¾ cup	120	15	0
Honey Almond Delight	1 cup	230	35	0
Honey Bunches of Oats				
Honey Roasted	¾ cup	120	15	5
with Almonds	¾ cup	130	30	5
Honeycomb	1⅓ cups	110	0	0
Honey Graham Oh's	¾ cup	110	20	5
Just Right				
Crunchy Nugget	1 cup	210	15	0
Fruit and Nut	1 cup	200	20	0
Kenmei Rice Bran	¾ cup	110	10	0
Kix	1⅓ cups	120	10	0
Berry Berry	¾ cup	120	10	0
Life	¾ cup	120	15	0
Cinnamon	1 cup	190	20	0
Lucky Charms	1 cup	120	10	0
Muesli				
Cranberry with almonds or				
walnuts	¾ cup	220	25	0
Raspberry with almonds	¾ cup	220	25	0
Swiss (Familia)				
Granola	½ cup	210	50	9
No Added Sugar	½ cup	200	30	5
Original Recipe	½ cup	210	30	5
Puffed Wheat	½ cup	170	45	9
Müeslix				
Crispy Blend	⅔ cup	200	25	0
Golden Crunch	¾ cup	210	50	9
Multi Bran Chex	1¼ cups	220	20	0
Natural Bran Flakes	⅔ cup	90	0	0

GRAINS AND PASTA

FOOD	AMOUNT	CALORIES		
		TOTAL	FAT	SAT-FAT
100% Natural	½ cup	190	25	9
Oats and Honey	½ cup	220	70	32
Oats, Honey, and Raisins	½ cup	220	70	32
Nut and Honey Crunch	⅔ cup	120	15	0
Nutri-Grain				
Almond Raisin	1¼ cups	200	25	0
Golden Wheat	¾ cup	100	5	0
Oat Squares	1 cup	220	25	5
Oatmeal Crisp				
with almonds	1 cup	230	50	5
with apples	1 cup	210	20	0
with raisins	1 cup	210	25	0
Product 19	1 cup	110	0	0
Puffed Rice	1 cup	50	0	0
Puffed Wheat	1¼ cups	50	0	0
Raisin Bran	1 cup	170	10	0
Raisin Nut Bran	1 cup	210	40	5
Raisin Squares	¾ cup	180	5	0
Reese's Peanut Butter Puffs	¾ cup	130	25	5
Rice Chex	1 cup	120	0	0
Rice Krispies	1¼ cups	110	0	0
Apple Cinnamon	¾ cup	110	0	0
Rice Krispies Treats	¾ cup	120	15	0
Shredded Wheat Spoon Size	1 cup	170	5	0
Shredded Wheat 'n Bran	1¼ cups	200	5	0
Smacks	¾ cup	110	5	0
Special K	1 cup	110	0	0
Sprinkle Spangle	1 cup	120	15	0
Toasted Oatmeal	¾ cup	120	10	0
Total	¾ cup	100	5	0
Corn Flakes	1⅓ cups	110	5	0
Raisin Bran	1 cup	180	15	0
Whole Grain	¾ cup	100	5	0
Triples	1 cup	120	10	0
Trix	1 cup	120	15	0
Wheat Chex	¾ cup	190	10	0
Wheaties	1 cup	110	10	0
Dunk-A-Balls	¾ cup	110	10	0
Honey Gold	¾ cup	110	5	0

Breakfast Cereals, Hot

If you are keeping track of total fat and you use butter or margarine, add 33
fat calories per teaspoon and 100 per tablespoon. If you use milk, add fat

GRAINS AND PASTA

FOOD	AMOUNT	CALORIES		
		TOTAL	FAT	SAT-FAT

calories depending on the type of milk (*see* **Breakfast Cereals, Cold**). If you are keeping track of saturated fat and you use butter, add 23 sat-fat calories per pat and 65 per tablespoon. If you use margarine, add 6 sat-fat calories per teaspoon and 18 per tablespoon. If you use milk, add sat-fat calories depending on the type of milk (*see* **Breakfast Cereals, Cold**).

FOOD	AMOUNT	TOTAL	FAT	SAT-FAT
Cream of Rice	1 oz dry	100	0	0
Cream of Wheat				
Mix 'n Eat, plain, cooked	1 pkt (1 oz)	100	0	0
regular, quick, instant,				
cooked	3 tbsp (33 g)	120	0	0
Farina (Pillsbury)	3 tbsp (28 g)	100	0	0
Grits (Quaker)	¼ cup	140	5	0
Instant				
Country Bacon	1 pkt (28 g)	100	5	0
Country Ham	1 pkt (28 g)	90	5	0
Original	1 pkt (28 g)	100	0	0
Real Butter	1 pkt (28 g)	100	15	0
Real Cheddar	1 pkt (28 g)	100	15	5
Sausage	1 pkt (28 g)	100	10	0
Malt-O-Meal, cooked	1 cup	120	0	0
Maypo	1 oz dry	100	9	NA
Oat Bran (Quaker)	½ cup	150	30	9
Oatmeal (Quaker)	½ cup dry	150	25	5
Ralston 100% Wheat	½ cup	130	10	0
Wheatena	⅓ cup	150	5	0
Flour				
All-Purpose (Pillsbury)	¼ cup	110	0	0
Bisquick, original (Betty				
Crocker)	⅓ cup	170	50	14
reduced-fat	⅓ cup	140	25	5
Brown rice	¼ cup	120	5	0
Buckwheat	¼ cup	100	10	0
Cake (Betty Crocker Softasilk)	¼ cup	100	0	0
Corn	1 cup	431	27	2
Cornmeal, yellow	¼ cup	120	10	0
Cornstarch	1 tbsp	29	0	0
Pastry	⅓ cup	100	5	0
Potato Starch	1 tbsp	30	0	0
Rye	¼ cup	100	5	0
Soy	½ cup	200	80	14

GRAINS AND PASTA

FOOD	AMOUNT	CALORIES		
		TOTAL	FAT	SAT-FAT
White	¼ cup	100	0	0
Whole-wheat	¼ cup	130	5	0
Grains (Cereal Grasses)				
Barley, pearl, light, uncooked	1 cup	700	18	4
Buckwheat groats (Kasha)	¼ cup	170	15	0
Bulgur, uncooked	1 cup	600	3	0
Couscous (no added fat)	1 cup prep.	190	5	0
Rice				
Brown				
raw	1 cup	666	32	9
cooked	1 cup	218	9	3
White				
raw	1 cup	676	6	2
cooked	1 cup	264	0	0
Instant, prepared	1 cup	161	0	0
Wild				
raw	1 cup	571	2	0
cooked	1 cup	166	1	0
Pastas (see also FROZEN, MICROWAVE, AND REFRIGERATED FOODS)				
Cooked				
Macaroni, spaghetti, shells				
noodles, etc.	1 cup	210	10	0
Barley egg	1 cup	220	25	9
Egg	1 cup	210	25	9
Spinach	1 cup	210	10	0
Whole-wheat	1 cup	210	15	0
Chow Mein Noodles				
Chung King	⅓ cup	140	65	9
Goodman's	⅔ cup	120	40	23
La Choy	½ cup	140	60	14
Refrigerated				
Celentano				
Broccoli Stuffed Shells	3 (280 g)	190	35	9
Contadina				
Angel's hair	1¼ cup	240	30	9
Fettucine	1¼ cups	250	30	9
Fettucine, cholesterol-free	1 cup	240	20	0
Linguine	1¼ cups	260	30	9
Ravioli, chicken and				
rosemary	1 cup	330	110	36

GRAINS AND PASTA

FOOD	AMOUNT	CALORIES		
		TOTAL	FAT	SAT-FAT
Refrigerated				
Contadina (*cont.*)				
Ravioli, garden vegetable	1 cup	240	45	**27**
Spinach tagliatelli	1¼ cups	270	35	**9**
Tortelloni, chicken and				
prosciutto	1¼ cups	360	120	**36**
Tortelloni, sausage and				
bell pepper	1 cup	330	90	**36**
DiGiorno				
Linguine	70 g	200	10	**0**
Tortelloni, mozzarella	1 cup	300	80	**45**
Mixed Pasta Dishes				
Fettuccine Alfredo	1 cup	880	610	**377**
Franco American				
Spaghetti with meatballs	1 cup	270	90	**45**
Hamburger Helper				
Beef Noodle	1 cup	240	80	**31**
Cheeseburger Macaroni	1 cup	300	130	**50**
Italian Rigatoni	1 cup	320	110	**38**
Lasagne	1 cup	310	100	**34**
Hormel				
Italian-Style Lasagna	1 bowl (284 g)	350	72	**36**
Macaroni and Cheese	1 cup	270	100	**54**
Noodles and Chicken				
(Hearty Helpings)	1 cup	250	100	**27**
Spaghetti	1 bowl (284 g)	240	23	**14**
Kid's Kitchen (Hormel)				
Cheezy Mac 'n Cheese	1 cup	260	100	**54**
Spaghetti and Franks	1 cup	270	100	**45**
Spaghetti and Mini				
Meatballs	1 cup	220	60	**36**
Kraft Pasta Dinners				
Deluxe	1 cup prep.	320	90	**56**
Dinomac and other kid				
dinners	1 cup prep.	410	170	**40**
Macaroni & Cheese				
Original and Mild White				
Cheddar	1 cup prep.	410	170	**40**
Legume (Vegetarian)				
Manicotti Florentine	1 pkg (312 g)	300	70	**9**

GRAINS AND PASTA

FOOD	AMOUNT	CALORIES		
		TOTAL	FAT	SAT-FAT
Lipton Pasta and Sauce				
Cheddar Broccoli	1 cup prep.	350	110	**36**
Rotini Primavera	1 cup prep.	320	100	**36**
Rice-A-Roni Noodle Roni				
Corkscrew Pasta	¾ cup prep.	420	220	**60**
Linguine Pasta with				
Parmesan Chicken	1 cup prep.	400	150	**45**
Rigatoni with Cheddar and				
Broccoli	1 cup prep.	400	170	**45**
Romano				
Tortelloni, cheese	142 g	310	90	**45**
Tortelloni, chicken	142 g	310	80	**36**
SpaghettiOs				
Meatballs	1 cup	260	100	**45**
Tuna Helper				
Cheesy Noodles	1 cup	290	110	**25**
Creamy Noodles	1 cup	300	130	**32**
Velveeta				
Rotini and Cheese	1 cup prep.	360	130	**83**
Shells and Cheese	1 cup prep.	410	130	**79**

Refrigerated Pasta Sauces: *see* **SAUCES, GRAVIES, AND DIPS.**

Miscellaneous
Pancakes (*see also* **FAST FOODS; FROZEN, MICROWAVE, AND REFRIGERATED FOODS;** and **RESTAURANT FOODS**)
Pancake Mix

Buttermilk (Hungry Jack)	3 4" pancakes	170	15	**0**
Extra Lights (Hungry Jack)	3 4" pancakes	180	20	**5**

Waffles: *see* **FAST FOODS; FROZEN, MICROWAVE, AND REFRIGERATED FOODS;** and **RESTAURANT FOODS.**

Wheat bran	1 cup	130	25	**4**
Wheat germ, toasted	1 tbsp	27	7	**1**
	1 cup	431	109	**19**

MEATS (BEEF, GAME, LAMB, PORK, AND VEAL)

The following cuts of beef are braised, roasted, or broiled, unless otherwise noted. *See also* **SAUSAGES AND LUNCHEON MEATS** for cold cuts made from beef and pork products and **FROZEN, MICROWAVE, AND REFRIGERATED FOODS.**

*Remember that most of the following calorie figures are for **only 1 ounce** of beef!*

FOOD	AMOUNT	CALORIES TOTAL	FAT	SAT-FAT
Beef				
Arm pot roast, braised				
lean and fat	1 oz	99	66	27
lean only	1 oz	68	25	11
Backribs	2 ribs (140 g)	370	220	99
Bottom round steak, braised				
lean and fat	1 oz	74	38	14
lean only	1 oz	67	25	9
Brisket flat half, braised				
lean and fat	1 oz	116	89	37
lean only	1 oz	74	40	17
Chuck steak, braised				
lean and fat	1 oz	108	78	32
lean only	1 oz	77	39	18
Club steak, broiled				
lean and fat	1 oz	129	104	50
lean only	1 oz	69	33	16
Flank steak, braised				
lean and fat	1 oz	73	39	18
lean only	1 oz	69	35	16
Ground beef, raw				
extra lean	1 oz	66	44	17
lean	1 oz	75	53	21
regular	1 oz	88	68	28
Ground beef, broiled, medium				
extra lean	1 oz	72	42	16
lean	1 oz	77	47	18
regular	1 oz	82	53	21
Ground beef, pan-fried, medium				
extra lean	1 oz	72	42	16
lean	1 oz	78	49	19
regular	1 oz	87	58	23
Porterhouse steak, broiled				
lean and fat	1 oz	85	54	22
lean only	1 oz	62	28	13

MEATS (BEEF, GAME, LAMB, PORK, AND VEAL)

FOOD	AMOUNT	CALORIES		
		TOTAL	FAT	SAT-FAT
Rib roast				
lean and fat	1 oz	108	81	**34**
lean only	1 oz	68	35	**17**
Round, broiled				
lean and fat	1 oz	78	47	**19**
lean only	1 oz	55	20	**7**
Rump roast				
lean and fat	1 oz	98	70	**33**
lean only	1 oz	59	24	**7**
Shortribs, braised				
lean and fat	1 oz	133	107	**45**
lean only	1 oz	84	46	**20**
Sirloin steak, broiled				
lean and fat	1 oz	79	46	**19**
lean only	1 oz	59	22	**12**
T-bone steak, broiled				
lean and fat	1 oz	92	63	**26**
lean only	1 oz	61	26	**11**
Tenderloin steak, broiled				
lean and fat	1 oz	75	44	**18**
lean only	1 oz	58	24	**9**
Top round, broiled				
lean and fat	1 oz	60	22	**8**
lean only	1 oz	54	16	**6**
Beef Dishes, Mixed				
Beef and vegetable stew	1 cup	220	99	**40**
Chili con carne, canned	1 cup	340	144	**52**
Lasagna	¹/₁₂ casserole	570	210	**142**
Spaghetti with meatballs and tomato sauce, canned	1 cup	260	90	**22**
Beef, Variety Meats and By-products				
Brain, simmered	1 oz	45	32	**7**
Liver, braised	1 oz	46	12	**5**
Liver Pâté	½ cup	289	204	**104**
	1 tbsp	36	26	**13**
Tongue, simmered	1 oz	81	53	**23**
Tripe	1 oz	28	10	**5**
Game				

*Remember that most of the following calorie figures are for **only 1 ounce** of game!*

Antelope, roasted	1 oz	42	7	**2**
Bear, simmered	1 oz	73	34	**NA**

MEATS (BEEF, GAME, LAMB, PORK, AND VEAL)

FOOD	AMOUNT	CALORIES		
		TOTAL	FAT	SAT-FAT
Beefalo, composite of cuts, roasted	1 oz	53	16	7
Bison, roasted	1 oz	41	6	2
Boar, wild, roasted	1 oz	45	11	3
Buffalo, water, roasted	1 oz	37	5	2
Caribou, roasted	1 oz	47	11	4
Deer, roasted	1 oz	45	8	3
Elk, roasted	1 oz	41	5	2
Goat, roasted	1 oz	41	8	2
Horse, roasted	1 oz	50	15	5
Moose, roasted	1 oz	38	2	1
Muskrat, roasted	1 oz	52	23	NA
Opossum, roasted	1 oz	63	26	NA
Rabbit				
domesticated, composite of cuts				
roasted	1 oz	44	16	5
stewed	1 oz	58	21	6
wild, stewed	1 oz	49	9	3
Raccoon, roasted	1 oz	72	37	NA
Squirrel, roasted	1 oz	39	9	1

Lamb

*Remember that most of the following calorie figures are for **only 1 ounce** of lamb!*

FOOD	AMOUNT	CALORIES		
Cubed, for stew or kabob (leg and shoulder), lean only				
braised	1 oz	63	22	8
broiled	1 oz	53	19	7
Foreshank, braised				
lean and fat	1 oz	69	34	14
lean only	1 oz	53	15	6
Ground lamb				
broiled	1 oz	81	50	26
Leg, whole (shank and sirloin), roasted				
lean and fat	1 oz	73	42	18
lean only	1 oz	54	20	7
Leg, shank half, roasted				
lean and fat	1 oz	64	32	13
lean only	1 oz	51	17	6

MEATS (BEEF, GAME, LAMB, PORK, AND VEAL)

| FOOD | AMOUNT | CALORIES | | |
		TOTAL	FAT	SAT-FAT
Leg, sirloin half, roasted				
lean and fat	1 oz	83	53	23
lean only	1 oz	58	23	8
Loin, roasted				
lean and fat	1 oz	88	60	25
lean only	1 oz	57	25	9
Chop, with bone, broiled				
lean and fat	1 chop (3½ oz)	357	265	145
lean only	1 chop (3½ oz)	189	74	37
Rib, broiled or roasted				
lean and fat	1 oz	102	76	33
lean only	1 oz	67	34	12
Chop, with bone, broiled				
lean and fat	1 chop (3½ oz)	398	315	148
lean only	1 chop (3½ oz)	212	105	40
Shoulder, whole (arm and blade)				
braised				
lean and fat	1 oz	97	63	27
lean only	1 oz	80	40	16

Pork

*Remember that many of the following calorie figures are for **only 1 ounce** of pork!*

FOOD	AMOUNT	TOTAL	FAT	SAT-FAT
Loin				
whole, broiled				
lean and fat, with bone	1 oz	98	69	25
	1 chop (104 g)	284	202	73
lean only, with bone	1 oz	73	39	13
	1 chop (104 g)	169	91	31
blade, pan-fried				
lean and fat, with bone	1 oz	117	94	34
	1 chop (104 g)	368	296	107
lean only, with bone	1 oz	85	51	19
	1 chop (89 g)	177	111	39
center loin, pan-fried				
lean and fat, with bone	1 oz	106	78	28
	1 chop (112 g)	333	244	88
lean only, with bone	1 oz	75	41	14
	1 chop (112 g)	178	96	33
center rib, broiled				
lean and fat, with bone	1 oz	97	67	24
	1 chop (104 g)	264	183	66

MEATS (BEEF, GAME, LAMB, PORK, AND VEAL)

FOOD	AMOUNT	CALORIES		
		TOTAL	FAT	SAT-FAT
Pork loin				
center rib, broiled (*cont.*)				
lean only, with bone	1 oz	73	38	13
	1 chop (104 g)	162	85	29
sirloin, broiled				
lean and fat, with bone	1 oz	94	64	23
	1 chop (106 g)	278	191	69
lean only, with bone	1 oz	69	35	12
	1 chop (106 g)	165	83	29
tenderloin, roasted				
lean only	1 oz	47	12	4
top loin, broiled				
lean and fat, with bone	1 oz	102	85	26
	1 chop (104 g)	295	211	76
lean only, with bone	1 oz	73	39	13
	1 chop (104 g)	165	86	30
Shoulder				
whole, roasted				
lean and fat	1 oz	92	65	24
lean only	1 oz	69	38	13
arm picnic, roasted				
lean and fat	1 oz	94	67	24
lean only	1 oz	65	32	11
blade, Boston, roasted				
lean and fat	1 oz	91	64	23
lean only	1 oz	73	43	15
Spareribs, cooked				
lean and fat	1 oz	113	77	30

Pork Products, Cured (*see also* **SAUSAGES AND LUNCHEON MEATS**)

FOOD	AMOUNT	TOTAL	FAT	SAT-FAT
Bacon, cooked	1 strip	36	28	10
Breakfast strips, cooked	1 strip	52	37	13
Canadian bacon, grilled	1 slice	43	18	6
Ham, boneless				
Extra lean (5% fat)	1 slice (28 g)	41	14	5
Regular (11% fat)	1 slice (28 g)	52	27	9
Ham, canned				
Extra lean (4% fat)	1 slice (28 g)	39	12	4
Regular (13% fat)	1 slice (28 g)	64	39	13

MEATS (BEEF, GAME, LAMB, PORK, AND VEAL)

		CALORIES		
FOOD	AMOUNT	TOTAL	FAT	SAT-FAT
Ham, center slice				
Country-style				
Lean and fat	1 oz	57	33	12
Lean	1 oz	55	21	1
Salt pork, raw	1 oz	212	205	75
Pork, Variety Meats and By-products				
Backfat, raw	1 oz	230	226	226
Chitterlings, simmered	1 oz	86	73	37
Feet				
pickled	1 oz	58	41	14
simmered, with bone	1 oz	55	32	11
Liver pâté	2 oz (56 g)	200	160	54
Tongue, simmered	1 oz	81	53	23
Tripe	1 oz	28	10	5
Veal				
*Remember that the following calorie figures are for **only 1 ounce** of veal!*				
Breast, lean and fat, braised	1 oz	86	54	26
Cubed, for stew (leg and shoulder)				
lean only, braised	1 oz	53	11	3
Cutlet, lean and fat, braised	1 oz	62	27	12
Ground, broiled	1 oz	49	19	8
Leg				
top round, lean and fat, braised	1 oz	60	16	6
top round, lean, braised	1 oz	57	13	5
Loin				
lean and fat, braised	1 oz	81	44	16
lean only, braised	1 oz	64	23	7
lean and fat, roasted	1 oz	61	31	16
lean only, roasted	1 oz	50	18	7
Rib				
lean and fat, braised	1 oz	71	32	13
lean only, braised	1 oz	62	20	7
lean and fat, roasted	1 oz	65	36	14
lean only, roasted	1 oz	50	19	6
Shoulder				
arm, lean and fat, braised	1 oz	67	26	10
arm, lean only, braised	1 oz	57	14	4

MEATS (BEEF, GAME, LAMB, PORK, AND VEAL)

FOOD	AMOUNT	CALORIES		
		TOTAL	FAT	SAT-FAT
Veal shoulder (*cont.*)				
blade, lean and fat, braised	1 oz	64	26	9
blade, lean, braised	1 oz	56	17	5
Sirloin				
lean and fat, braised	1 oz	72	34	13
lean only, braised	1 oz	58	17	5

NUTS AND SEEDS

FOOD	AMOUNT	CALORIES		
		TOTAL	FAT	SAT-FAT
Nuts				
Almonds, shelled				
slivered	1 cup	795	630	60
whole, dry-roasted	1 oz (24 nuts)	167	132	13
Almond butter				
plain	1 tbsp	101	85	8
honey-cinnamon	1 tbsp	96	75	7
Almond paste	1 oz	127	69	7
	1 cup	1012	556	53
Beechnuts, dried	1 oz	164	128	15
Brazil nuts, shelled, dried	1 oz (8 med nuts)	186	169	41
Butternuts, dried	1 oz	174	146	3
Cashew nuts				
dry-roasted	1 oz (18 med nuts)	163	118	23
	1 cup	787	572	113
oil-roasted	1 oz (18 med nuts)	163	123	24
	1 cup	748	564	112
jumbo	12 nuts (30 g)	190	130	27
Cashew butter, plain	1 oz	167	126	25
	1 tbsp	94	71	14
Chestnuts, Chinese				
raw	1 oz	64	3	0
dried	1 oz	103	5	1
boiled and steamed	1 oz	44	2	0
roasted	1 oz	68	3	0

NUTS AND SEEDS

| FOOD | AMOUNT | CALORIES | | |
		TOTAL	FAT	SAT-FAT
Chestnuts, European				
raw, unpeeled	1 oz	60	6	1
raw, peeled	1 oz	56	3	1
dried, unpeeled	1 oz	106	11	2
dried, peeled	1 oz	105	10	2
boiled and steamed	1 oz	37	4	1
roasted	1 oz (3 nuts)	70	6	1
	1 cup	350	28	5
Chestnuts, Japanese				
raw	1 oz	44	1	0
dried	1 oz	102	3	0
boiled and steamed	1 oz	16	1	0
roasted	1 oz	57	2	0
Coconut meat				
dried, creamed	1 oz	194	177	157
dried, sweetened, flaked	1 oz	135	82	73
	1 cup	351	214	190
dried, toasted	1 oz	168	120	107
fresh frozen with sugar	2 tbsp	45	25	18
fresh, shredded or grated	1 oz	101	86	76
	1 cup	283	241	214
Coconut cream				
fresh	1 tbsp	49	47	42
	1 cup	792	749	664
canned	1 tbsp	36	30	27
	1 cup	568	472	419
Coconut milk				
fresh	1 tbsp	35	32	29
	1 cup	552	515	457
canned	1 tbsp	30	29	26
	1 cup	445	434	385
frozen	1 tbsp	30	28	25
	1 cup	486	449	398
Filberts (hazelnuts)				
dried	1 oz	179	160	12
	1 cup, chopped	727	648	48
dry-roasted	1 oz	188	169	12
oil-roasted	1 oz	187	163	12
Hickory nuts, dried	1 oz	187	165	18
Macadamia nuts				
dried	1 oz	199	188	28

NUTS AND SEEDS

FOOD	AMOUNT	CALORIES		
		TOTAL	FAT	SAT-FAT
Macadamia nuts (*cont.*)				
oil-roasted	1 oz (24 halves)	204	196	**29**
	1 cup	962	923	**139**
Mixed nuts				
dry-roasted, with peanuts	1 oz	169	131	**18**
	1 cup	814	634	**85**
oil-roasted, with peanuts	1 oz	175	144	**22**
	1 cup	876	720	**112**
oil-roasted, without peanuts	1 oz	175	144	**23**
	1 cup	886	728	**118**
Peanuts, shelled				
dry-roasted	1 oz (35 kernels)	161	126	**17**
	1 cup	827	646	**90**
oil-roasted	1 oz (35 kernels)	165	126	**18**
	1 cup	841	642	**89**
Planters				
Hot Spicy (to heat)	37 pieces (28 g)	160	120	**18**
Snack Mix (to heat)	¼ cup	140	70	**9**
Sweet 'n Crunchy	18 pieces (28 g)	140	60	**9**
Peanut butter, smooth	2 tbsp	190	148	**24**
Peter Pan Smart Choice, reduced fat	2 tbsp	190	110	**18**
Pecans				
dried	1 oz	190	173	**14**
dry-roasted	1 oz (14 halves)	187	165	**13**
oil-roasted	1 oz	195	182	**15**
Pine nuts	1 oz	160	144	**27**
Pistachios				
dried	1 oz	164	124	**16**
dry-roasted	1 oz (47 kernels)	172	135	**17**
Walnuts, black, dried	1 oz (14 halves)	172	145	**9**
	1 cup	759	637	**41**
English or Persian, dried	1 oz (14 halves)	182	158	**14**
	1 cup	770	668	**60**
Walnut halves	⅓ cup	210	190	**18**
Walnut pieces	¼ cup	190	170	**18**

NUTS AND SEEDS

FOOD	AMOUNT	TOTAL	FAT	SAT-FAT
		CALORIES		
Seeds				
Poppy	1 tsp	15	11	**NA**
	1 tbsp	66	51	**NA**
Pumpkin and squash				
whole, roasted	1 oz	127	50	**9**
kernels, dried	1 oz	154	117	**22**
kernels, roasted	1 oz	148	108	**20**
Sesame, kernels, dried	1 tbsp	47	39	**6**
	1 cup	882	739	**104**
Sunflower				
in shell, roasted	1 oz	86	59	**8**
shelled	1 oz	80	59	**8**
dried	1 oz	162	127	**13**
dry-roasted	1 oz	165	127	**13**
	1 tbsp	66	51	**4**
	1 cup	745	574	**60**
oil-roasted	1 oz	175	147	**15**
	1 cup	830	698	**73**
toasted	1 oz	176	145	**15**
	1 cup	829	685	**72**
Tahini	1 tbsp	90	72	**10**
Watermelon, dried	1 oz	158	121	**25**

POULTRY

See also **SAUSAGES AND LUNCHEON MEATS** for cold cuts made from poultry products and **FROZEN, MICROWAVE, AND REFRIGERATED FOODS.**

*Remember that many of the following calorie figures are for **only 1 ounce** of poultry!*

FOOD	AMOUNT	TOTAL	FAT	SAT-FAT
		CALORIES		
Chicken				
Back				
meat and skin				
raw	½ back (99 g)	316	256	**74**
	1 oz	90	73	**21**
fried, batter-dipped	½ back (120 g)	397	237	**63**
	1 oz	94	56	**15**
fried, flour-coated	½ back (72 g)	238	134	**36**
	1 oz	94	53	**14**
roasted	½ back (53 g)	159	100	**28**
	1 oz	85	54	**15**

POULTRY

FOOD	AMOUNT	CALORIES		
		TOTAL	FAT	SAT-FAT
Chicken back (*cont.*)				
meat only				
raw	½ back (51 g)	70	27	7
	1 oz	39	15	4
fried	½ back (58 g)	167	80	22
	1 oz	82	39	10
roasted	½ back (51 g)	70	27	7
	1 oz	39	15	4
Breast				
meat and skin				
raw	1 breast (145 g)	250	121	35
	1 oz	49	24	7
fried, batter-dipped	1 breast (140 g)	364	166	44
	1 oz	74	34	9
fried, flour-coated	1 breast (98 g)	218	78	22
	1 oz	63	23	6
roasted	1 breast (98 g)	193	69	19
	1 oz	56	20	6
meat only				
raw	1 breast (118 g)	129	13	4
	1 oz	31	3	1
fried	1 breast (86 g)	161	36	10
	1 oz	53	12	3
roasted	1 breast (86 g)	129	13	4
	1 oz	31	3	1
Drumstick				
meat and skin				
raw	1 drumstick (73 g)	117	57	16
	1 oz	46	22	6
fried, batter-dipped	1 drumstick (72 g)	193	102	27
	1 oz	76	40	10
fried, flour-coated	1 drumstick (49 g)	120	60	16
	1 oz	69	35	9
roasted	1 drumstick (52 g)	112	52	14
	1 oz	61	28	8

POULTRY

FOOD	AMOUNT	CALORIES		
		TOTAL	FAT	SAT-FAT
Drumstick (*cont.*)				
meat only				
raw	1 drumstick			
	(62 g)	74	19	5
	1 oz	34	9	2
fried	1 drumstick			
	(42 g)	82	31	8
	1 oz	55	21	5
roasted	1 drumstick			
	(44 g)	74	19	5
	1 oz	34	9	2
Gizzard				
raw	1 gizzard (37 g)	44	14	4
	1 oz	33	11	3
simmered	1 cup	222	48	14
	1 oz	43	9	3
Ground				
Fresh (Perdue)	1 oz	48	30	9
Frozen (Longacre)	1 oz	55	30	9
Leg				
meat and skin				
raw	1 leg (167 g)	312	182	51
	1 oz	53	31	9
fried, batter-dipped	1 leg (158 g)	431	230	61
	1 oz	77	41	11
fried, flour-coated	1 leg (112 g)	285	145	39
	1 oz	72	37	10
roasted	1 leg (114 g)	265	138	38
	1 oz	66	34	9
meat only				
raw	1 leg (130 g)	156	45	11
	1 oz	34	10	2
fried	1 leg (94 g)	195	79	21
	1 oz	59	24	6
roasted	1 leg (95 g)	156	45	11
	1 oz	34	10	2
Liver				
chopped chicken livers	1 tbsp	28	17	4
raw	1 liver (32 g)	40	11	4
	1 oz	35	10	3
simmered	1 cup	219	69	23
	1 oz	44	14	5

POULTRY

| FOOD | AMOUNT | CALORIES | | |
		TOTAL	FAT	SAT-FAT
Chicken neck				
meat and skin				
raw	1 neck (50 g)	148	118	33
	1 oz	84	67	18
fried, batter-dipped	1 neck (52 g)	172	110	29
	1 oz	94	60	16
fried, flour-coated	1 neck (36 g)	119	76	21
	1 oz	94	60	16
simmered	1 neck (38 g)	94	62	17
	1 oz	70	46	13
meat only				
raw	1 neck (20 g)	31	16	4
	1 oz	44	22	6
fried	1 neck (22 g)	50	23	6
	1 oz	65	30	8
simmered	1 neck (18 g)	32	13	3
	1 oz	44	21	5
Thigh				
meat and skin				
raw	1 thigh (94 g)	199	129	36
	1 oz	60	39	11
fried, batter-dipped	1 thigh (86 g)	238	128	34
	1 oz	78	42	11
fried, flour-coated	1 thigh (62 g)	162	84	23
	1 oz	74	38	11
roasted	1 thigh (62 g)	153	86	24
	1 oz	70	40	11
meat only				
raw	1 thigh (69 g)	82	24	6
	1 oz	34	10	3
fried	1 thigh (52 g)	113	48	13
	1 oz	62	26	7
roasted	1 thigh (52 g)	82	24	6
	1 oz	34	10	3
Wing				
meat and skin				
raw	1 wing (49 g)	109	70	20
	1 oz	63	41	11
fried, batter-dipped	1 wing (49 g)	159	96	26
	1 oz	92	56	15
fried, flour-coated	1 wing (32 g)	103	64	17
	1 oz	91	57	15

POULTRY

| FOOD | AMOUNT | CALORIES | | |
		TOTAL	FAT	SAT-FAT
Wing				
meat and skin (*cont.*)				
roasted	1 wing (34 g)	99	60	17
	1 oz	82	50	14
meat only				
raw	1 wing (29 g)	36	9	2
	1 oz	36	9	2
fried	1 wing (20 g)	42	16	5
	1 oz	60	23	6
roasted	1 wing (21 g)	36	9	2
	1 oz	36	9	2
Chicken Dishes, Mixed (*see also* **FROZEN, MICROWAVE, AND REFRIGERATED FOODS.**)				
Chicken à la king	1 cup	470	306	116
Chicken and noodles	1 cup	365	162	46
Chicken potpie	⅓ pie	545	279	93
Duck, domesticated				
meat and skin				
raw	½ duck (634 g)	2561	2245	754
	1 oz	115	100	33
roasted	½ duck (382 g)	1287	975	332
	1 oz	96	72	25
meat only				
raw	½ duck (303 g)	399	162	63
	1 oz	37	15	6
roasted	½ duck (221 g)	399	162	63
	1 oz	37	15	6
liver, raw	1 liver (44 g)	60	18	6
	1 oz	39	12	4
Duck, wild				
meat and skin, raw	½ duck (270 g)	571	369	125
	1 oz	60	39	13
breast meat only, raw	1 breast (83 g)	102	32	10
	1 oz	35	11	3
Goose, domesticated				
meat and skin				
raw	½ goose (1319 g)	4893	3991	1161
	1 oz	105	86	25

POULTRY

FOOD	AMOUNT	CALORIES		
		TOTAL	FAT	SAT-FAT
Goose meat and skin (*cont.*)				
roasted	½ goose (774 g)	2362	1527	**479**
	1 oz	86	56	**18**
meat only				
raw	½ goose (766 g)	1237	492	**192**
	1 oz	46	18	**7**
roasted	½ goose (591 g)	1237	492	**192**
	1 oz	46	18	**7**
liver, raw	1 liver (94 g)	125	36	**14**
	1 oz	38	11	**4**
Pheasant				
meat and skin, raw	½ pheasant (400 g)	723	335	**97**
	1 oz	51	24	**7**
meat only, raw	½ pheasant (352 g)	470	115	**39**
	1 oz	38	9	**3**
breast meat only, raw	1 breast (182 g)	243	53	**18**
	1 oz	38	8	**3**
leg meat only, raw	1 leg (107 g)	143	41	**14**
	1 oz	38	11	**4**
Quail				
meat and skin, raw	1 quail (109 g)	210	118	**33**
	1 oz	54	31	**9**
meat only, raw	1 quail (92 g)	123	38	**11**
	1 oz	38	12	**3**
breast meat only, raw	1 breast (56 g)	69	15	**4**
	1 oz	35	8	**2**
Squab (pigeon)				
meat and skin, raw	1 squab (199 g)	584	426	**151**
	1 oz	83	61	**21**
meat only, raw	1 squab (168 g)	239	113	**30**
	1 oz	40	19	**5**
breast meat only, raw	1 breast (101 g)	135	41	**11**
	1 oz	38	12	**3**

POULTRY

FOOD	AMOUNT	CALORIES		
		TOTAL	FAT	SAT-FAT
Turkey				
Back				
meat and skin				
raw	½ back (183 g)	275	120	**35**
	1 oz	43	18	**5**
roasted	½ back (130 g)	265	120	**35**
	1 oz	58	26	**8**
meat only				
raw	½ back (150 g)	180	47	**16**
	1 oz	34	9	**3**
roasted	½ back (96 g)	180	47	**16**
	1 oz	34	9	**3**
Breast				
meat and skin				
raw	1 oz	35	7	**2**
roasted	1 oz	43	8	**2**
meat only				
raw	1 oz	31	2	**1**
roasted	1 oz	31	2	**1**
Cutlet, braised	1 oz	31	2	**1**
Ground				
Fresh				
Perdue	1 oz	40	20	**6**
Shady Brook	1 oz	43	20	**6**
Frozen				
Longacre	1 oz	53	33	**7**
Leg				
meat and skin				
raw	1 leg (349 g)	412	112	**34**
	1 oz	33	9	**3**
roasted	1 leg (245 g)	418	119	**37**
	1 oz	48	14	**4**
meat only				
raw	1 leg (329 g)	356	70	**24**
	1 oz	31	6	**2**
roasted	1 leg (224 g)	355	70	**24**
	1 oz	31	6	**2**
Wing				
meat and skin				
raw	1 wing (128 g)	203	89	**24**
	1 oz	45	20	**5**

POULTRY

FOOD	AMOUNT	CALORIES		
		TOTAL	FAT	SAT-FAT
Turkey wing				
meat and skin (*cont.*)				
roasted	1 wing (90 g)	186	80	**22**
	1 oz	59	25	**7**
meat only				
raw	1 wing (90 g)	96	9	**3**
	1 oz	30	3	**1**
roasted	1 wing (60 g)	96	9	**3**
	1 oz	30	3	**1**

RESTAURANT FOODS

FOOD	AMOUNT	CALORIES		
		TOTAL	FAT	SAT-FAT
Au Bon Pain				
Breads				
Bagels				
Cinnamon Raisin	1	280	9	**<9**
Plain, Onion, or Sesame	1	270	9	**<9**
Loaf				
Baguette	1	810	18	**<9**
Cheese	1	1670	261	**81**
Four Grain	1	1420	99	**<9**
Onion Herb	1	1430	117	**<9**
Parisienne	1	1490	36	**<9**
Muffins				
Blueberry	1	390	99	**36**
Bran	1	390	99	**27**
Carrot	1	450	198	**45**
Corn	1	460	153	**27**
Cranberry Walnut	1	350	117	**18**
Oat Bran Apple	1	400	90	**18**
Pumpkin	1	410	144	**18**
Whole Grain	1	440	144	**18**
Rolls				
Alpine	1	220	27	**<9**
Country Seed	1	220	36	**<9**
Hearth	1	250	18	**<9**
Petit Pain	1	220	<9	**<9**
Pumpernickel	1	210	18	**<9**
Rye	1	230	18	**<9**

RESTAURANT FOODS

FOOD	AMOUNT	CALORIES		
		TOTAL	FAT	SAT-FAT
Breads				
Rolls (*cont.*)				
3-Seed Raisin	1	250	36	<9
Vegetable	1	230	45	<9
Sandwich				
Braided Roll	1 roll	387	99	27
Croissant	1 roll	300	126	72
French	1 roll	320	<9	<9
Hearth	1 roll	370	27	<9
Multigrain	2 slices	391	27	9
Pita Pocket	1 pocket	80	<9	NA
Rye	2 slices	374	36	9
Cookies				
Chocolate Chip	1 serving	280	135	81
Chocolate Chunk Pecan	1 serving	290	153	54
Oatmeal Raisin	1 serving	250	81	27
Peanut Butter	1 serving	290	135	54
White Chocolate Chunk				
Pecan	1 serving	300	153	54
Croissants				
Dessert				
Almond	1	420	225	108
Apple	1	250	90	54
Blueberry Cheese	1	380	180	108
Chocolate	1	400	216	126
Cinnamon Raisin	1	390	117	72
Coconut Pecan	1	440	207	108
Hazelnut Chocolate	1	480	252	126
Plain	1	220	90	54
Strawberry or Raspberry				
Cheese	1	400	180	108
Sweet Cheese	1	420	207	126
Hot Filled				
Ham and Cheese	1	370	180	108
Spinach and Cheese	1	290	144	90
Turkey and Cheddar	1	410	198	117
Turkey and Havarti	1	410	189	117
Salads				
Chicken Tarragon Garden	1	310	135	18
Cracked Pepper Chicken				
Garden	1	100	18	<9
Garden, small	1	20	<9	<9

RESTAURANT FOODS

FOOD	AMOUNT	CALORIES		
		TOTAL	FAT	SAT-FAT
Salads (*cont.*)				
Garden, large	1	40	<9	<9
Grilled Chicken Garden	1	110	18	<9
Shrimp Garden	1	102	18	<9
Tuna Garden	1	350	225	36
Salad Dressings				
Balsamic Vinaigrette	2¼ oz	311	297	45
Champagne Vinaigrette	2¼ oz	251	234	36
County Blue Cheese	2¼ oz	325	279	54
Honey with Poppy Seed	2¼ oz	351	315	54
Low-Cal Italian	2¼ oz	68	54	<9
Olive Oil Caesar	2¼ oz	255	144	NA
Parmesan and Pepper	2¼ oz	235	189	45
Sesame French	2¼ oz	339	243	36
Tomato Basil	2¼ oz	66	<9	0
Sandwich Fillings				
Cheese				
Brie	1 serving	300	216	135
Cheddar	1 serving	110	81	45
Herb	1 serving	290	261	162
Provolone	1 serving	155	113	66
Swiss	1 serving	330	216	135
Meat				
Albacore Tuna Salad	1 serving	310	216	36
Bacon	1 serving	140	108	36
Chicken Tarragon	1 serving	270	135	18
Country Ham	1 serving	150	63	27
Cracked Pepper Chicken	1 serving	120	18	<9
Grilled Chicken	1 serving	130	36	<9
Roast Beef	1 serving	180	72	36
Smoked Turkey	1 serving	100	9	<9
Soups (*see also* **SOUPS,** *Homemade or Restaurant*)				
Beef Barley	1 cup	74	18	<9
	1 bowl	112	23	9
Chicken Noodle	1 cup	79	9	<9
	1 bowl	119	15	<9
Clam Chowder	1 cup	289	162	81
	1 bowl	433	243	126
Cream of Broccoli	1 cup	201	153	72
	1 bowl	302	234	108
Garden Vegetarian	1 cup	29	<9	<9
	1 bowl	44	<9	<9

RESTAURANT FOODS

| FOOD | AMOUNT | CALORIES | | |
		TOTAL	FAT	SAT-FAT
Soups (*cont.*)				
Minestrone	1 cup	105	9	<9
	1 bowl	158	15	<9
Split Pea	1 cup	176	9	<9
	1 bowl	264	15	<9
Tomato Florentine	1 cup	61	9	<9
	1 bowl	92	15	<9
Vegetarian Chili	1 cup	139	27	<9
	1 bowl	208	36	<9
Chinese Restaurant				
Barbecued pork (not fried)	1 whole dish	1374	986	355
Barbecued spareribs	1 whole dish	1863	1232	480
Beef with vegetables	1 whole dish	1572	1068	263
Chicken with cashews	1 whole dish	1765	1075	186
Chicken with vegetables	1 whole dish	1224	652	102
Chinese Noodle soup	1 serving	265	81	NA
Egg roll	1	152	103	30
Hot and sour soup	1 serving	165	72	NA
Hunan shrimp (not fried)	1 whole dish	1068	755	100
Kung pao beef	1 whole dish	2458	1706	444
Kung pao chicken	1 whole dish	1806	1134	158
Kung pao shrimp	1 whole dish	1068	755	115
Moo shu pork	1 whole dish	1383	1053	258
Orange beef	1 whole dish	1710	1216	342
Pork with vegetables	1 whole dish	1574	1219	338
Sweet and sour pork	1 whole dish	1845	1509	389
Sweet and sour shrimp	1 whole dish	1069	805	130
Szechuan pork	1 whole dish	1694	1339	356
Velvet corn soup	1 serving	115	27	NA
Wonton soup	1 serving	283	108	NA
International House of Pancakes (IHOP)				
Pancakes				
Buttermilk	1 (56 g)	108	28	6
Buckwheat	1 (63 g)	134	45	11
Country Griddle	1 (63 g)	134	34	9
Egg	1 (56 g)	102	45	11
Harvest Grain 'n Nut	1 (63 g)	160	74	12
Foods prepared with Eggstro'dnaire				
Broccoli and Mushroom Omelette	1	310	62	NA

RESTAURANT FOODS

		CALORIES		
FOOD	AMOUNT	TOTAL	FAT	SAT-FAT
Foods prepared with Eggstro'dnaire (*cont.*)				
Breakfast Burrito	1	456	109	**NA**
Chicken Fajita Burrito	1	523	89	**NA**
French Toast	1 piece	99	18	**NA**
Waffles				
Regular	1 (112 g)	305	133	**30**
Belgian				
Regular	1 (168 g)	408	177	**100**
Harvest Grain 'n Nut	1 (168 g)	445	251	**107**
Italian Restaurant				
Appetizers				
Antipasto	1½ lbs	629	423	**132**
Entrees				
Eggplant Parmigiana with spaghetti	2½ cups	1208	558	**145**
Fettuccine Alfredo	2½ cups	1498	873	**434**
Lasagna	2 cups	958	477	**192**
Linguine with red clam sauce	3 cups	892	207	**36**
Linguine with white clam sauce	3 cups	907	261	**45**
Spaghetti with meat sauce	3 cups	918	225	**92**
Spaghetti with meatballs	3½ cups	1155	351	**92**
Spaghetti with sausage	2½ cups	1043	351	**94**
Spaghetti with tomato sauce	3½ cups	849	153	**34**
Veal Parmigiana with spaghetti	1½ cups	1064	396	**128**
Side Dishes				
Fried calamari	3 cups	1037	630	**83**
Garlic bread	8 oz	822	360	**90**
Spaghetti with tomato sauce	1½ cups	409	72	**16**
Mexican Restaurant				
Appetizers				
Beef and cheese nachos with sour cream and guacamole	1 serving	1362	801	**250**
Cheese quesadilla with sour cream and guacamole	1 serving	900	531	**220**
Cheese Nachos	1 serving	807	500	**225**

RESTAURANT FOODS

FOOD	AMOUNT	CALORIES		
		TOTAL	FAT	SAT-FAT
Entrees				
Beef burrito	1 serving	833	360	121
with beans, rice, sour cream, and guacamole	1 serving	1639	711	248
Beef chimichanga	1 serving	802	423	113
with beans, rice, sour cream, and guacamole	1 serving	1607	774	241
Beef enchilada	1 serving	324	171	67
two enchiladas with beans and rice	1 serving	1253	522	140
Chicken fajitas and flour tortillas	1 serving	839	216	54
with beans, rice, sour cream, and guacamole	1 serving	1661	567	173
Chile rellenos	1 serving	487	342	45
two chile rellenos with beans and rice	1 serving	1578	864	173
Chicken enchilada	1 serving	329	162	103
two enchiladas with beans and rice	1 serving	1264	513	270
Chicken taco	1 serving	219	99	27
two tacos with beans and rice	1 serving	1042	378	119
Taco salad				
with sour cream and guacamole	1 serving	1099	639	177
Side Dishes				
Rice	¾ cup	229	34	5
Refried beans	¾ cup	375	146	60
Tortilla chips	50 chips	645	432	81
Swiss Chalet				
Apple pie	1 serving	413	171	36
Back rib	½ rib	405	234	81
	full rib	810	468	162
Caesar Salad Appetizer	1 serving	345	171	18
Caesar Salad Entree	1 serving	454	342	36
Chicken				
white (with skin)	¼ chicken	381	198	36
white (skinless)	¼ chicken	225	72	18
dark (with skin)	¼ chicken	313	153	45
dark (skinless)	¼ chicken	232	90	27

RESTAURANT FOODS

FOOD	AMOUNT	CALORIES		
		TOTAL	FAT	SAT-FAT
Chicken (with skin)	½ chicken	694	351	**81**
Chicken Pot Pie	1 pie	494	216	**45**
Chicken Salad and Roll	1 serving	466	198	**36**
Roll	1 roll	116	9	**0**

SALAD BAR FOODS

FOOD	AMOUNT	CALORIES		
		TOTAL	FAT	SAT-FAT
Bacon bits	1 tbsp	105	30	**0**
Baked beans	½ cup	160	36	**<9**
Breadsticks, sesame	2	20	<9	**NA**
Cheese, shredded Cheddar	2 tbsp	110	81	**54**
Cheese nachos	2 tbsp	70	45	**NA**
Chow mein noodles	½ cup	140	60	**14**
Cole slaw	½ cup	180	108	**20**
Cottage cheese (4% fat)	½ cup	110	43	**23**
Croutons	2 tbsp	30	10	**0**
Puddings				
Bread pudding	½ cup	170	36	**NA**
Chocolate mousse	½ cup	160	45	**NA**
Chocolate pudding	½ cup	140	27	**NA**
Lemon mousse	½ cup	160	45	**NA**
Rice pudding	½ cup	135	18	**NA**
Vanilla pudding	½ cup	140	27	**NA**
Salads				
Macaroni	½ cup	280	162	**NA**
Pasta				
with broccoli	½ cup	150	81	**NA**
chicken	½ cup	215	144	**NA**
fiesta	½ cup	190	90	**NA**
seafood	½ cup	245	171	**NA**
tuna	½ cup	240	153	**NA**
Polynesian	½ cup	160	45	**NA**
Potato	½ cup	135	45	**14**
Red skin potato	½ cup	150	72	**14**
Three-bean	½ cup	130	18	**NA**
Tuna	½ cup	190	85	**NA**

SALAD BAR FOODS

FOOD	AMOUNT	CALORIES		
		TOTAL	FAT	SAT-FAT
Salad dressings	1 tbsp	60–90	50–72	**9–18**
	4 tbsp	240–360	200–288	**36–72**
Soup, prepared from canned soup (*see also* **SOUPS,** *Homemade or Restaurant*)				
Bean and ham	¾ cup	145	36	**NA**
Beef barley	¾ cup	95	18	**NA**
Beef stew	¾ cup	85	9	**NA**
Chicken corn noodle	¾ cup	85	9	**NA**
Chicken rice	¾ cup	85	9	**NA**
Chili con carne with beans	¾ cup	170	45	**NA**
Clam chowder, New				
England–style	¾ cup	180	45	**NA**
Crab	¾ cup	55	18	**NA**
Cream of broccoli	¾ cup	95	45	**NA**
Sunflower seeds	1 oz	180	144	**20**
Tofu	½ cup	90	36	**7**
Tortilla chips	1 oz	140	54	**9**
Turkey, diced	2 tbsp	60	45	**NA**
Toppings for Home-Prepared Salads				
Bac·Os (Betty Crocker)	1 tbsp	30	10	**0**
Bac'n Pieces (McCormick)	1½ tbsp	30	10	**0**
Real Bacon Bits (Hormel)	1 tbsp	90	45	**9**
Salad Crispins, Mini Croutons				
(Hidden Valley)	1 tbsp	35	10	**0**

SAUCES, GRAVIES, AND DIPS

FOOD	AMOUNT	CALORIES		
		TOTAL	FAT	SAT-FAT
Sauces				
Barbecue				
Masterpiece	2 tbsp	40–60	0	**0**
Honey Dijon	2 tbsp	50	10	**0**
Open Pit	2 tbsp	50	5	**0**
Bearnaise	1 tbsp	53	48	**29**
	½ cup	423	383	**232**
Browning and Seasoning	1 tbsp	15	0	**0**
Cheese	1 tbsp	31	21	**14**
	½ cup	250	170	**110**

SAUCES AND GRAVIES

FOOD	AMOUNT	CALORIES		
		TOTAL	FAT	SAT-FAT
Clam, white	½ cup	120	80	14
Cooking sauces				
Uncle Ben's				
Sauce for Beef with				
Mushrooms	½ cup	70	10	0
Sauce for Country				
Chicken	½ cup	130	80	45
Sauce for Pepper Steak	½ cup	70	15	0
Sweet and Sour	½ cup	120	0	0
Campbell's Simmer Chef				
Creamy Mushroom and				
Herb	½ cup	110	80	18
Golden Honey Mustard	½ cup	150	20	0
Hearty Onion and				
Mushroom	½ cup	50	10	0
Old Country Cacciatore	½ cup	110	35	9
Oriental Sweet and Sour	½ cup	110	10	0
Cream	1 tbsp	28	22	14
	½ cup	225	175	110
Curry Cream	1 tbsp	40	31	20
	½ cup	317	250	160
Hollandaise	1 tbsp	82	80	47
	½ cup	660	627	377
Horseradish (Kraft)	1 tbsp	20	15	0
Louis	1 tbsp	63	60	14
	½ cup	504	480	112
Nacho Cheese (Kaukauna)	2 tbsp	90	60	18
Pasta, refrigerated				
Contadina				
Alfredo (light)	½ cup	190	120	63
Pesto with Basil	¼ cup	310	270	45
Pesto with Sun-dried				
Tomatoes	¼ cup	250	220	36
DiGiorno				
Alfredo	¼ cup	220	200	126
Marinara	½ cup	100	40	9
Romano				
Alfredo	3½ oz	140	90	54
Soy	1 tbsp	11	0	0
Spaghetti				
Healthy Choice				
Traditional	½ cup	50	5	5

SAUCES AND GRAVIES

FOOD	AMOUNT	CALORIES TOTAL	FAT	SAT-FAT
Spaghetti (cont.)				
Prego				
Flavored with Meat	½ cup	160	50	**14**
Garden Combination	½ cup	90	10	**5**
Marinara	½ cup	110	50	**14**
Mushroom and Diced Onion	½ cup	120	35	**14**
Mushroom and Diced Tomato	½ cup	110	35	**9**
Mushroom and Extra Spices	½ cup	120	35	**9**
Mushroom and Green Pepper	½ cup	100	35	**9**
Onion and Garlic	½ cup	120	9	**9**
Three Cheese	½ cup	100	20	**5**
Tomato, Onion, and Garlic	½ cup	120	55	**14**
Traditional	½ cup	150	50	**18**
Ragú				
All Chunky Garden Style	½ cup	120	40	**5**
Garlic and Basil	½ cup	90	25	**0**
Light Garden Harvest	½ cup	50	0	**0**
Light Pasta Sauce	½ cup	60	15	**0**
Vegetable Primavera	½ cup	110	35	**5**
Tartar				
fat-free (Kraft)	2 tbsp	25	0	**0**
regular (Hellman's)	1 tbsp	70	70	**9**
Tomato, canned	1 cup	74	0	**0**
White	1 tbsp	24	17	**11**
	½ cup	195	138	**88**
Worcestershire	1 tbsp	0	0	**0**
Gravies				
Beef, canned	½ cup	62	25	**13**
Franco-American				
Chicken	¼ cup	45	35	**9**
Heinz				
Classic Chicken	¼ cup	30	15	**0**
Fat-Free, all	¼ cup	15	0	**0**
Rich Mushroom	¼ cup	20	5	**0**
Roasted Turkey	¼ cup	25	10	**0**
Savory Brown	¼ cup	25	10	**0**
Zesty Brown	¼ cup	20	5	**0**

SAUCES AND GRAVIES

FOOD	AMOUNT	CALORIES TOTAL	FAT	SAT-FAT
Dips				
Bean (Fritos)	2 tbsp (35 g)	40	10	5
Cheddar Cheese, mild (Herr's)	2 tbsp (30 g)	45	25	14
Jalapeño (Frito-Lay)	2 tbsp (34 g)	50	30	9
Jalapeño (Herr's)	2 tbsp (30 g)	30	25	9
French Onion				
Bacon (Lucerne)	2 tbsp	60	45	23
Frito-Lay's	2 tbsp (33 g)	60	45	27
Green Onion (Lucerne)	2 tbsp	50	45	18
Guacamole	2 tbsp	50	30	5
Hummus with tahini	2 tbsp	57	30	0
Salsa				
Chunky (Herr's)	2 tbsp (31 g)	12	0	0
Chunky (Utz)	2 tbsp (30 g)	60	0	0
Dip (Pace)	2 tbsp (31.8 g)	10	0	0
Dip (Tostistos)	2 tbsp (33 g)	15	0	0
Mexican (Kaukauna)	2 tbsp (28 g)	15	0	0
Mild (Rojo's)	2 tbsp (29 g)	10	0	0
Salsa and Cream Cheese (Kaukauna)	2 tbsp (28 g)	70	50	27
Salsa con Queso (Tostistos)	2 tbsp (34 g)	40	20	5
Southwest, mild (Safeway)	2 tbsp (28 g)	10	0	0

SAUSAGES AND LUNCHEON MEATS

FOOD	AMOUNT	CALORIES TOTAL	FAT	SAT-FAT
Bacon	2 slices (11 g)	60	45	18
Hickory-smoked (Smithfield)	2 slices (15 g)	90	70	27
Thick-sliced (Gwaltney)	1 slice (8 g)	45	35	9
Turkey (Louis Rich)	1 slice (14 g)	30	20	5
Barbecue loaf, pork, beef	28 g	49	23	8
	1 slice (22 g)	40	18	7
Beerwurst, beer salami				
beef	28 g	92	75	31
	1 slice (22 g)	75	61	25
pork	28 g	67	48	16
	1 slice (22 g)	55	39	13

SAUSAGES AND LUNCHEON MEATS

FOOD	AMOUNT	CALORIES		
		TOTAL	FAT	SAT-FAT
Berliner, pork, beef	28 g	65	44	15
	1 slice (22 g)	53	36	13
Bockwurst, raw	28 g	87	70	26
	1 link (64 g)	200	161	59
Bologna				
Beef (Oscar Mayer)	1 slice (28 g)	90	70	36
Chicken (Gwaltney)	1 slice (32 g)	80	60	36
Chicken, pork, and beef				
(Thorn Apple)	1 slice (37 g)	120	90	18
Pork	1 slice (28 g)	70	51	18
Pork and beef (Oscar				
Mayer)	1 slice (28 g)	90	70	27
Pork, chicken, and beef				
(Oscar Mayer)	1 slice (28 g)	90	70	27
Light	1 slice (28 g)	60	35	14
Pork and turkey (Gwaltney)	1 slice (38 g)	120	100	36
Turkey (Louis Rich)	1 slice (28 g)	50	35	9
Bratwurst, pork, beef	28 g	92	71	25
	1 link (70 g)	226	175	63
Bratwurst, pork, cooked	28 g	85	66	24
	1 link (84 g)	256	198	71
Braunschweiger, pork	28 g	102	82	28
	1 slice (17 g)	65	52	18
Breakfast strips, beef, cured				
cooked	1 slice (11 g)	51	35	15
Cheese dog	1 frank (45 g)	150	120	45
Chicken breast				
Deli Thin				
Fat-free (Oscar Mayer)	4 slices (52 g)	40	0	0
Oven-roasted (Louis Rich)	5 slices (55 g)	60	15	5
Chicken roll, white meat				
(Tyson)	3 slices (55 g)	90	50	18
Chipped beef	28 g	50	20	9
Corned beef brisket				
Cooked	28 g	71	48	16
Loaf, jellied	1 slice (28 g)	43	16	7
Thorn Apple Valley	84 g	190	150	63
Cured beef				
Oven-roasted (Hillshire				
Farms)	6 slices (57 g)	50	5	0
Dried beef, cured (beef jerky)	28 g	47	10	4

SAUSAGES AND LUNCHEON MEATS

FOOD	AMOUNT	CALORIES		
		TOTAL	FAT	SAT-FAT
Dutch brand loaf, pork, beef	1 slice (28 g)	68	45	16
Frankfurter				
Beef	1 frank (57 g)	190	150	63
Healthy Choice Low-Fat				
Beef Franks	1 frank (50 g)	60	15	5
Quarter-pound (Hebrew				
National)	1 frank (114 g)	350	300	108
Chicken (Wampler-				
LongAcre)	1 frank (56 g)	120	100	27
Pork and Turkey (Oscar				
Mayer)	1 frank (45 g)	150	120	45
Pork, Turkey, and Beef				
Light (Oscar Mayer)	1 frank (57 g)	110	80	27
Healthy Choice	1 frank (57 g)	70	15	5
Turkey				
Louis Rich	1 frank (57 g)	110	70	23
Extra Lean (Jennie-O)	1 frank (45 g)	45	20	5
Ham (see also **MEATS**, *Pork*				
Products, Cured)				
Baked (Oscar Mayer)	3 slices (63 g)	60	10	5
Boiled (Oscar Mayer)	3 slices (63 g)	70	15	5
Chopped	28 g	68	48	16
	1 slice (21 g)	50	36	12
Cured (Hormel)	85 g	100	45	14
Danish (Plumrose)	2 slices (56 g)	65	25	9
Deli Thin				
Baked Ham	4 slices (52 g)	50	10	0
Honey Ham	4 slices (52 g)	50	15	5
Minced	28 g	75	53	18
	1 slice (21 g)	55	39	14
Salad spread	28 g	61	40	13
	1 tbsp	32	21	7
Smoked				
Esskay	85 g	120	50	18
Hickory-Smoked	3 slices (89 g)	160	100	36
Oscar Mayer	3 slices (63 g)	60	20	9
Smok-a-Roma	57 g	120	70	27
Turkey ham (see Turkey cold				
cuts)				
Ham and cheese loaf or roll	1 slice (28 g)	73	52	19
Ham and cheese spread	28 g	69	47	22
	1 tbsp	37	25	12

SAUSAGES AND LUNCHEON MEATS

| FOOD | AMOUNT | CALORIES | | |
		TOTAL	FAT	SAT-FAT
Headcheese, pork	1 slice (28 g)	60	40	13
Honey loaf, pork, beef	1 slice (28 g)	36	11	4
Honey roll sausage, beef	28 g	52	27	10
	1 slice (22 g)	42	22	8
Kielbasa, pork, beef (Eckrich)	28 g	90	75	27
	1 slice (25 g)	81	64	23
Knockwurst, beef (Hebrew National)	1 link (85 g)	260	210	81
Lebanon bologna, beef	28 g	64	38	16
	1 slice (22 g)	52	31	13
Liver cheese, pork	28 g	86	65	23
Liver pudding, pork	45 g	170	110	9
Liverwurst (Braunschweiger)				
Jones	1 slice (56 g)	150	110	36
Oscar Mayer	1 slice (56 g)	190	160	54
Luncheon meat				
beef, loaved	1 slice (28 g)	87	67	29
beef, thin-sliced	28 g	35	8	3
	5 slices (21 g)	26	6	2
pork, beef	1 slice (28 g)	100	82	30
pork, canned	28 g	95	77	28
	1 slice (21 g)	70	57	20
Luxury loaf, pork	1 slice (28 g)	40	12	4
Mortadella, beef, pork	28 g	88	65	24
	1 slice (14 g)	47	34	13
Mother's loaf, pork	28 g	80	57	20
	1 slice (21 g)	59	42	15
Olive loaf	1 slice (28 g)	70	45	15
Pastrami				
beef	1 slice (28 g)	99	74	27
turkey	1 slice (28 g)	40	16	9
Pâté				
Chicken liver	1 tbsp	26	15	4
Goose liver	28 g	131	112	NA
	1 tbsp	60	51	NA
Pork	28 g	100	80	27
Peppered beef (Carl Buddig)	71 g	100	45	18
Peppered loaf, pork, beef	1 slice (28 g)	42	16	6
Pepperoni (Hormel)	15 slices (28 g)	140	120	54
	1 sausage (252 g)	1248	993	364

SAUSAGES AND LUNCHEON MEATS

FOOD	AMOUNT	CALORIES		
		TOTAL	FAT	SAT-FAT
Pickle and pimento loaf (Oscar Mayer)	1 slice (28 g)	70	50	18
Picnic loaf, pork, beef	1 slice (28 g)	66	42	15
Pork cracklins (fried pork fat with skin)	½ oz (14 g)	80	50	9
Potted meat	¼ cup (58 g)	110	80	27
Salami				
Beef (Hebrew National)	56 g	170	130	54
Cotto (Oscar Mayer)	2 slices (46 g)	100	80	32
Dry or hard, pork	28 g	115	86	30
Sandwich spread, pork, beef	28 g	67	44	15
	1 tbsp	35	23	8
Sausage				
Beef (Jones Dairy Farm)	2 links (45 g)	170	140	NA
Biscuits (Jimmy Dean)	2 (96 g)	330	190	63
Blood	28 g	107	88	34
	1 slice (25 g)	95	78	30
Ham (Smithfield)	48 g	180	140	54
Italian, cooked, pork	28 g	92	66	23
	1 link (5/lb)	216	155	55
	1 link (4/lb)	268	192	68
Italian Turkey (Shady Brook Farms)	1 link (64 g)	100	45	14
Liver, liverwurst, pork	28 g	93	73	27
	1 slice (17 g)	59	46	17
Luncheon, pork and beef	28 g	74	53	19
	1 slice (22 g)	60	43	16
New England brand, pork, beef	28 g	46	19	6
	1 slice (22 g)	37	16	5
Polish, pork	28 g	92	73	26
	1 sausage (8 oz)	739	587	211
Pork				
Bob Evans	2 patties, pan-fried (53 g)	230	180	63
Country	28 g	120	100	36
Hot				
Gwaltney	39 g	150	130	45
Jamestown	36 g	170	140	45
Links (Parks)	2 links (42 g)	170	150	54
Smoked	1 link (85 g)	290	230	81

SAUSAGES AND LUNCHEON MEATS

		CALORIES		
FOOD	AMOUNT	TOTAL	FAT	SAT-FAT
Sausage (*cont.*)				
Pork and beef, cooked	1 patty (28 g)	112	92	33
	1 link (13 g)	52	33	15
Smoked link				
pork	28 g	110	81	29
	1 link (67 g)	265	194	69
	1 link (16 g)	62	46	16
pork and beef	28 g	95	77	27
	1 link (67 g)	229	186	65
	1 link (16 g)	54	44	15
Summer, beef	3 slices (57 g)	180	140	63
Vienna (Hormel)	28 g	70	60	36
Scrapple (Parks)	¼" slice (55 g)	110	60	23
Tongue, beef				
raw	28 g	63	41	18
simmered	28 g	80	53	23
Tripe, beef, raw	28 g	28	10	5
Turkey breast, processed				
Oven-Roasted (Oscar Mayer)	3 slices (63 g)	70	15	0
Fat-Free Deli Thin (Oscar Mayer)	4 slices (52 g)	40	0	0
Smoked white (Louis Rich)	1 slice (28 g)	30	10	0
Turkey cold cuts				
Bacon (Louis Rich)	1 slice (14 g)	30	20	5
Bologna (Louis Rich)	1 slice (28 g)	50	35	9
Ham				
Chopped	1 slice (28 g)	40	20	9
Jennie-O	56 g	80	40	7
Louis Rich	1 slice (28 g)	35	10	0
Pastrami	1 slice (28 g)	40	16	9
Salami (Louis Rich)	1 slice (28 g)	45	25	9
Cotted Salami (Louis Rich)	1 slice (28 g)	90	50	18
Turkey roll				
Light and dark meat	1 slice (28 g)	42	18	5
Light meat	1 slice (28 g)	42	18	5

SNACK FOODS

FOOD	AMOUNT	CALORIES		
		TOTAL	FAT	SAT-FAT
Breadsticks				
Grissini-style, garlic (Stella D'oro)	3 (15 g)	60	0	0
Thin Bread Sticks (Pepperidge Farm)				
Cheddar Cheese	7 (16 g)	70	25	9
Chips and Crisps				
Bagel Chips				
New York Style	31 g	140	30	5
Planet	55 g	150	0	0
Bugles				
Crisp-baked	1½ cups	130	25	5
Original	1⅓ cups	160	80	72
Cheese Curls (Weight Watchers)	1 pkg (14 g)	70	25	9
Cheese Puffs Super Cheese (Safeway)	30 pieces (28 g)	160	100	9
Cheese Corn Curls	25 pieces (30 g)	150	70	18
Cheese Twists	1 cup (30 g)	150	100	18
Cheetos	21 pieces (28 g)	150	80	18
Cheez'n Breadsticks (Kraft)	1 unit (32 g)	130	60	36
Cheez'n Crackers (Kraft)	1 unit (31 g)	130	70	36
Corn Chips	20 chips (30 g)	170	80	14
Fritos	32 chips (28 g)	160	90	14
King-Size Corn Chips	12 chips (28 g)	160	90	14
Scoops	10 chips (28 g)	150	80	14
Jax (Bachman)	25 pieces (30 g)	150	70	9
Crunchy	⅔ cup	170	110	18
PB'n Grahamsticks (Kraft)	1 unit (32 g)	170	90	23
Pop Chips (Betty Crocker)	1½ cups	130	30	5
Pita Chips (Shra-Lins)	1 serving (14 g)	60	18	9
Potato Chips				
Lay's	18 chips (28 g)	150	90	23
Bar-B-Q	15 chips (28 g)	150	90	18
Sour Cream and Onion	22 chips (28 g)	150	90	23
Wavy Lay's Au-Gratin	13 chips (28 g)	150	90	23
Mr. Phipps				
Sour Cream 'n Onion	22 chips (28 g)	130	35	5
Pringles				
Original	14 crisps (28 g)	160	90	23
Right Crisps	16 crisps (28 g)	140	60	18
Sour Cream and Onion	14 crisps (28 g)	160	90	23

SNACK FOODS

FOOD	AMOUNT	CALORIES		
		TOTAL	FAT	SAT-FAT
Potato Chips (*cont.*)				
Ruffles (Frito-Lay)	12 chips (28 g)	150	90	27
Cheddar and Sour Cream	13 chips (28 g)	160	90	23
Ranch	13 chips (28 g)	150	80	23
Safeway				
Barbecue Ripple Chips	18 chips (28 g)	140	90	23
Utz	20 chips (28 g)	150	80	18
Bar-B-Q Ripple Cut	20 chips (28 g)	150	80	18
Grandma Utz's				
Handcooked	20 chips (28 g)	150	80	27
Kettle Classics Crunchy	20 chips (28 g)	150	80	14
Ripple Cut	20 chips (28 g)	150	80	18
Sour Cream and Onion				
Ripple Cut	20 chips (28 g)	160	90	27
Potato Sticks (Durkee)	¾ cup	160	90	14
Pretzel Chips (Mr. Phipps)				
Original	16 chips (28 g)	120	20	0
Fat-free	16 chips (28 g)	100	0	0
Tortilla Chips				
Doritos	15 chips (28 g)	140	60	9
Guiltless Gourmet	22 chips (28 g)	110	15	0
Mr. Phipps				
Tortilla Crisps, original	29 crisps (30 g)	130	40	5
Tortilla Crisps, nacho				
cheese	28 crisps (31 g)	140	40	9
Safeway Tortilla Chips				
Blue corn	14 chips (28 g)	140	60	14
Extra cheese	13 chips (28 g)	140	60	14
White corn	7 chips (28 g)	140	60	14
Yellow and white corn	8 chips (28 g)	140	70	9
Tostitos	6 chips (28 g)	130	50	9
Utz	17 chips (28 g)	140	60	9
Nacho Tortilla	17 chips (28 g)	140	60	9
Crackers				
Austin				
Cheese Crackers on Cheese	6 (39 g)	210	100	27
Cheese Crackers and Peanut				
Butter	6 (39 g)	210	90	23
Toasty Crackers and Peanut				
Butter	6 (39 g)	210	90	23
Delicious				
Crispy Bacon	11 (30 g)	150	60	14

SNACK FOODS

FOOD	AMOUNT	CALORIES		
		TOTAL	FAT	SAT-FAT
Delicious crackers (*cont.*)				
Hearty Wheat	13 (31 g)	140	50	**14**
Real Cheddar Cheese	11 (30 g)	140	50	**14**
Sesame Wheat	13 (31 g)	150	60	**14**
Snack	9 (31 g)	150	60	**14**
Tangy Onion	11 (30 g)	140	50	**14**
Devonsheer				
Melba Rounds				
Garlic	5 (15 g)	60	10	**0**
Honey bran	5 (15 g)	50	0	**0**
Onion	5 (15 g)	50	0	**0**
Plain	5 (15 g)	50	0	**0**
Sesame	5 (15 g)	60	20	**5**
12 Grain	5 (15 g)	50	0	**0**
Vegetable	5 (15 g)	50	0	**0**
Melba Toast				
Plain	3 (14 g)	50	0	**0**
Sesame	3 (14 g)	50	10	**0**
Rye	3 (14 g)	50	0	**0**
Keebler				
Club				
Garlic Bread	4 (14 g)	60	15	**5**
Original	4 (14 g)	70	25	**9**
Cracker Paks				
Club and Cheddar	1 pkg (36 g)	190	100	**23**
Toast and Peanut Butter	1 pkg (39 g)	190	80	**18**
Munch 'ems				
Cheddar	28 (30 g)	140	50	**9**
Ranch	28 (30 g)	130	45	**9**
Seasoned Original	28 (30 g)	130	45	**9**
Sour Cream and Onion	28 (30 g)	140	50	**9**
Toasteds Complements				
Buttercrisp	9 (29 g)	140	60	**14**
Onion	9 (29 g)	140	50	**9**
Rye	9 (29 g)	140	60	**9**
Sesame	9 (29 g)	140	60	**9**
Wheat	9 (29 g)	140	60	**14**
Reduced Fat	10 (28 g)	120	30	**9**
Town House				
Original	5 (16 g)	80	40	**9**
Reduced-fat	5 (16 g)	70	20	**5**

SNACK FOODS

FOOD	AMOUNT	CALORIES		
		TOTAL	FAT	SAT-FAT
Keebler crackers (*cont.*)				
Wheatables				
Ranch	26 (30 g)	150	70	**18**
All other flavors	26 (30 g)	150	60	**18**
Zesta Saltines				
Fat-free	5 (14 g)	50	0	**0**
Original	5 (15 g)	60	15	**5**
Lu				
Milk Lunch New England				
Biscuits	4 (32 g)	140	35	**9**
Manischewitz crackers				
Matzo				
American	1 board (28 g)	110	15	**5**
Premium Gold Unsalted				
Tops	1 sheet (31 g)	140	40	**23**
Snack Bits	15 bits (28 g)	130	35	**23**
Mrs. Wright's (Safeway)				
Cheddar Cheese Snack	28 (30 g)	150	60	**18**
Chicken Flavored Snack	11 (31 g)	160	80	**18**
Garden Vegetable	13 (31 g)	150	60	**14**
Onion Snack	11 (31 g)	140	50	**14**
Oyster and Soup	21 (30 g)	120	30	**0**
Saltine	5 (15 g)	60	15	**5**
Sesame Cheddar Snack	13 (31 g)	150	60	**14**
Sesame Snack	9 (31 g)	160	60	**18**
Sesame Wheat Snack	13 (31 g)	150	60	**14**
Snack	10 (15 g)	70	20	**9**
Unsalted Tops	5 (15 g)	60	15	**5**
Wheat Snack	13 (31 g)	140	50	**14**
Wheatstone	8 (28 g)	130	50	**14**
Nabisco				
Better Cheddars	22 (30 g)	150	70	**18**
Reduced-fat	24 (30 g)	140	50	**14**
Bugs Bunny Graham Snacks				
Chocolate	13 (30 g)	140	40	**9**
Cinnamon	13 (30 g)	140	35	**5**
Cheese Nips	29 (30 g)	150	60	**14**
Cheese Tid-Bit	32 (30 g)	150	70	**14**
Chicken in a Biskit	14 (30 g)	160	80	**14**
Garden Crisps	15 (30 g)	130	30	**5**

SNACK FOODS

FOOD	AMOUNT	CALORIES		
		TOTAL	FAT	SAT-FAT
Nabisco crackers (cont.)				
Harvest Crisps				
5-Grain	13 (31 g)	130	30	5
Nabs				
Cheese Crackers with				
Peanut Butter	1 pkg (40 g)	200	100	18
Toasted, with Peanut				
Butter	1 pkg (40 g)	200	100	18
Oysterettes	19 (15 g)	60	20	5
Premium Saltines				
Fat-Free	5 (15 g)	60	0	0
Low-Sodium	5 (14 g)	60	10	0
Original	5 (14 g)	60	15	0
Unsalted Tops	5 (14 g)	60	15	0
with Multi-Grain	5 (14 g)	60	15	0
Rice crackers	½ cup (30 g)	110	0	0
Ritz crackers	5 (16 g)	80	35	5
Ritz Bits				
Mini Ritz	48 (30 g)	160	80	14
Peanut Butter				
Sandwiches	14 (31 g)	160	80	14
Cheese Ritz with Peanut				
Butter	1 pkg (40 g)	210	110	23
with Real Cheese	1 pkg (40 g)	210	110	27
Whole-Wheat	5 (15 g)	70	20	0
SnackWell's (see listing after Ry-Krisp)				
Sociables	7 (15 g)	80	35	5
Swiss Cheese	15 (29 g)	140	60	14
Teddy Grahams				
Cinnamon	24 pieces (30 g)	140	40	9
Honey	24 pieces (30 g)	140	40	9
Toasted Oat Thins	18 (30 g)	140	50	9
Triscuit Wafers	7 wafers (31 g)	140	45	9
Deli-style Rye	7 wafers (32 g)	140	45	9
Garden Herb	6 wafers (28 g)	130	40	9
Reduced Fat	7 wafers (32 g)	120	30	5
Wheat 'n Bran	7 wafers (32 g)	140	45	9
Uneeda Biscuits Unsalted				
Tops	2 (15 g)	60	15	0
Vegetable Thins	14 (31 g)	160	80	14

SNACK FOODS

FOOD	AMOUNT	CALORIES		
		TOTAL	FAT	SAT-FAT
Nabisco crackers (*cont.*)				
Waverly	5 (15 g)	70	30	**9**
Wheat Thins				
Multigrain	17 (30 g)	130	35	**5**
Original	16 (29 g)	140	50	**9**
Reduced Fat	18 (31 g)	130	35	**5**
Wheatsworth Stone Ground				
Wheat	5 (16 g)	80	30	**5**
Pepperidge Farm				
Swirled Bread Crisps, garlic				
and butter	1 oz (28 g)	140	50	**9**
Distinctive				
Butter Thins	4 (15 g)	70	25	**9**
Hearty Wheat	3 (16 g)	80	30	**0**
Quartet	3 (13 g)	60	20	**0**
Symphony	4 (17 g)	80	30	**5**
Three Cracker	3 (14 g)	70	20	**0**
Goldfish				
Cheddar Cheese	55 (30 g)	140	50	**14**
Original	55 (30 g)	140	60	**18**
Parmesan Cheese	60 (30 g)	140	50	**14**
Pizza	55 (30 g)	140	60	**14**
Real Vanilla	19 (30 g)	150	60	**23**
Reduced sodium cheddar				
cheese	60 (30 g)	150	60	**14**
Sesame Snack Sticks				
Sesame	9 (31 g)	150	50	**5**
Three-Cheese	9 (31 g)	140	45	**18**
Quaker				
Honey Nut Mini Rice Cakes	5 (14 g)	50	0	**0**
Rice Cakes	1 cake	35	0	**0**
Ry-Krisp				
Natural	2 (15 g)	60	0	**0**
SnackWell's (Nabisco)				
Cheese	38 (30 g)	130	20	**5**
Cinnamon Graham Snacks	20 (30 g)	110	0	**0**
Classic Golden	6 (14 g)	60	10	**0**
Cracked Pepper	7 (15 g)	60	0	**0**
Wheat	5 (15 g)	60	0	**0**
Sunshine				
Cheez-It	27 (30 g)	160	80	**18**
Hot and Spicy	26 (30 g)	160	80	**14**
White Cheddar	26 (30 g)	160	80	**18**

SNACK FOODS

FOOD	AMOUNT	CALORIES		
		TOTAL	FAT	SAT-FAT
Sunshine (*cont.*)				
Hi-Ho, all flavors	9 (31 g)	160	80	14
Krispy Saltines				
Mild Cheddar	5 (15 g)	60	20	5
Original	5 (14 g)	60	10	0
Soup and Oyster	17 (15 g)	60	15	0
Fruit Snacks				
Fruit by the Foot	1 roll (21 g)	80	15	0
Fruit Gushers	1 pouch (14 g)	90	10	0
Fruit Jammers	1 pouch (28 g)	100	10	5
Fruit Roll-ups	1 roll (14 g)	50	5	0
Troll	1 pouch (28 g)	90	0	0
Trolls in Trouble	1 pouch (28 g)	80	15	5
Weight Watchers	1 pkg (14 g)	50	0	0
Granola Bars				
Carnation Breakfast Bars				
Chewy Chocolate Chip	1 bar (36 g)	150	50	23
Chewy Peanut Butter	1 bar (36 g)	140	45	18
Kellogg's				
Chewy Granola Chocolate				
Chunk	1 bar (28 g)	110	20	5
Low-Fat Granola Bar	1 bar (21 g)	80	15	0
Nutrigrain Cereal Bar				
Oat and Fruit	1 bar (37 g)	140	35	9
Kudos				
Chocolate Chip	1 bar (28 g)	130	45	23
Chocolate Chunk with nuts	1 bar (20 g)	90	30	9
Honey Nut	1 bar (20 g)	90	30	9
Nutty Fudge	1 bar (28 g)	130	50	23
Nature Valley Low-fat Chewy	1 bar (28 g)	110	20	0
Quaker Chewy				
Apple Berry	1 bar (28 g)	120	35	9
Chocolate Chip	1 bar (28 g)	120	30	14
Peanut Butter and				
Chocolate Chip	1 bar (28 g)	120	40	14
S'mores	1 bar (28 g)	120	35	14
Trail Mix	1 bar (28 g)	120	45	9
Quaker Low-fat, all flavors	1 bar (21 g)	80	15	0

SNACK FOODS

| FOOD | AMOUNT | CALORIES | | |
		TOTAL	FAT	SAT-FAT
Sunfelt				
Almond	1 bar (28 g)	130	60	**18**
Chocolate Chip	1 bar (35 g)	160	60	**27**
Oatmeal Raisin or Raisin	1 bar (35 g)	150	50	**18**
Oats and Honey	1 bar (28 g)	120	45	**18**
Lunch Packs				
Lunch 'n Munch (Hillshire Farm)				
Smoked Turkey Breast	1 pkg (128 g)	400	320	**81**
Lunchables (Oscar Mayer)				
Delux Variety Pack				
Turkey and Ham with cheese	1 pkg (145 g)	360	180	**99**
Chicken and Turkey with cheese	1 pkg (145 g)	380	190	**90**
Fun Pack				
Bologna	1 pkg (318 g)	530	260	**126**
Ham	1 pkg (318 g)	450	180	**90**
Turkey	1 pkg (318 g)	430	170	**81**
Ham and Cheddar	1 pkg (128 g)	340	180	**99**
Lean Turkey and Cheddar	1 pkg (128 g)	360	200	**99**
With dessert				
Chicken and Monterey Jack	1 pkg (176 g)	378	160	**81**
Popcorn				
Air-popped, no added fat	1 cup popped	30	0	**0**
Commercially Popped				
Bachman All Natural				
Air-Popped	2¾ cups	170	100	**9**
Cheese Popcorn	3 cups	160	80	**9**
with white Cheddar cheese	2½ cups	160	80	**9**
Boston's				
Caramel Popcorn	⅔ cup	120	20	**0**
Lite Popcorn	4 cups	140	50	**5**
Crunch 'n Munch Buttery Toffee				
Popcorn with Peanuts	⅔ cup	140	35	**9**
Fiddle Faddle Caramel				
Popcorn with peanuts	¾ cup	140	50	**27**
Smartfood, Butter-flavored	3 cups	150	80	**18**

SNACK FOODS

| FOOD | AMOUNT | CALORIES | | |
		TOTAL	FAT	SAT-FAT
Popcorn, commercially popped (*cont.*)				
Utz				
Butter	2 cups	160	110	18
Caramel Corn Clusters	1¼ cups	160	20	0
Cheese	2 cups	120	80	14
White Cheddar Cheese	2 cups	150	70	14
Weight Watchers (Smart Snackers)				
Butter	1 pkg (19 g)	90	20	0
Butter Toffee	1 pkg (26 g)	110	25	9
Caramel	1 pkg (26 g)	110	10	9
White Cheddar Cheese	1 pkg (19 g)	100	35	0
Microwave				
Jolly Time Light	5 cups popped	120	50	9
Newman's Own Oldstyle				
Picture Show	3½ cups popped	170	100	18
Orville Redenbacker's				
Butter, snack-size	1 bag (50 g)	210	130	18
Natural	1 cup popped	30	18	0
Reden Budders	2 tbsp (36 g)	150	90	23
Smart Pop, butter	3 tbsp (45 g)	100	15	0
Pop·Secret				
Original Butter	4 cups popped	170	110	27
Buttery Burst	4 cups popped	170	100	27
Video Club Generic				
Butter Flavor Light	5 c	170	60	9
Natural	4½ c	200	110	23
Movie Theater				
Popped in coconut oil	kids (5 cups)	300	180	126
	sm (7 cups)	398	243	171
	med (11 cups)	647	387	279
	med (16 cups)	901	540	387
	lg (20 cups)	1161	693	495
Popped in coconut oil with butter topping	kid's (5 cups)	472	333	198
	sm (7 cups)	632	450	261
	med (11 cups)	910	639	369
	med (16 cups)	1221	873	504
	lg (20 cups)	1642	1134	657

SNACK FOODS

FOOD	AMOUNT	CALORIES		
		TOTAL	FAT	SAT-FAT
Popped in Canola shortening	sm (7 cups)	361	198	**63**
	med (11 cups)	627	342	**108**
	lg (16 cups)	850	468	**144**
Pop-Tarts				
Kellogg's				
Apple cinnamon	1 tart (52 g)	210	50	**9**
Blueberry	1 tart (52 g)	210	60	**9**
Brown sugar cinnamon	1 tart (50 g)	220	80	**9**
Chocolate fudge	1 tart (52 g)	200	40	**9**
Frosted blueberry or cherry	1 tart (52 g)	200	50	**9**
Frosted brown sugar cinnamon	1 tart (50 g)	210	70	**9**
Frosted choc vanilla creme	1 tart (52 g)	200	50	**9**
Frosted chocolate fudge	1 tart (52 g)	200	40	**9**
Frosted strawberry	1 tart (52 g)	200	40	**9**
Nutri-Grain, all flavors	1 bar (37 g)	140	35	**5–9**
S'Mores	1 tart (52 g)	200	50	**5**
Strawberry	1 tart (52 g)	210	50	**9**
Pretzels				
Buttermilk Ranch Pretzels (Snyders of Hanover)	⅓ cup	130	45	**9**
Cheez'n Pretzels	1 unit (24 g)	110	50	**36**
Hard (Wege)	1 pretzel (30 g)	110	10	**0**
Honey Mustard Pretzel Bits	11 pieces (28 g)	140	70	**9**
Honey Mustard and Onion				
Snyders of Hanover	⅓ cup	130	95	**0**
Utz	⅓ cup	80	50	**9**
Nibs	½ cup	110	15	**0**
Oat bran (Weight Watchers)	1 pkg (42 g)	170	25	**0**
Party Mix	25 pieces (30 g)	150	70	**9**
Petites	18 (30 g)	120	10	**10**
Sourdough Hard (Snyders of Hanover)	1 pretzel (28 g)	111	0	**0**
Cheddar Cheese	1 pretzel (28 g)	160	70	**9**
Stix (Snyders of Hanover)	32 sticks	100	10	**0**
Thin (Rold Gold)	10 (28 g)	110	0	**0**
Wheel (Utz)	20 (28 g)	110	9	**0**

SNACK FOODS

FOOD	AMOUNT	CALORIES		
		TOTAL	FAT	SAT-FAT
Snack Mixes				
Cheerios Snack Mix				
Cheddar Cheese	¾ cup	130	45	**9**
Original	¾ cup	130	45	**9**
Chex Mix (Ralston)				
Traditional	⅔ cup	150	45	**9**
Zesty Ranch	½ cup	130	40	**9**
Doo Dads Snack Mix	½ cup	150	60	**9**
Fiesta Fun Mix	½ cup	300	180	**27**
Gold Fish (Pepperidge Farm)				
Honey Mustard	½ cup	180	90	**14**
Nutty Deluxe	½ cup	180	80	**14**
Original	½ cup	170	70	**14**
Roasted Peanuts	½ cup	170	70	**14**
Seasoned	½ cup	170	70	**9**
Zesty Cheddar	½ cup	180	90	**14**
Party Mix				
Oriental	½ cup	300	180	**27**
Pastamore	½ cup	260	100	**18**
Sesame Walnut	½ cup	300	180	**27**
Smokehouse	½ cup	260	160	**18**
Swiss Mix	½ cup	380	160	**72**
Trail Mix	½ cup	300	160	**27**
Deluxe Super	½ cup	300	120	**45**
Tropical	½ cup	300	120	**72**
Vending Machine Foods (Lance)				
Cakes				
Brownies	1¾ oz/pkg	200	81	**9**
Dunking Sticks	5½ oz/pkg	380	180	**54**
Fig Cake	2⅛ oz/pkg	210	27	**9**
Oatmeal Cake	2 oz/pkg	240	99	**27**
Raisin Cake	2 oz/pkg	230	90	**27**
Candy				
Chocolaty Peanut Bar	2 oz/pkg	320	162	**54**
Peanut Bar	1¾ oz/pkg	260	126	**27**
Chips, etc.				
Cheese Balls	1⅛ oz/pkg	190	117	**27**
Corn Chips				
BBQ	1¾ oz/pkg	260	144	**36**
Plain	1¾ oz/pkg	270	153	**27**

SNACK FOODS

FOOD	AMOUNT	CALORIES		
		TOTAL	FAT	SAT-FAT
Crunchy Cheese Twists	1½ oz/pkg	260	144	36
Gold-n-Chee	1⅜ oz/pkg	180	81	18
6-pak tray	6 oz/pkg	780	432	54
Jalapeno Cheese Tortilla Chips	1⅛ oz/pkg	160	72	18
Nacho Tortilla Chips	1⅛ oz/pkg	160	72	18
Popcorn				
Cheese	⅞ oz/pkg	130	72	9
Plain	1 oz/pkg	160	90	18
Pork Skins				
BBQ	½ oz/pkg	80	45	18
Plain	½ oz/pkg	80	45	18
Potato Chips				
BBQ	1⅛ oz/pkg	190	108	27
Cajun-style	2 oz/pkg	320	180	36
Plain	1⅛ oz/pkg	190	135	36
Sour Cream and Onion	1⅛ oz/pkg	190	108	27
Pretzel Twists	1½ oz/pkg	150	9	0
Cookies				
Apple-Cinnamon	2 oz/pkg	240	72	18
Apple-Oatmeal	1.65 oz/pkg	190	63	18
Blueberry	2 oz/pkg	240	72	18
Bonnie Sandwich	1³⁄₁₆ oz/pkg	160	63	18
Choc-O-Lunch	1⁵⁄₁₆ oz/pkg	180	63	18
	4½ oz/pkg	585	203	41
Choc-O-Mint	1¼ oz/pkg	180	90	27
Coated Graham	1⁵⁄₁₆ oz/pkg	200	90	36
Fig Bar	1½ oz/pkg	150	18	9
Fudge–Chocolate Chip	2 oz/pkg	260	90	36
Malt	1¼ oz/pkg	190	99	18
Nekot	1½ oz/pkg	210	90	18
Nut-O-Lunch	4½ oz/pkg	630	243	81
Oatmeal Cookies	2 oz/pkg	260	90	18
Peanut Butter Creme-Filled	1¾ oz/pkg	240	90	27
Soft Chocolate Chip	2 oz/pkg	260	90	36
Strawberry	2 oz/pkg	240	72	18
Van-O-Lunch	1⁵⁄₁₆ oz/pkg	180	63	18
	4½ oz/pkg	630	162	41
Crackers				
Captain's Wafers with Cream Cheese and Chives	1⁵⁄₁₆ oz/pkg	170	81	18

SNACK FOODS

FOOD	AMOUNT	CALORIES		
		TOTAL	FAT	SAT-FAT
Cheese-on-Wheat	1⁵⁄₁₆ oz/pkg	180	81	**18**
Lanchee	1¼ oz/pkg	180	99	**18**
Nip-Chee	1⁵⁄₁₆ oz/pkg	130	81	**18**
Peanut Butter Wheat	1⁵⁄₁₆ oz/pkg	190	99	**18**
Rye-Chee	1⁷⁄₁₆ oz/pkg	190	81	**18**
Spicy Gold-n-Chee	10 oz/pkg	1400	540	**180**
Thin Wheat Snacks	10 oz/pkg	1600	720	**180**
Toastchee	1⅜ oz/pkg	190	99	**18**
Toasty	1¼ oz/pkg	180	90	**18**
Nuts				
Cashews	1⅛ oz/pkg	190	135	**27**
long tube	2½ oz/pkg	400	288	**54**
Peanuts				
Honey-toasted	1⅜ oz/pkg	230	153	**27**
Roasted (shell)	1¾ oz/pkg	190	135	**27**
Salted	1⅛ oz/pkg	190	135	**27**
tube	3 oz/pkg	480	360	**72**
Pistachios	1⅛ oz/pkg	180	126	**18**
Pie				
Pecan Pie	3 oz/pkg	350	135	**27**

SOUPS

If you are keeping track of total fat calories and your soup is made with whole milk, add 100 fat calories and 206 total calories per can. With 2% milk, add 58 fat calories and 166 total calories per can. If you are keeping track of saturated fat and your soup is made with whole milk, add 62 sat-fat calories and 206 total calories per can. With 2% milk, add 37 sat-fat calories and 166 total calories per can.

FOOD	AMOUNT	CALORIES		
		TOTAL	FAT	SAT-FAT
Canned				
Condensed, prepared with water				
Campbell				
Bean with Bacon	1 cup prep.	180	45	**18**
Beef Broth	1 cup prep.	15	0	**0**
Beef Noodle	1 cup prep.	70	25	**9**

SOUPS

FOOD	AMOUNT	CALORIES		
		TOTAL	FAT	SAT-FAT
Campbell (cont.)				
Broccoli Cheese	1 cup prep.	110	60	27
Cheddar Cheese	1 cup prep.	150	90	45
Chicken Alphabet	1 cup prep.	80	20	9
Chicken Broth	1 cup prep.	30	20	5
Chicken and Dumplings	1 cup prep.	80	25	9
Chicken Gumbo	1 cup prep.	60	15	5
Chicken Noodle	1 cup prep.	70	25	9
Chicken NoodleO's	1 cup prep.	80	25	9
Chicken and Stars	1 cup prep.	70	20	5
Chicken with Rice	1 cup prep.	70	25	9
Chicken Vegetable	1 cup prep.	80	20	5
Chicken Won Ton	1 cup prep.	45	10	0
Consomme Beef	1 cup prep.	25	0	0
Cream of Asparagus	1 cup prep.	110	60	18
Cream of Celery	1 cup prep.	110	60	23
Cream of Chicken	1 cup prep.	130	70	27
Cream of Mushroom	1 cup prep.	110	60	23
Cream of Mushroom (Healthy Request)	1 cup prep.	70	30	9
Cream of Potato	1 cup prep.	90	25	14
Cream of Shrimp	1 cup prep.	100	60	18
Creamy Chicken Mushroom	1 cup prep.	130	80	23
Double Noodle	1 cup prep.	100	25	9
French Onion	1 cup prep.	70	25	0
Golden Mushroom	1 cup prep.	80	25	9
Green Pea	1 cup prep.	180	25	9
Homestyle Chicken Noodle	1 cup prep.	70	25	14
Italian Tomato	1 cup prep.	100	5	0
Manhattan Clam Chowder	1 cup prep.	70	20	5
Minestrone	1 cup prep.	90	20	9
New England Clam Chowder	1 cup prep.	90	25	5
Old-Fashioned Tomato Rice	1 cup prep.	120	20	5
Old-Fashioned Vegetable	1 cup prep.	70	25	5
Split Pea with Ham and Bacon	1 cup prep.	180	30	18
Tomato (Healthy Request)	1 cup prep.	90	20	5
Tomato Bisque	1 cup prep.	130	25	14
Turkey Noodle	1 cup prep.	80	25	9
Turkey Vegetable	1 cup prep.	80	25	9
Vegetable	1 cup prep.	90	15	5

SOUPS

FOOD	AMOUNT	CALORIES		
		TOTAL	FAT	SAT-FAT
Campbell (*cont.*)				
Vegetable Beef	1 cup prep.	80	20	9
Vegetarian Vegetable	1 cup prep.	90	20	0
Pepperidge Farm				
Gazpacho	⅔ cup	70	20	0
Ready to Serve				
Campbell's				
Chunky				
Beef	10¾ oz	200	50	18
Chicken Mushroom				
Chowder	1 cup	210	110	36
Hearty Vegetable with				
Pasta	1 cup	130	25	5
New England Clam				
Chowder	10¾ oz	300	160	63
Sirloin Burger	1 cup	190	80	32
Vegetable	10¾ oz	160	35	9
Healthy Request				
Chicken Broth	1 cup	20	0	0
Hearty Chicken Vegetable	1 cup	120	20	9
Home Cookin'				
Bean and Ham	1 cup	160	25	9
Chicken Noodle	10¾ oz	130	30	14
Old-Fashioned				
Vegetable Beef	1 cup	150	45	14
Progresso Pasta Soups				
Hearty Penne in Chicken				
Broth	1 cup	70	10	0
Hearty Vegetable and Rotini	1 cup	110	10	0
Dehydrated				
Knorr's				
Black Bean	1 pkg (53 g)	200	10	0
Chicken Flavor Vegetable	1 pkg (30 g)	100	0	0
Hearty Lentil	1 pkg (57 g)	220	0	0
Navy Bean	1 pkg (38 g)	140	0	0
Potato Leek	1 pkg (34 g)	120	0	0

SOUPS

| FOOD | AMOUNT | CALORIES | | |
		TOTAL	FAT	SAT-FAT
Nissin Top Ramen				
Cup Noodles Ramen Noodle Soup				
Chicken flavor	1 pkg (64 g)	300	110	54
Oodles of Noodles, all flavors	½ pkg (43 g)	200	70	36
Soup Starter (Borden)				
Beef Vegetable	⅛ pkg (28 g dry)	90	5	0
Chicken Noodle	⅛ pkg (24 g dry)	80	5	0
The Spice Hunter				
Hunan Noodle	1 pkg (29 g)	110	10	0
Szechwan Noodle	1 pkg (33 g)	130	5	0
Homemade or Restaurant				
Cream of Mushroom	1 cup	170	155	98
French Onion	1 cup	350	125	65
Gazpacho	1 cup	111	80	11
New England Clam Chowder	1 cup	230	145	65
Vichyssoise	1 cup	315	210	140
Mix				
Matzo Ball	2 tbsp	80	0	0

SWEETS

| FOOD | AMOUNT | CALORIES | | |
		TOTAL	FAT	SAT-FAT
Brownies				
Fudge (Little Debbie)	2 (61 g)	270	120	23
Low-fat (Hostess)	1 (40 g)	140	25	5
Nonfat (Entenmann's)	1 (40 g)	110	0	0
with Nuts	1 (40 g)	180	80	18
without Nuts	1 (40 g)	160	60	18
Brownie mixes				
Betty Crocker				
Fudge	1 (34 g)	200	80	16
White Chocolate Swirl	1 (33 g)	180	70	25
Duncan Hines				
Chocolate Lover's	1 (31 g)	160	60	11

SWEETS

FOOD	AMOUNT	CALORIES		
		TOTAL	FAT	SAT-FAT
Pillsbury				
Cream Cheese Swirl	1 (30 g)	190	80	23
Fudge	1 (30 g)	200	80	14
Hot Fudge	1 (31 g)	160	60	18
Buns				
Breakfast	1 (55 g)	170	25	9
Butterfly	1 (55 g)	190	35	9
Cinnamon Raisin				
(Entenmann's)	1 (61 g)	160	0	0
Honey (Morton)	1 (64 g)	250	90	23
Hot Cross	1	168	56	16
Rum	1 (55 g)	190	45	9
Sticky	1 (55 g)	210	70	14
Entenmann's	1 (71 g)	270	100	18
Cakes (Bakery, Homemade, and Restaurant)				
Almond Danish coffee cake	⅛ cake (57 g)	230	100	18
Almond poppy seed loaf	⅕ cake (80 g)	330	130	23
Angel food	¹⁄₁₂ cake	125	0	0
Angel food loaf	2″ slice (55 g)	150	5	0
Angel food ring	⅙ cake (47 g)	130	5	0
Apple Danish coffee cake	⅛ cake (57 g)	160	60	18
Baked Alaska	¹⁄₁₂	263	112	60
Banana nut loaf	2″ slice (76 g)	270	120	27
Bavarian chocolate	2 × 2″ square			
	(80 g)	340	180	63
Black Forest	1 slice (80 g)			
	(7″ diam.)	330	170	41
Blueberry cheese coffee cake	⅛ cake (57 g)	170	70	18
Boston cream	⅙ cake (113 g)	320	120	27
Carrot	1 slice (80 g)			
	(7″ diam.)	300	130	36
Cheesecake	¹⁄₁₂ cake	280	162	89
Blueberry-topped	⅙ cake (113 g)	350	180	81
French	4″ wedge (125 g)	370	200	54
Cherry pudding	⅛ cake (74 g)	290	130	23
Chocolate crunch ring	⅛ cake (71 g)	310	140	36
Chocolate fudge	1 slice (80 g)			
	(7″ diam.)	300	140	32
Chocolate marble loaf	⅕ cake (80 g)	340	150	32

SWEETS

FOOD	AMOUNT	CALORIES		
		TOTAL	**FAT**	**SAT-FAT**
Chocolate sheet cake				
with vanilla icing	1 slice (80 g)	320	160	**36**
Cinnamon sticks	1 stick (57 g)	200	60	**14**
Cupcake	1 (80 g)	340	140	**36**
Devil's food fudge	⅙ cake (85 g)	340	140	**36**
Devil's food layer with white	2½" wedge			
icing	(80 g)	360	170	**45**
Fruitcake	1 slice (125 g)	470	171	**32**
German chocolate	¹⁄₁₆ cake			
	(10" diam.)	521	277	**27**
Golden coconut	1 slice (80 g)			
	(7" diam.)	320	160	**36**
Hazelnut torte	¹⁄₁₆ torte	315	187	**56**
Ladyfingers	12 (85 g)	280	35	**14**
Lemon crunch ring	⅛ cake (71 g)	270	110	**23**
Lemon Supreme	1 slice (80 g)			
	(7" diam.)	320	160	**36**
Pecan cinnamon ring	⅛ cake (71 g)	300	130	**23**
Pecan twirls sweet rolls	2 twirls (56 g)	220	80	**9**
Pound	2" slice (80 g)	300	140	**45**
Strawberry cheese Danish				
coffee cake	⅛ cake (57 g)	170	80	**18**
Yellow layer				
with chocolate icing	2½" wedge			
	(80 g)	320	140	**36**
with white icing	2½" wedge			
	(80 g)	350	170	**45**

Cakes and Snack Cakes, by Brand Name
Entenmann's

FOOD	AMOUNT	TOTAL	FAT	SAT-FAT
All Butter Pound Loaf	¼ cake (85 g)	330	130	**81**
Apple Puffs	1 puff (85 g)	260	110	**27**
Assorted Rugelach	1 piece (21 g)	100	60	**41**
Cheese Coffee Cake	⅑ cake (54 g)	190	70	**42**
Cheese Crumb Babka	¹⁄₁₀ danish (57 g)	220	90	**42**
Cheese-Filled Crumb Coffee				
Cake	⅛ cake (57 g)	210	90	**36**
Cinnamon Filbert Ring	⅙ danish (61 g)	270	150	**27**
Cinnamon Rugelach	1 piece (21 g)	100	60	**32**
Crumb Coffee Cake	¹⁄₁₀ cake (57 g)	250	110	**27**

SWEETS

FOOD	AMOUNT	CALORIES		
		TOTAL	FAT	SAT-FAT
Entenmann's Fat-and-Cholesterol-Free				
Apple Spice	⅕ cake (79 g)	200	0	0
Banana Crunch	⅕ cake (85 g)	220	0	0
Banana Loaf	⅙ cake (76 g)	190	0	0
Blueberry Crunch	⅙ cake (76 g)	180	0	0
Chocolate Crunch	⅕ cake (79 g)	210	0	0
Chocolate Loaf	⅕ cake (85 g)	210	0	0
Golden Chocolatey Chip Loaf	⅕ cake (85 g)	220	0	0
Golden Loaf	¼ cake (85 g)	220	0	0
Lemon Twist	⅛ danish (53 g)	130	0	0
Marble Loaf	⅙ cake (71 g)	200	0	0
Mocha Iced Chocolate	⅙ cake (85 g)	200	0	0
Pineapple Crunch	⅙ cake (76 g)	190	0	0
Raspberry Cheese Pastry	⅑ cake (54 g)	140	0	0
Raspberry Twist	⅛ danish (53 g)	140	0	0
Hostess				
Blueberry Muffin Loaf	1 muffin (108 g)	440	170	27
Cinnamon Crumb, low-fat	2 cakes (51 g)	150	10	0
Cup Cakes with Creamy Filling	2 cakes (91 g)	330	100	45
Cup Cakes, reduced-fat	2 cakes (77 g)	240	25	5
HoHos	3 cakes (85 g)	370	160	108
Suzy Q's	1 cake (58 g)	220	80	36
Twinkies	2 cakes (77 g)	280	80	27
Little Debbie				
Apple Delights	1 cake (35 g)	140	40	14
Apple Streusel Coffee Cake	2 cakes (57 g)	220	70	9
Chocolate Chip Snack Cake	2 cakes (68 g)	290	130	27
Creme-Filled Snack Cake	2 cakes (71 g)	300	130	23
Devil Square	1 wrap (62 g)	260	110	27
Fudge Round	1 cake (34 g)	140	50	9
Marshmallow Pie	1 pie (39 g)	160	50	27
Marshmallow Supreme	1 cake (32 g)	130	45	9
Oatmeal Creme Pie	1 pie (38 g)	170	70	14
Oatmeal Light	1 wrap (38 g)	140	50	9
Strawberry Shortcake Roll	1 roll (61 g)	230	70	14
Swiss Cake Roll	2 cakes (61 g)	250	110	27
Zebra Cake	2 cakes (74 g)	320	150	27

SWEETS

| FOOD | AMOUNT | CALORIES | | |
		TOTAL	FAT	SAT-FAT
Pepperidge Farm				
Chocolate Fudge	⅙ cake (80 g)	300	140	**45**
Chocolate Mousse	⅛ cake (73 g)	250	100	**27**
Classic Carrot	⅛ cake (80 g)	350	190	**36**
Devil's Food	⅙ cake (80 g)	290	122	**45**
Sara Lee				
All Butter Pound Cake	⅙ cake (76 g)	310	150	**81**
Butter Streusel Coffee Cake	⅙ cake (54 g)	220	110	**54**
Crumb Coffee Cake	⅛ cake (57 g)	220	80	**14**
Double Chocolate Layer	⅛ cake (79 g)	260	110	**99**
Flaky Coconut Layer	⅛ cake (81 g)	280	130	**·108**
French Cheesecake	⅙ cake (111 g)	350	190	**127**
Original Cream Cheesecake	¼ cake (121 g)	350	160	**81**
Pecan Coffee Cake	⅙ cake (54 g)	220	110	**'54**
Strawberry French Cheesecake	⅙ cake (123 g)	320	130	**81**
Strawberry Shortcake	⅛ cake (71 g)	180	70	**45**
Tastykake				
Butterscotch Krimpets	3 cakes (85 g)	320	70	**18**
Chocolate Cupcakes	2 cakes (60 g)	220	60	**14**
Chocolate Junior Yellow Layer	1 cake (94 g)	360	120	**23**
Chocolate Kandy Kakes	4 cakes (76 g)	360	150	**90**
Creme-Filled Chocolate				
Cupcake	2 cakes (64 g)	200	25	**9**
Butter Cream–Iced	2 cakes (64 g)	250	70	**18**
Chocolate-Iced	2 cakes (64 g)	250	70	**18**
Creme-Filled Koffee Kake	2 cakes (57 g)	240	80	**18**
Fudge Bar	1 bar (43 g)	170	60	**9**
Koffee Kake	1 cake (71 g)	270	80	**14**
Oatmeal Raisin Bar	1 bar (43 g)	190	60	**14**
Peanut Butter Kandy Kake	4 cakes (76 g)	370	170	**81**
Tasty Minis, Creme-Filled Chocolate Cupcakes				
Butter Creme–Iced	4 cakes (57 g)	240	80	**18**
Chocolate-Iced	4 cakes (57 g)	240	80	**18**
Koffee Kake	4 cakes (51 g)	210	80	**14**
Vanilla Cupcake, Chocolate-Iced	4 cakes (57 g)	220	70	**14**
Weight Watchers				
Double Fudge	1 dessert (78 g)	190	40	**9**

SWEETS

FOOD	AMOUNT	CALORIES		
		TOTAL	FAT	SAT-FAT
Cake Mixes				
Angel food	¹⁄₁₂ cake	140	0	0
Betty Crocker				
Peanut Butter–Chocolate Swirl	¹⁄₁₂ cake	240	90	23
Duncan Hines				
Butter Recipe	¹⁄₁₀ cake	320	140	63
Caramel, Raspberry, White, Yellow, Fudge Marble, or Spice	¹⁄₁₂ cake	250	100	23
Devil's Food	¹⁄₁₂ cake	290	130	27
Pillsbury				
Banana Bread	¹⁄₁₂ loaf	170	50	9
Blueberry Bread	¹⁄₁₂ loaf	180	60	0
Butter Recipe	¹⁄₁₂ cake	260	110	54
Chocolate Caramel Nut	¹⁄₁₆ cake	290	170	36
Date Bread	¹⁄₁₂ loaf	160	25	0
Devil's Food	¹⁄₁₂ cake	270	130	27
Double Hot Fudge	¹⁄₁₆ cake	310	150	63
Funfetti	¹⁄₁₂ cake	240	80	18
Lemon	¹⁄₁₀ cake	310	120	27
Strawberry Cream Cheese	¹⁄₁₆ cake	300	150	41
Yellow	¹⁄₁₂ cake	260	110	27
Candy				
Almond Joy	1 pkg (49 g)	240	120	81
Andes				
Creme de Menthe Thins	8 pieces (38 g)	200	110	90
Toasted Coconut Thins	8 pieces (38 g)	210	120	99
Baby Ruth	1 bar (59.5 g)	280	110	63
Fun size	2 bars (42 g)	200	80	45
Butterfinger, fun size	2 bars (42 g)	200	70	36
Caramels				
Chocolate (Riesen)	5 pieces (40 g)	180	60	27
Creams (Goetze's)	3 pieces (36 g)	135	30	9
Plain				
Brach's	4 pieces (37 g)	150	35	9
Kraft	5 pieces (41 g)	170	30	9
Carob peanut clusters	1 piece (28 g)	150	90	36
Carob raisins	40 pieces (41 g)	160	45	36
Chocolate-covered peanuts	15 pieces (40 g)	220	120	54
Chocolate-covered peanut clusters	3 pieces (43 g)	230	130	63

SWEETS

FOOD	AMOUNT	CALORIES		
		TOTAL	FAT	SAT-FAT
Chocolate-covered fudge mix	14 pieces (40 g)	190	70	**36**
Chocolate Mint Pattie (Brach)	3 pieces (36 g)	140	26	**18**
Dots	12 pieces (43 g)	150	0	**0**
Fondant (mints, candy corn, other)	1 oz	105	0	**0**
French burnt peanuts	28 pieces (40 g)	190	80	**9**
Good and Plenty	33 pieces (40 g)	130	0	**0**
Gumdrops	1 oz	100	0	**0**
Gummi Bears	10 pieces (40 g)	140	0	**0**
Halvah (Joyva)				
Chocolate-covered	½ bar (57 g)	380	210	**45**
Chocolate-flavored	½ bar (57 g)	390	230	**36**
Marble	½ bar (57 g)	390	230	**36**
Hard	1 oz	110	0	**0**
Heath Sensations	⅓ bag (43 g)	220	120	**63**
Hershey's Chocolate				
Cookies 'n' Mint	1 bar (43 g)	230	110	**54**
Hugs	8 pieces (38 g)	210	110	**72**
Kisses	8 pieces (39 g)	210	110	**72**
with almonds	8 pieces (38 g)	210	120	**63**
Milk Chocolate	1 bar (43 g)	230	120	**81**
with Almonds	1 bar (41 g)	230	130	**63**
Miniatures	5 pieces (42 g)	230	130	**72**
Hot Tamales	19 pieces (40 g)	150	0	**0**
Jellybeans	1 oz	105	0	**0**
Jordan almonds	13 pieces (42 g)	200	70	**9**
Jujy Fruits	15 pieces (40 g)	160	0	**0**
Kit Kat	1 bar (42 g)	220	110	**72**
Licorice sticks	4 pieces (37 g)	120	0	**0**
M & M's				
Peanut	1 bag (49.3 g)	250	120	**45**
Plain	1 bag (47.9 g)	230	90	**54**
Semi-Sweet Mini	1 tbsp (14 g)	70	35	**18**
Malted Milk Balls	17 pieces (40 g)	180	60	**60**
Marshmallows (Kraft)	5 pieces (34 g)	110	0	**0**
Mighty Malts	10 pieces (42 g)	200	60	**60**
Milk Chocolate–Covered Jots	39 pieces (40 g)	190	60	**36**
Milk Chocolate Peanut Jots	17 pieces (40 g)	200	90	**27**
Milk Duds	13 pieces (40 g)	170	50	**36**
Milky Way	1 bar (61 g)	280	100	**45**
Mr. Goodbar	1 bar (42 g)	280	160	**63**
Mounds Bar	1 bar (53 g)	250	120	**99**

SWEETS

FOOD	AMOUNT	CALORIES		
		TOTAL	FAT	SAT-FAT
Necco Mints	2 pieces (6 g)	24	0	**0**
Nerds	1 box (11 g)	40	0	**0**
Nestlé				
Crunch, fun size	4 bars (39 g)	200	90	**54**
Milk Chocolate Giant Bar	¼ bar (35 g)	190	100	**54**
Nonpareils (dark chocolate)	17 pieces (41 g)	200	80	**54**
Pastel Mints (Petite)	¼ cup	210	100	**18**
Payday	1 bar (52 g)	240	110	**90**
Peanut brittle	40 g	180	40	**9**
Peanut Butter Cups (Estee)	5 candies (38 g)	200	110	**63**
Peanut Chews (Goldenberg's)	3 pieces (37 g)	180	80	**18**
Planters				
Chocolate Crisp, bite-size	13 pieces (30 g)	140	60	**18**
Peanut Butter Chocolate	4 pieces (42 g)	230	130	**45**
Peanut Butter Crisp	12 pieces (31 g)	150	70	**14**
Raisinets (Nestlé)	¼ cup	200	70	**36**
Raisins, chocolate-covered	34 pieces (40 g)	170	60	**45**
Reese's				
Miniatures	5 pieces (39 g)	210	110	**45**
NutRageous	1 bar (45 g)	250	140	**36**
Peanut Butter Cup	2 cups	240	130	**54**
Rolo	1 package (54 g)	260	110	**81**
Skittles (all flavors)	¼ cup	170	15	**0**
	1 bag (61.5 g)	250	25	**5**
Snickers	1 bar (59 g)	280	120	**45**
Peanut Butter	1 bar (57 g)	310	180	**63**
3 Musketeers	1 bar (60.4 g)	260	70	**36**
Fun size	2 bars (33.2 g)	140	40	**23**
Tootsie Roll				
Midgie	6 pieces (40 g)	160	25	**5**
Pop	1 pop (17 g)	60	0	**0**
Snack Bar	2 bars (28 g)	110	20	**0**
Whitman's				
Bars				
Cookies-n-Cream	1 bar (28 g)	150	80	**63**
Super Extra Crispy	1 bar (21 g)	120	60	**27**
Super Extra Dark	1 bar (28 g)	140	80	**54**
Super Extra Milk	1 bar (28 g)	160	90	**45**
Sampler				
Assorted Chocolates	3 pieces (40 g)	200	100	**54**
Assorted Creams	3 pieces (40 g)	180	70	**45**

SWEETS

FOOD	AMOUNT	CALORIES		
		TOTAL	FAT	SAT-FAT
Whitman's				
Sampler (*cont.*)				
Dark Chocolate	3 pieces (40 g)	200	90	**54**
Milk Chocolate	3 pieces (40 g)	200	90	**54**
Nut, Chewy, and Crisp	3 pieces (40 g)	200	110	**54**
Whoppers Malted Milk Balls	7 pieces (45 g)	210	80	**63**
Yogurt-covered				
Almond	11 pieces (42 g)	210	120	**63**
Peanut	17 pieces (41 g)	210	120	**54**
Pretzel	⅓ cup	140	45	**36**
Raisin	30 pieces (41 g)	180	60	**45**
York Peppermint Pattie	1 bar (42 g)	170	35	**23**
	3 pieces (41 g)	170	35	**23**
Cookies and Bars				
Assorted				
Biscotti	1 piece (30 g)	270	20	**5**
Mundle Bread	2 pieces (30 g)	140	50	**14**
Archway cookies				
Apple-Filled Oatmeal	1 (28 g)	110	30	**5**
Apple n' Raisin	1 (30 g)	130	40	**9**
Chocolate Chip and Toffee	1 (29 g)	140	60	**14**
Coconut Macaroon	1 (23 g)	90	45	**36**
Frosty Lemon	1 (28 g)	120	45	**9**
Fruit Bar	1 (28 g)	90	0	**0**
Gingersnap	5 (30 g)	130	40	**9**
Granola	2 (28 g)	100	0	**0**
Lemon Snap	5 (30 g)	150	70	**14**
Oatmeal	1 (27 g)	110	25	**9**
Date-Filled	1 (28 g)	110	35	**9**
Iced	1 (28 g)	120	45	**9**
Raisin	1 (28 g)	100	0	**0**
Ruth's Golden	1 (28 g)	120	40	**9**
Old-Fashioned Molasses	1 (27 g)	120	30	**9**
Raspberry-Filled	1 (28 g)	110	40	**9**
Rocky Road	1 (28 g)	130	60	**14**
Delicious cookies				
Animal Cracker	9 (28 g)	130	45	**14**
Assorted Sandwiches	2 (26 g)	120	45	**18**
Assorted Sugar Wafers	4 (29 g)	160	80	**18**
Banana Rama	2 (25 g)	120	40	**18**
Butter Thin	10 (29 g)	110	45	**18**

SWEETS

FOOD	AMOUNT	CALORIES		
		TOTAL	FAT	SAT-FAT
Delicious cookies (cont.)				
Chocolate Chip Thin	10 (29 g)	110	45	**18**
Coconut Bar	3 (28 g)	140	60	**27**
Coconut Sandwich	3 (33 g)	150	50	**27**
Cookie Legend				
Chocolate Chip	3 (31 g)	150	60	**18**
Fudge Graham	2 (25 g)	120	50	**36**
Fudge Mint	4 (28 g)	140	60	**36**
Pecan Shortbread	2 (36 g)	180	90	**14**
Duplex Sandwich	2 (26 g)	120	45	**18**
English Toffee made with				
Heath	2 (30 g)	145	72	**18**
Fig Bar	2 (36 g)	115	35	**9**
Ginger Snap	4 (29 g)	130	30	**5**
Graham				
Cinnamon	2 (27 g)	130	45	**5**
Honey Graham	2 (27 g)	120	30	**9**
Land O Lakes Frosted Butter	2 (35 g)	180	90	**9**
Lemon Sandwich	3 (33 g)	150	50	**27**
Musselman's Apple Sauce				
Oatmeal	2 (32 g)	130	35	**9**
Oatmeal	2 (28 g)	120	45	**9**
Iced	2 (28 g)	120	40	**9**
Peanut Butter Sandwich	3 (33 g)	155	50	**27**
Shortbread	5 (30 g)	140	50	**27**
Skippy and Welch's Peanut				
Butter and Jelly Sandwich	1 (26 g)	120	60	**14**
Strawberry Sandwich	3 (33 g)	150	50	**27**
Sugar	2 (28 g)	130	40	**9**
Vanilla Sandwich	2 (26 g)	120	45	**18**
Vanilla Wafer	8 (28 g)	110	15	**9**
Entenmann's cookies				
Chocolate Chip	3 (30 g)	140	60	**18**
Entenmann's Fat-and-				
Cholesterol-Free				
Chocolate Brownie	2 (24 g)	80	0	**0**
Estee cookies				
Chocolate Chip	4 (31 g)	150	60	**18**
Chocolate Sandwich	3 (34 g)	160	50	**14**
Oatmeal Raisin	4 (34 g)	130	40	**9**
Peanut Butter Sandwich	3 (34 g)	160	60	**9**

SWEETS

| FOOD | AMOUNT | CALORIES | | |
		TOTAL	FAT	SAT-FAT
Vanilla	4 (28 g)	140	50	9
Vanilla Sandwich	3 (34 g)	160	50	9
Famous Amos cookies				
Chocolate Chip	4 (30 g)	130	50	18
Fifty 50 cookies				
Chocolate Chip	4 (32 g)	170	90	27
Frookie cookies				
Apple Cinnamon Oat Bran	2 (21 g)	100	35	5
Chocolate Chip	2 (21 g)	90	45	5
Dream Cream				
Strawberry Yogurt Cream				
Wafer	2 (15 g)	70	36	18
Vanilla Yogurt Cream				
Wafer	2 (15 g)	70	36	18
Fig Fruits	2 (30 g)	110	18	0
Honey Graham	2 (30 g)	110	25	5
Oatmeal Raisin	2 (21 g)	90	30	5
Keebler cookies				
Chocolate Chip				
Chips Deluxe	1 (16 g)	80	40	14
Chips Deluxe Bakery				
Crisp	3 (36 g)	180	80	27
Chocolate Lover's	1 (17 g)	90	40	23
Rainbow Chips Deluxe	1 (16 g)	80	35	18
Soft Batch	1 (16 g)	80	35	9
Chocolate Fudge Sandwich	1 (17 g)	80	35	9
Coconut Chocolate Drop	1 (16 g)	80	45	18
Elfin Delight				
Caramel Apple Oatmeal	1 (18 g)	70	15	9
Chocolate Sandwich				
with Fudge Creme	3 (34 g)	150	30	9
with Vanilla Creme	3 (34 g)	150	30	9
Creme Sandwich	3 (35 g)	150	30	9
E. L. Fudge				
Butter-Flavored Chocolate				
Sandwich	3 (34 g)	170	70	18
Chocolate Sandwich with				
Vanilla Creme Filling	3 (35 g)	170	70	18
Fudge Sandwich	3 (34 g)	160	60	18
Fudge Vanilla Creme	1 (17 g)	80	30	9
French Vanilla Creme	1 (17 g)	80	30	9

SWEETS

FOOD	AMOUNT	CALORIES		
		TOTAL	FAT	SAT-FAT
Keebler cookies (*cont.*)				
Fudge 'n Caramel	2 (24 g)	120	50	36
Fudge Stick	3 (29 g)	150	70	41
Fudge Stripe	3 (32 g)	160	70	41
Graham crackers				
Chocolate	8 (31 g)	140	50	14
Cinnamon Crisp	8 (30 g)	140	40	9
Cinnamon Crisp (low-fat)	8 (28 g)	110	10	5
Deluxe Fudge-Covered	3 (28 g)	140	60	41
Honey	8 (31 g)	150	50	14
Honey (low-fat)	9 (31 g)	120	15	5
Grasshopper	4 (30 g)	150	60	45
PB Fudgebutter	2 (24 g)	130	70	36
Pecan Sandie	1 (16 g)	80	45	9
Sweet Spot	1 pkg (23 g)	120	50	27
Toffee Sandie	2 (26 g)	130	70	18
Vanilla Wafer	8 (31 g)	150	60	18
Little Debbie cookies				
Figaroo	2 (43 g)	160	35	5
Fudge Macaroo	1 (29 g)	140	70	36
Lemon Stix	1 (44 g)	220	90	23
Nutty Bar	2 (57 g)	290	150	27
Oatmeal Light	1 (38 g)	140	50	9
Peanut Butter Bar	2 (54 g)	270	130	23
Peanut Butter Natural	1 wrap (44 g)	230	120	18
Star Crunch	1 (31 g)	140	60	9
Supreme	1 (32 g)	130	45	9
Lu cookies				
The Little Schoolboy	2 (25 g)	130	60	27
Le Petit-Beurre	4 (33 g)	150	35	18
Mrs. Wright's cookies				
Animal	6 (28 g)	130	45	14
Chocolate Chip	2 (31 g)	160	70	27
Chocolate Devil's Food	2 (34 g)	120	10	0
Creme Wafer	5 (28 g)	140	60	14
Devil's Food Sandwich				
Creme	2 (30 g)	140	50	9
Dutch Apple Bar	2 (35 g)	120	15	5
Fig Bar	2 (35 g)	120	30	9
Whole-Wheat	2 (35 g)	120	30	9

SWEETS

FOOD	AMOUNT	CALORIES		
		TOTAL	FAT	SAT-FAT
Ginger Lotta Snap	6 (30 g)	130	35	9
Graham				
Fudge	1 (24 g)	120	50	36
Honey Graham	4 (28 g)	130	30	0
Lemon Sandwich Creme	2 (30 g)	130	40	9
Oatmeal	2 (26 g)	130	50	14
Striped Shortbread	2 (27 g)	140	70	36
Sugar	2 (28 g)	140	60	18
Vanilla Sandwich Creme	2 (30 g)	140	60	18
Murray cookies				
Assortment	5 (27 g)	120	45	14
Butter	8 (30 g)	130	40	9
Duplex Creme	3 (28 g)	130	60	14
Lemon Creme	3 (28 g)	130	60	14
Sugar Wafer	6 (33 g)	130	20	0
Vanilla Creme	3 (28 g)	130	60	14
Vanilla Wafer	8 (28 g)	120	25	9
Nabisco cookies				
Apple Newtons, fat-free	2 (29 g)	100	0	0
Barnum's Animal Cracker	12 (31 g)	140	35	5
Biscos Sugar Wafer	3 (28 g)	140	60	14
Brown Edge Wafer	5 (29 g)	140	50	14
Cameo Creme Sandwich	2 (28 g)	130	40	9
Chips Ahoy!	3 (32 g)	160	70	23
Chewy	3 (36 g)	170	70	23
Chunky	1 (17 g)	80	40	27
reduced-fat	3 (32 g)	150	50	14
Sprinkled	3 (36 g)	170	70	23
Chocolate Teddy Graham	24 (30 g)	140	40	9
Cranberry Newtons, fat-free	2 (29 g)	100	0	0
Famous Chocolate Wafer	5 (32 g)	140	35	14
Fig Newton	2 (31 g)	110	25	9
fat-free	2 (29 g)	100	0	0
Fudge-Striped Shortbread	3 (32 g)	160	70	14
Ginger Snap	4 (28 g)	120	25	5
Grahams				
Cinnamon	5 (32 g)	140	25	5
Honey	4 (28 g)	120	25	5
Fudge-Covered	3 (28 g)	140	60	14
Lorna Doone Shortbread	4 (29 g)	140	60	9
Mallomars	2 (26 g)	120	45	27

SWEETS

FOOD	AMOUNT	CALORIES		
		TOTAL	FAT	SAT-FAT
Nabisco cookies (cont.)				
Marshmallow Twirl	1 (30 g)	130	50	**14**
Mystic Mint Sandwich	1 (17 g)	90	35	**9**
Nilla Wafers	8 (32 g)	140	40	**9**
Nutter Butter				
Bites	10 (30 g)	150	60	**14**
Peanut Creme Patties	5 (31 g)	160	80	**14**
Peanut Butter Sandwich	2 (28 g)	130	50	**9**
Oatmeal	1 (17 g)	80	30	**5**
Iced Oatmeal	1 (17 g)	80	25	**5**
Oreos				
Chocolate Sandwich	3 (33 g)	160	60	**14**
Double Stuf Chocolate				
Sandwich	2 (28 g)	140	60	**14**
Fudge-Covered	1 (21 g)	110	50	**14**
Mini Oreo	9 (30 g)	140	60	**14**
White Fudge–Covered	1 (21 g)	110	50	**14**
Pinwheels	1 (30 g)	130	45	**23**
Raspberry Newton, fat-free	1 (20 g)	70	0	**0**
Social Tea Biscuit	6 (28 g)	120	30	**5**
SnackWell's (*see listing after* **Safeway Select Cookies**)				
Strawberry Newton	1 (20 g)	70	0	**0**
Vanilla Sandwich	3 (35 g)	170	70	**18**
Pepperidge Farm cookies				
Beacon Hill	1 (26 g)	130	60	**18**
Bordeaux	4 (28 g)	130	50	**23**
Milk Chocolate	3 (32 g)	160	80	**32**
Brussels	3 (30 g)	150	60	**27**
Charleston	1 (26 g)	130	60	**23**
Chesapeake Chocolate				
Chunk Pecan	1 (26 g)	140	70	**14**
Chessmen	3 (26 g)	120	45	**27**
Chocolate Chip	3 (28 g)	140	60	**23**
Dessert Favorite	3 (33 g)	170	80	**27**
Fruitful				
Apricot Raspberry Cup	3 (32 g)	140	50	**18**
Cherry Cobbler	1 (17 g)	70	25	**9**
Peach Tart	2 (30 g)	120	25	**9**
Raspberry Tart	2 (30 g)	120	25	**9**
Strawberry Cup	3 (32 g)	140	50	**18**
Geneva	3 (31 g)	160	80	**32**
Ice Cream Favorite	5 (33 g)	180	90	**23**

SWEETS

FOOD	AMOUNT	CALORIES		
		TOTAL	FAT	SAT-FAT
Lido	1 (17 g)	90	40	14
Milano	3 (34 g)	180	90	41
Double Chocolate	2 (28 g)	150	70	27
Hazelnut	2 (25 g)	130	70	18
Milk Chocolate	3 (35 g)	180	90	32
Mint	2 (26 g)	140	70	32
Orange	2 (26 g)	140	70	23
Nantucket Chocolate				
Crunch	1 (26 g)	130	60	27
Old-Fashioned				
Brownie Chocolate Nut	3 (30 g)	160	80	27
Chocolate Chip	3 (28 g)	140	60	23
Ginger Man	4 (27 g)	120	35	9
Lemon Nut Crunch	3 (31 g)	170	80	18
Oatmeal Raisin	3 (34 g)	160	60	14
Shortbread	2 (26 g)	140	70	23
Sugar	3 (30 g)	140	60	14
Party Favorites Assortment	3 (32 g)	170	80	27
Santa Fe Oatmeal Raisin	1 (26 g)	120	40	9
Sausalito Milk Chocolate				
Macademia	1 (26 g)	140	70	18
Soft-Baked				
Chocolate Chunk	1 (26 g)	130	50	23
Milk Chocolate				
Macademia	1 (26 g)	130	60	23
Oatmeal Raisin	1 (26 g)	110	40	9
Tahoe White Chunk				
Macademia	1 (26 g)	130	70	27
Rippin' Good cookies				
Assorted Creme Wafers	3 (28 g)	140	60	14
Chocolate Chip	3 (32 g)	150	60	18
Chocolate Chip Sandwich	2 (31 g)	150	60	18
Coconut Bar	3 (26 g)	130	50	23
Cookie Jar Assortment	3 (33 g)	150	60	18
Duplex Sandwich	3 (34 g)	160	50	14
Frosted Fudgie	3 (32 g)	140	50	14
Granola and Peanut Butter				
Sandwich	2 (31 g)	150	60	23
Holly Jolly Wafer	4 (33 g)	170	80	45
Iced Spice	3 (32 g)	130	25	5
Lemon Crisp	3 (32 g)	160	70	14

SWEETS

FOOD	AMOUNT	CALORIES		
		TOTAL	FAT	SAT-FAT
Rippin' Good cookies (*cont.*)				
Macaroon Sandwich	2 (31 g)	150	60	23
Mini Bits Striped Daintie	13 (30 g)	140	50	27
Oatmeal	3 (32 g)	150	50	14
Iced	3 (36 g)	150	40	9
Striped	2 (28 g)	150	70	36
Peanut Butter Sandwich	2 (31 g)	150	50	14
Sugar	3 (32 g)	150	60	14
Toffee 'n Creme Sandwich	2 (31 g)	150	60	14
Vanilla Sandwich	3 (34 g)	160	50	14
Safeway Select cookies				
Biscotti				
Chocolate dipped in				
Dark Chocolate	2 (38 g)	170	80	36
White Chocolate	2 (38 g)	170	80	36
The Original	2 (38 g)	150	60	23
dipped in Dark				
Chocolate	2 (38 g)	170	70	36
Very Chocolate	2 (32 g)	160	70	14
Very Peanut Butter				
Chocolate Chip Oatmeal	2 (32 g)	160	80	14
Very Raisin Oatmeal	2 (32 g)	150	50	14
SnackWell's Cookies				
(Nabisco)				
Chocolate Chip	13 (29 g)	130	30	14
Chocolate Sandwich	2 (25 g)	100	20	5
Creme Sandwich	2 (26 g)	110	20	5
Double Fudge Cookie Cake				
Fat-free	1 (16 g)	50	0	0
Oatmeal Raisin	2 (27 g)	110	25	0
Stella D'Oro cookies				
Fruit Delight	1 (23 g)	70	0	0
Fruit Slice	1 (17 g)	50	0	0
Sunshine cookies				
Almond Crescent	4 (31 g)	150	50	15
Fig Bar	2 (28 g)	110	25	5
Ginger Snap	7 (29 g)	130	40	9
Golden Fruit				
Apple Biscuit	1 (20 g)	70	10	0

SWEETS

FOOD	AMOUNT	CALORIES		
		TOTAL	FAT	SAT-FAT
Golden Fruit (*cont.*)				
Cranberry Biscuit	1 (20 g)	70	10	0
Raisin Biscuit	1 (20 g)	70	10	0
Graham				
Cinnamon	2 (31 g)	140	50	14
Honey	2 (28 g)	120	40	9
Hydrox Chocolate Sandwich				
Creme	3 (31 g)	150	60	18
Reduced-fat	3 (31 g)	130	35	9
Lemon Cooler	5 (30 g)	140	50	14
Oatmeal	3 (35 g)	170	60	14
Iced	2 (29 g)	130	45	27
Oh! Berry Strawberry Wafer	8 (28 g)	100	0	0
Peanut Butter Sugar Wafer	4 (32 g)	170	80	18
Sugar Wafer	3 (26 g)	130	60	14
Sunshine Classic				
Chocolate Chip	1 (19 g)	100	50	23
Chocolate Chip				
Shortbread	1 (19 g)	100	60	18
Chocolate Chip with				
Walnuts	1 (19 g)	100	50	23
Chocolate Chocolate Chip	1 (19 g)	90	50	18
Vanilla Wafer	7 (31 g)	150	60	14
Vienna Finger	2 (29 g)	140	50	14
Reduced-fat	2 (29 g)	130	30	5
Twix cookies				
Chocolate Caramel	1 (29 g)	140	60	23
Chocolate Peanut Butter	1 (25 g)	130	70	27
Weight Watchers Smart				
Snackers cookies				
Chocolate Chip	2 (30 g)	140	45	18
Chocolate Sandwich	3 (31 g)	140	35	9
Oatmeal Raisin	2 (30 g)	140	15	0
Vanilla Sandwich	3 (31 g)	120	25	9
Cookies and Bars, Mixes				
Apple Streusel (Pillsbury)	1 bar	150	50	14
Cheesecake Bar				
Lemon (Pillsbury)	1 bar	170	90	32
Strawberry Swirl (Betty				
Crocker)	1 bar	210	110	32
Oreo Bar (Pillsbury)	1 bar	150	50	14

SWEETS

FOOD	AMOUNT	CALORIES		
		TOTAL	FAT	SAT-FAT
Cookies, Ready-to-Make				
Chocolate Chip (Pillsbury)	2	140	60	**14**
Sugar (Pillsbury)	2	130	45	**14**
Danish Pastry				
Almond or pecan	1 (55 g)	220	100	**18**
Blueberry	1 (55 g)	190	80	**18**
Cheese	1 (110 g)	380	170	**45**
Cherry Cheese	1 (100 g)	360	140	**45**
Coconut	1 (55 g)	210	80	**27**
Danish Ring				
Pecan	⅛ ring (57 g)	230	100	**23**
Walnut	⅛ ring (55 g)	240	120	**23**
Danish Twist (Entenmann's)				
Cinnamon	⅙ danish (61 g)	260	130	**27**
Raspberry	⅙ danish (53 g)	220	100	**27**
Lemon-filled	1 (100 g)	350	140	**32**
Orange Danish (Pillsbury, ready-to-make)	1 (41 g)	140	50	**14**
Donuts				
Bakery				
Apple raisin rosebud	1 (55 g)	220	90	**23**
Carrot cake	1 (80 g)	340	160	**41**
Chocolate-iced yellow cake	1 (55 g)	230	90	**27**
Cinnamon rosebud	1 (64 g)	260	110	**36**
Custard creme–filled	1 (65 g)	240	130	**63**
Glazed (Krispy Kreme)	1 (38 g)	180	100	**27**
Glazed yeast-raised	1 (55 g)	240	130	**36**
Honey wheat	1 (80 g)	340	150	**36**
Lemon custard–filled	1 (65 g)	190	140	**36**
Old-fashioned	1 (62 g)	270	140	**36**
Sour cream	1 (80 g)	340	160	**36**
Entenmann's				
Crumb-Topped donuts	1 (60 g)	260	110	**27**
Devil's Food Crumb	1 (60 g)	250	110	**32**
Rich Frosted	1 (57 g)	280	170	**54**
Hostess				
Cinnamon Donettes	4 (61 g)	240	90	**36**
Frosted	1 (40 g)	180	100	**63**
Powdered Donettes	4 (61 g)	250	100	**36**
Little Debbie				
Donut Sticks	1 stick (47 g)	210	110	**27**

SWEETS

FOOD	AMOUNT	CALORIES		
		TOTAL	FAT	SAT-FAT
Dumplings, Turnovers, and Strudel				
Apple Dumpling (Pepperidge Farm)	1 (85 g)	290	99	**23**
Apple-filled pastry	1 (64 g)	190	45	**9**
Apple fritter	1 (70 g)	300	130	**32**
Apple strudel	1 piece (64 g)	200	90	**27**
Apple turnover (Pepperidge Farm)	1 (89 g)	330	130	**27**
Apricot-filled pastry	1 roll (64 g)	200	50	**9**
Apricot strudel	1 piece (64 g)	220	100	**27**
Custard-filled pastry	1 (64 g)	190	40	**9**
Peach Dumpling (Pepperidge Farm)	1 (85 g)	320	99	**23**
Toaster Strudel				
Pillsbury (all flavors)	1 (54 g)	180	60	**14**
Frosting				
Betty Crocker				
Creamy Deluxe, Vanilla	2 tbsp	140	45	**14**
Frosting Partner				
Cream cheese frosting/ strawberry topping	2 tbsp	130	35	**14**
Dark chocolate frosting/ raspberry topping	2 tbsp	130	45	**14**
Milk chocolate frosting/ fudge topping	2 tbsp	140	50	**23**
Vanilla frosting/lemon topping	2 tbsp	130	35	**14**
Duncan Hines				
Caramel	2 tbsp	140	50	**14**
Vanilla, Raspberries, and Cream	2 tbsp	140	50	**14**
Pillsbury				
Chocolate Fudge	2 tbsp	140	50	**14**
Milk Chocolate	2 tbsp	140	50	**14**
Frozen Custard				
Kohr Brothers				
Light, Vanilla and Chocolate	4 fl oz	130	50	**36**
Frozen Yogurt, Grocery Store Freezer Compartment				
Ben and Jerry's				
Cherry Garcia	½ cup	170	30	**18**

SWEETS

| FOOD | AMOUNT | CALORIES | | |
		TOTAL	FAT	SAT-FAT
Breyers				
Chocolate Chip Cookie				
Dough	½ cup	170	45	**18**
Colombo				
Shoppe Style				
Bavarian Chocolate				
Chunk	½ cup	170	50	**27**
Cappuccino Coffee Bean	½ cup	170	40	**23**
Caramel Pecan Chunk	½ cup	170	40	**18**
Chocolate Chip Cookie				
Dough	½ cup	170	45	**27**
Old World Chocolate	½ cup	120	15	**9**
Toffee Bar Crunch	½ cup	180	60	**36**
Vanilla Chocolate Twist	½ cup	120	15	**9**
White Chocolate Almond	½ cup	200	70	**45**
Slender Scoops, all flavors	½ cup	90–100	0	**0**
Dannon				
Light Nonfat, all flavors	½ cup	80–90	0	**0**
Pure Indulgence				
Crunchy Expresso	½ cup	160	40	**27**
Vanilla	½ cup	130	20	**9**
Elan Low-Fat				
Vanilla	½ cup	130	25	**14**
Häagen-Dazs				
Chocolate	½ cup	160	25	**14**
Coffee	½ cup	160	25	**14**
Strawberry Cheesecake				
Craze	½ cup	220	70	**36**
Vanilla	½ cup	160	25	**14**
Häagen-Dazs Bars				
Piña Colada	1 bar (70 g)	90	10	**5**
Raspberry and Vanilla	1 bar (71 g)	90	10	**0**
Kemp's				
Chocolate	½ cup	110	25	**18**
Fudge Marble	½ cup	110	0	**0**
Peach	½ cup	90	0	**0**
Pralines and Caramel	½ cup	150	35	**18**
Strawberry	½ cup	90	0	**0**
Vanilla	½ cup	120	25	**18**
Stonyfield Farm				
Chocolate Mint Chip	4 fl oz	140	30	**27**
Decaf French Roast	4 fl oz	100	0	**0**

SWEETS

FOOD	AMOUNT	CALORIES		
		TOTAL	FAT	SAT-FAT
Double Raspberry	4 fl oz	120	0	0
Mocha Almond Fudge	4 fl oz	150	35	0
Very Vanilla	4 fl oz	100	0	0
TCBY				
Honey Almond Vanilla	½ cup	150	25	14
Strawberry White Chocolate				
Almond Crunch	½ cup	130	20	14
Triple Chocolate Brownie	½ cup	150	25	14
TCBY Yog-A-Bar				
Vanilla	1 bar (63 g)	160	80	54
Vanilla Crunch	1 bar (67 g)	200	110	63
Vanilla with Heath Toffee	1 bar (67 g)	190	100	63

Frozen Yogurt, Yogurt or Ice Cream Shop
Colombo (These figures are for 1 fl oz. Ask the server for the number of ounces in your serving.)

Lite (nonfat)	1 fl oz	25	0	0
Low-fat	1 fl oz	28	4	2
Peanut butter low-fat	1 fl oz	30	6	1
ICBIY				
Nonfat	sm (6¾ fl oz)	135	0	0
	med (9⅓ fl oz)	187	0	0
	lg (12 fl oz)	240	0	0
Original	sm (6¾ fl oz)	182	43	NA
	med (9⅓ fl oz)	251	59	NA
	lg (12 fl oz)	324	76	NA
TCBY				
Nonfat	sm (5 fl oz)	138	0	0
	med (7 fl oz)	193	0	0
	lg (9 fl oz)	248	0	0
Original	sm (5 fl oz)	163	38	23
	med (7 fl oz)	228	53	32
	lg (9 fl oz)	293	68	41

Ice Cream
Ben & Jerry's

Ice Cream				
Aztec Harvests Coffee	½ cup	250	130	90
Deep Dark Chocolate	½ cup	250	130	81
Double Chocolate Fudge				
Swirl	½ cup	250	140	81
Mocha Fudge	½ cup	250	150	81
Vanilla	½ cup	230	150	90

SWEETS

FOOD	AMOUNT	CALORIES		
		TOTAL	FAT	SAT-FAT
Ben & Jerry's				
Ice Cream (*cont.*)				
Vanilla Bean	½ cup	230	150	**90**
White Russian	½ cup	240	140	**90**
Peace Pops				
Chocolate Chip Cookie				
Dough	1 (145 g)	510	270	**117**
English Toffee Crunch	1 (135 g)	420	250	**162**
Breyers				
Strawberry	½ cup	130	60	**36**
Viennetta				
Chocolate	1 slice	190	100	**72**
All other flavors	1 slice	190	100	**63**
Dove Bar				
Dark Chocolate Chocolate	1 (79 g)	270	150	**99**
Dark Chocolate Vanilla	1 (78 g)	260	150	**99**
French Vanilla Bite-Size	5 (103 g)	370	210	**135**
Milk Chocolate Vanilla	1 (77 g)	260	150	**99**
Vanilla	1 (98 g)	230	200	**126**
Edy's Grand				
Ice Cream				
Cherry Chocolate Chip	½ cup	150	80	**45**
Chocolate	½ cup	140	80	**45**
Chocolate Chip Cookie				
Dough	½ cup	170	80	**45**
Chocolate Fudge Sundae	½ cup	140	70	**36**
Cookies 'n Cream	½ cup	160	80	**45**
Crunchy Cone	½ cup	160	80	**54**
Ice Cream Sandwich	½ cup	150	70	**45**
Malt Ball 'n Fudge	½ cup	150	70	**45**
Strawberry	½ cup	120	50	**36**
Vanilla Bean	½ cup	150	80	**54**
Light Ice Cream				
Almond Praline	½ cup	110	35	**18**
Cheesecake Chunk	½ cup	120	45	**27**
Chocolate Chip Cookie				
Dough	½ cup	120	40	**23**
Chocolate Fudge Mousse	½ cup	110	35	**23**
Cookies 'n Cream	½ cup	110	40	**23**
French Silk	½ cup	120	45	**27**
Rocky Road	½ cup	120	40	**23**

SWEETS

FOOD	AMOUNT	CALORIES		
		TOTAL	FAT	SAT-FAT
Tangerine Dream	½ cup	100	35	18
Vanilla	½ cup	100	35	23
Eskimo Pie				
Chocolate-Coated Vanilla				
Bar	1 bar (75 ml)	150	90	54
Eskimo Pie	2½ fl oz (75 ml)	150	90	54
with Crisped Rice	1 bar (52 g)	160	100	54
Sandwich	1 (96 ml)	170	60	18
Good Humor				
Candy Center Crunch	1 bar (88.7 ml)	260	170	126
Chocolate Chip Cookie				
Sandwich	1 (118 ml)	300	120	72
Chocolate Eclair	1 bar (89 ml)	170	80	27
King Cone	1 cone (136 ml)	300	90	54
Original Ice Cream Bar	1 bar (89 ml)	190	90	72
Popsicle (Twister)	1 piece (52 ml)	45	0	0
Sidewalk Sundae	1 cone (118 ml)	280	140	90
Strawberry Shortcake	1 bar (89 ml)	160	80	36
Toasted Almond	1 bar (89 ml)	190	80	36
Häagen-Dazs				
Exträas				
Caramel Cone Explosion	1 bar (93 g)	350	210	126
Iced Cappuccino	1 bar (96 g)	330	220	126
Strawberry Cheesecake				
Craze	½ cup	290	160	90
Ice Cream				
Butter Pecan	½ cup	320	220	99
Chocolate	½ cup	270	160	99
Chocolate Chocolate Chip	½ cup	300	180	108
Coffee	½ cup	270	160	99
Cookies and Cream	½ cup	270	160	99
Macadamia Brittle	½ cup	300	180	99
Rum Raisin	½ cup	270	160	90
Strawberry	½ cup	250	150	90
Vanilla Fudge	½ cup	280	160	99
Vanilla Swiss Almond	½ cup	310	190	99
Ice Cream Bar				
Vanilla and Almonds	1 bar (106 g)	370	240	126
Vanilla and Dark				
Chocolate	1 bar (112 g)	390	240	162

SWEETS

| FOOD | AMOUNT | CALORIES | | |
		TOTAL	FAT	SAT-FAT
Häagen-Dazs				
Ice Cream Bar (*cont.*)				
Vanilla and Milk				
Chocolate	1 bar (100 g)	330	220	**126**
Sherbet				
Raspberry Sorbet and				
Cream	½ cup	190	80	**45**
Heath				
Ice Cream Bar	1 bar (49 g)	160	110	**72**
Healthy Choice Low-Fat				
Ice Cream				
Cappuccino Chocolate				
Chunk	½ cup	120	20	**9**
Fudge Brownie	½ cup	120	20	**9**
Peanut Butter Cookie				
Dough 'n Fudge	½ cup	120	20	**9**
Praline and Caramel	½ cup	130	20	**5**
Rocky Road	½ cup	140	20	**9**
Vanilla	½ cup	100	20	**14**
Klondike				
Chocolate	1 piece (148 ml)	280	180	**126**
Gold	5 fl oz (148 ml)	390	230	**135**
Krispy	1 piece (148 ml)	300	180	**117**
Krunch	1 piece (89 ml)	200	110	**72**
Lite				
Original	1 piece (74 ml)	110	50	**36**
Sandwiches	1 piece (83 ml)	100	20	**14**
Vanilla (The Original)	1 piece (148 ml)	290	180	**126**
Vanilla Ice Cream Sandwich	1 piece (148 ml)	250	80	**54**
Lucerne				
Vanilla Ice Cream	½ cup	150	70	**45**
Mattus' Low-Fat Ice Cream				
Caramel Crunch	½ cup	190	27	**9**
Chocolate	½ cup	160	27	**18**
Chocolate Chocolate Cookie	½ cup	170	27	**18**
Coffee	½ cup	170	27	**18**
Cookies and Cream	½ cup	190	27	**9**
Honey Vanilla	½ cup	160	27	**18**
Len and Cherries	½ cup	170	27	**9**
Vanilla	½ cup	170	27	**18**
Milky Way				
Ice Cream Bar, Dark	1 bar (51 g)	170	80	**36**

SWEETS

FOOD	AMOUNT	CALORIES		
		TOTAL	FAT	SAT-FAT
Milky Way				
Ice Cream Bar, Dark	1 bar (51 g)	170	80	36
Low Fat Milk Shake	1 cup	220	30	18
Nestlé				
Bon Bon	9 pieces (103 g)	370	230	135
Cool Creation				
Ice Pop	1 pop (65 g)	50	0	0
Mickey Mouse Ice Cream Bar	1 bar (44 g)	110	60	27
Special Movie Edition Ice Cream Cone	1 cone (85 g)	280	120	81
Surprise Ice Pop	1 pop (64 g)	60	0	0
Crunch				
reduced-fat	1 bar (50 g)	130	60	45
Vanilla	1 bar (60 g)	200	120	81
Drumstick Sundae Cone				
Vanilla	1 cone (103 g)	350	180	99
Vanilla Caramel	1 cone (108 g)	360	180	108
Flintstones Push-Up				
Cool Cream Sherbet Treat	1 tube (60 g)	90	20	9
Original Sherbet Treat	1 tube (64 g)	100	20	9
Pebbles Ice Cream Treat	1 tube (50 g)	120	60	36
Snickers				
Ice Cream Bar	4 bars (108 g)	390	220	81
Trix				
Pops	1 bar (53 g)	40	0	0
Weight Watchers				
Chocolate Mousse	2 bars (82 g)	70	10	5
English Toffee Crunch Bar	1 bar (41 g)	120	60	32
Orange Vanilla Treat	2 bars (80 g)	70	10	5
Vanilla Sandwich Bar	1 bar (68 g)	160	35	18
Weight Watchers Sweet Celebrations				
Brownie à la Mode	1 dessert (91 g)	190	40	9
Chocolate Chip Cookie Dough Sundae	½ cup (77 g)	180	35	14
Double Fudge Brownie Parfait	1 parfait (109 g)	190	25	18
Praline Toffee Crunch Parfait	1 parfait (104 g)	190	25	18

SWEETS

FOOD	AMOUNT	CALORIES		
		TOTAL	FAT	SAT-FAT
Ice Cream Cones				
Cake	1 cone	16	9	<9
Sugar	1 cone	60	9	<9
Ice Cream Toppings				
Hershey's				
Candy Bar Sprinkles	2 tbsp	140	45	27
Chocolate Chips	1 oz	140	72	45
Coconut	2 tbsp	58	37	33
Reese's Sprinkles	2 tbsp	160	70	45
Juice Bars				
Fruit 'n Juice, all flavors (Dole)	1 bar	70	0	0
Fruit Juice Bar, all flavors (Dole)	1 bar	45	0	0
Pies (Bakery, Homemade, or Restaurant)				
Apple	⅙ pie (104 g)	280	120	36
Boston cream	⅟₁₂ pie	370	153	83
Cherry	⅙ pie (104 g)	310	120	32
Cherry Beehive (Entenmann's)	⅕ pie (130 g)	270	0	0
Coconut custard	¼ pie (139 g)	410	200	81
Dutch apple	⅙ pie (104 g)	290	110	27
Lemon meringue	⅙ pie (113 g)	290	120	36
Peach	⅙ pie (104 g)	300	100	23
Pecan	⅙ pie (113 g)	440	200	45
Sweet potato	⅙ pie (104 g)	270	80	23
Snack Pies				
Hostess				
Apple Fruit	1 pie (122 g)	410	170	81
Blueberry Fruit	1 pie (122 g)	400	150	72
Cherry Fruit	1 pie (122 g)	430	170	81
Tastykake				
Chocolate-Iced Tasty-Klair	1 pie (113 g)	410	180	45
French Apple	1 pie (120 g)	360	110	27
Pies, Frozen				
Mrs. Smith's				
Bake and Serve				
Apple	⅙ pie (123 g)	270	100	18
Apple Cranberry	⅙ pie (123 g)	280	100	18
Blackberry	⅙ pie (123 g)	280	100	18

SWEETS

FOOD	AMOUNT	CALORIES		
		TOTAL	FAT	SAT-FAT
Bake and Serve *(cont.)*				
Blueberry	⅙ pie (123 g)	260	100	**18**
Cherry	⅙ pie (123 g)	270	100	**18**
Coconut Custard	⅕ pie (142 g)	280	110	**45**
Dutch Apple Crumb	⅙ pie (123 g)	310	110	**23**
Mince	⅙ pie (123 g)	300	100	**18**
Pumpkin Custard	¹⁄₁₀ pie (130 g)	230	60	**18**
Handy-to-Serve				
Pecan	⅕ pie (136 g)	520	210	**36**
Old-Fashioned				
Apple	⅛ pie (131 g)	370	160	**32**
Cherry	⅛ pie (131 g)	320	120	**23**
Peach	⅛ pie (131 g)	310	120	**23**
Ready-to-Serve				
Apple	⅕ pie (69 g)	310	120	**23**
Boston Creme	⅛ pie (131 g)	170	50	**14**
French Silk Chocolate	⅕ pie (136 g)	410	190	**54**
Lemon Meringue	⅕ pie (136 g)	300	70	**18**
Pecan	⅕ pie (136 g)	520	210	**36**
Thaw and Serve				
Banana Cream	¼ pie (96 g)	250	80	**23**
Chocolate Cream	¼ pie (96 g)	290	130	**36**
Lemon Cream	¼ pie (96 g)	270	120	**27**
Thaw and Serve Smart-Style				
All fruit flavors	⅙ pie (95 g)	180	25	**5**
Blueberries and Cheese				
Yogurt	⅙ pie (80 g)	160	45	**14**
Peaches and Cheese Yogurt	⅙ pie (80 g)	170	45	**14**
Strawberries and Banana				
Yogurt	⅙ pie (80 g)	160	27	**5**
Sara Lee				
Chocolate Cream	⅕ pie (136 g)	500	280	**144**
Coconut Cream	⅕ pie (136 g)	480	280	**126**
Lemon Meringue	⅙ pie (142 g)	350	100	**23**
Pie, Mixes				
No Bake Chocolate Silk Pie				
(Jell-O)	⅙ pie (45 g)	310	140	**54**
Pie Crusts				
Graham Cracker (Keebler				
Ready)	⅛ 9″ crust	110	45	**9**

SWEETS

FOOD	AMOUNT	CALORIES		
		TOTAL	FAT	SAT-FAT
Hershey's Chocolate (Keebler Ready)	⅛ 9″ crust	110	45	9
2 pie-crust shell				
Mrs. Smith's	⅛ 9″ crust	80	35	9
Richford	⅛ 9″ crust	80	45	18
2 pie-crust shell, deep-dish pie				
Mrs. Smith's	⅛ 9″ crust	90	50	9
Puddings				
Chocolate				
Fat-free	4 oz	100	0	0
Hershey's Kisses	4 oz	180	50	14
Jell-O	4 oz	160	45	18
Snack Pack (Hunt's), all flavors	4 oz	150–160	50	14
Tapioca (Swiss Miss)	4 oz	140	35	9
Vanilla (Swiss Miss)	4 oz	160	50	14
Puddings, Restaurant				
Caramel bavarian cream	½ cup	246	128	73
Chocolate mousse	½ cup	324	199	115
Crème caramel	1 cup	303	125	27
Custard, baked	1 cup	305	125	61
Sugars, Syrups, etc.				
Honey	1 tbsp	65	0	0
Jams, Jellies, and Preserves	1 tbsp	55	0	0
Molasses	1 tbsp	43	0	0
Sugar				
Brown, firmly packed	1 tbsp	51	0	0
	½ cup	410	0	0
White				
Granulated	1 tsp	16	0	0
	½ cup	385	0	0
Powdered, sifted	1 cup	385	0	0
Syrups				
Chocolate (Hershey's)	2 tbsp	100	9	0
Corn	1 tbsp	61	0	0
Maple	1 tbsp	61	0	0

SWEETS

| FOOD | AMOUNT | CALORIES | | |
		TOTAL	FAT	SAT-FAT
Miscellaneous				
Baklava (Apollo)	4½ pieces (125 g)	540	280	**45**
Carob Chips	1 oz (2⅔ tbsp)	140	63	**52**
Chocolate				
baking, unsweetened	1 oz	145	135	**81**
chips	1 oz	140	72	**45**
semi-sweet	30 chips (15 g)	70	35	**23**
Chocolate Eclairs	1	239	122	**40**
Custard cream puffs	1	303	163	**63**
Escalloped Apples (Stouffer's)	⅔ cup	180	25	**0**
Gelatin dessert	½ cup	70	0	**0**
Puff Pastry, frozen (Pepperidge Farm)				
Sheets	⅙ sheet (41 g)	200	100	**23**
Shells	1 shell (47 g)	230	130	**27**

VEGETABLES AND VEGETABLE PRODUCTS

See also **FROZEN, MICROWAVE, AND REFRIGERATED FOODS.**

| FOOD | AMOUNT | CALORIES | | |
		TOTAL	FAT	SAT-FAT
Alfalfa seeds, sprouted, fresh	1 cup	10	0	**0**
Artichoke				
fresh	1 medium	65	0	**0**
	1 large	83	0	**0**
cooked	1 medium	53	0	**0**
hearts				
canned in water	½ cup	35	0	**0**
marinated, undrained	½ cup	190	135	**18**
Asparagus				
fresh	½ cup	15	0	**0**
	4 spears	13	0	**0**
cooked	½ cup	22	0	**0**
	4 spears	15	0	**0**
Baked beans, canned				
Brown Sugar and Bacon (Campbell's)	½ cup	170	25	**9**

VEGETABLES AND VEGETABLE PRODUCTS

FOOD	AMOUNT	CALORIES		
		TOTAL	FAT	SAT-FAT
Baked beans, canned (*cont.*)				
Plain or Vegetarian in Tomato Sauce	½ cup	117	5	2
(Campbell's)	½ cup	130	20	9
Pork 'n Beans (Hanover)	½ cup	120	15	5
with beef	½ cup	160	42	20
with franks	½ cup	184	76	27
with pork	½ cup	134	18	7
and sweet sauce	½ cup	141	17	7
and tomato sauce	½ cup	124	12	5
Bamboo shoots				
fresh	1 cup	41	0	0
cooked	1 cup	15	0	0
canned	1 cup	25	0	0
Beans				
Black				
dry	1 cup	661	25	6
boiled	1 cup	227	8	2
Great Northern				
dry	1 cup	621	19	6
boiled	1 cup	210	7	2
canned	1 cup	300	9	3
Kidney				
dry	1 cup	613	14	2
boiled	1 cup	225	8	1
canned	1 cup	208	7	1
Kidney, California red				
dry	1 cup	607	0	0
boiled	1 cup	219	0	0
Kidney, red				
dry	1 cup	619	18	3
boiled	1 cup	225	8	1
canned	1 cup	216	8	1
Kidney, royal red				
dry	1 cup	605	7	1
boiled	1 cup	218	3	0
Lima, baby				
fresh	1 cup	216	6	1
boiled	1 cup	188	5	1
Lima, large				
fresh	1 cup	176	11	3

VEGETABLES AND VEGETABLE PRODUCTS

		CALORIES		
FOOD	AMOUNT	TOTAL	FAT	SAT-FAT
Beans				
Lima, large (*cont.*)				
boiled	1 cup	208	6	1
canned	1 cup	186	4	1
Navy				
dry	1 cup	697	24	6
boiled	1 cup	259	9	2
canned	1 cup	296	10	3
Pink				
dry	1 cup	721	21	6
boiled	1 cup	252	7	2
Pinto				
dry	1 cup	656	20	4
boiled	1 cup	235	8	2
canned	1 cup	186	7	1
Refried				
canned (Del Monte)	1 cup	260	32	10
Mexican restaurant	¾ cup	375	146	60
Snap				
fresh	1 cup	34	0	0
cooked	1 cup	44	0	0
canned	1 cup	36	0	0
Soy				
dry	1 cup	774	334	48
boiled	1 cup	298	139	20
Soy products				
miso	1 cup	565	150	22
tofu	1 piece (2½ × 2¾ × 1 in)	88	50	7
White, small				
dry	1 cup	723	23	4
boiled	1 cup	253	10	1
Yellow				
fresh	1 cup	676	46	12
boiled	1 cup	254	17	4
Beets				
fresh	1 cup slices	60	0	0
	2 beets	71	0	0
cooked	1 cup slices	52	0	0
	2 beets	31	0	0
canned, drained	1 cup	54	0	0

VEGETABLES AND VEGETABLE PRODUCTS

| FOOD | AMOUNT | CALORIES | | |
		TOTAL	FAT	SAT-FAT
Black-eyed or cowpeas,				
cooked	1 cup	190	0	0
Broadbeans				
fresh	1 cup	511	21	3
boiled	1 cup	186	6	1
canned	1 cup	183	5	0
Broccoli				
fresh	1 cup chopped	24	0	0
	1 spear	42	0	0
cooked	1 cup chopped	46	0	0
	1 spear	53	0	0
Brussels sprouts, cooked	1 cup	60	0	0
	1 sprout	8	0	0
Cabbage				
fresh	1 cup shredded	16	0	0
	1 head	215	0	0
cooked	1 cup shredded	32	0	0
	1 head	270	0	0
Cabbage, Chinese				
fresh	1 cup shredded	9	0	0
cooked	1 cup shredded	20	0	0
Cabbage, red				
fresh	1 cup shredded	19	0	0
cooked	1 cup shredded	32	0	0
Cabbage, Savoy				
fresh	1 cup shredded	19	0	0
cooked	1 cup shredded	35	0	0
Carob flour	1 tbsp	14	0	0
Carrots				
fresh	1	31	0	0
	1 cup shredded	48	0	0
cooked	1 cup sliced	70	0	0
Carrot juice	1 cup	98	0	0
Cauliflower, fresh or cooked	3 flowerets	13	0	0
	1 cup pieces	24	0	0
Celery, fresh	1 stalk	6	0	0
	1 cup dices	18	0	0
Chard, Swiss				
fresh	1 cup chopped	6	0	0
	1 leaf	9	0	0
cooked	1 cup chopped	35	0	0

VEGETABLES AND VEGETABLE PRODUCTS

		CALORIES		
FOOD	AMOUNT	TOTAL	FAT	SAT-FAT
Chickpeas or garbanzos				
dry	1 cup	729	109	11
boiled	1 cup	269	38	4
canned	½ cup	110	18	3
Chili with beans, canned	1 cup	286	126	54
Coleslaw (see also **FAST** **FOODS**)				
made with mayonnaise	1 cup	171	161	34
Collard greens, cooked	1 cup chopped	27	0	0
Corn				
cooked	1 ear	85	9	1
	1 cup kernels	178	15	3
canned, cream style	1 cup	186	10	1
popped (see **SNACKS**)				
Cucumber, fresh	1 cucumber	39	0	0
	1 cup slices	14	0	0
Dandelion greens				
fresh	1 cup chopped	25	0	0
cooked	1 cup chopped	35	0	0
Eggplant				
fresh	1 eggplant	27	0	0
cooked	1 cup cubes	27	0	0
Endive, fresh	1 cup chopped	8	0	0
	1 head	86	0	0
Garlic, fresh	1 clove	4	0	0
Kale				
fresh	1 cup chopped	33	0	0
cooked	1 cup chopped	41	0	0
Leeks				
fresh	1	76	0	0
	¼ cup	16	0	0
cooked	1	38	0	0
	¼ cup	8	0	0
Lentils				
dry	1 cup	649	17	2
boiled	1 cup	231	7	1
Lettuce, fresh				
Boston butterhead	1 head (5-in)	21	0	0
crisphead, iceberg	1 head (6-in)	70	0	0
	1 wedge	20	0	0
	1 cup chopped	5	0	0

VEGETABLES AND VEGETABLE PRODUCTS

		CALORIES		
FOOD	AMOUNT	TOTAL	FAT	SAT-FAT
Lettuce, fresh (*cont.*)				
looseleaf, romaine	1 cup	10	0	**0**
Mushrooms				
fresh, sliced or chopped	1 cup	20	0	**0**
	1 lb	127	0	**0**
cooked	1 cup	42	0	**0**
canned	1 cup	38	0	**0**
Mushrooms, shiitake				
dried	4	44	0	**0**
cooked	4	44	0	
	1 cup	80	0	**0**
Okra				
fresh	8 pods	36	0	**0**
	1 cup	38	0	**0**
cooked	8 pods	27	0	**0**
	1 cup	50	0	**0**
Onions				
fresh	1 cup	54	0	**0**
cooked	1 cup	58	0	**0**
fried onion rings, frozen	7 rings	285	168	**54**
Onions, green, fresh	1 cup	26	0	**0**
Parsley, fresh	10 sprigs	3	0	**0**
Parsnips				
fresh	1 cup	100	0	**0**
cooked	1 cup	126	0	**0**
Peas, green				
fresh	1 cup	118	0	**0**
cooked	1 cup	134	0	**0**
Peas, split				
fresh	1 cup	671	21	**0**
boiled	1 cup	231	7	**0**
Peas and carrots, canned	1 cup	96	6	**0**
Peas and onions, canned	1 cup	122	8	**0**
Peppers				
hot chili, fresh	1	18	0	**0**
	½ cup	30	0	**0**
jalapeño	½ cup	17	0	**0**
sweet, fresh	1	18	0	**0**
	½ cup	12	0	**0**
sweet, cooked	1	13	0	**0**
	½ cup	12	0	**0**

VEGETABLES AND VEGETABLE PRODUCTS

		CALORIES		
FOOD	AMOUNT	TOTAL	FAT	SAT-FAT
Potatoes				
au gratin	1 cup	320	167	**104**
baked in skin	1 (2 per lb)	145	0	**0**
	1 lb	325	0	**0**
boiled in skin	1	173	0	**0**
	1 (3 per lb)	104	0	**0**
	1 cup	118	0	**0**
	1 lb	345	0	**0**
boiled, pared before cooking	1 (2 per lb)	146	0	**0**
	1 (3 per lb)	88	0	**0**
	1 cup	101	0	**0**
	1 lb	295	0	**0**
Fried, frozen				
French fries (*see also* **FAST FOODS**)				
Act II Microwave	1 box (88 g)	240	110	**23**
Ore Ida potatoes				
Crispers	17 (84 g)	220	110	**18**
Dinner Fries	8 (84 g)	110	30	**9**
Golden Crinkles	16 (84 g)	120	35	**9**
Tater Tots	9 (84 g)	160	70	**14**
Zesties	12 (84 g)	160	80	**14**
Potato puff	1	16	7	**3**
	½ cup	138	60	**28**
Frozen, other preparations				
hashed brown	½ cup	170	81	**38**
mashed				
with whole milk	½ cup	81	6	**3**
with whole milk and butter	½ cup	111	40	**22**
Ore Ida potatoes				
Mashed, butter flavor	½ cup	80	20	**5**
Onion Tater Tots	9 (84 g)	150	60	**14**
Potato Wedges with skins	9 (84 g)	110	25	**9**
Potatoes O'Brien	¾ cup	60	0	**0**
Twice-Baked				
Cheddar cheese	1 (140 g)	200	80	**27**
Sour Cream and Chives	1 (140 g)	180	60	**36**
Potato chips (*see* **SNACK FOODS**)				

VEGETABLES AND VEGETABLE PRODUCTS

FOOD	AMOUNT	CALORIES		
		TOTAL	FAT	SAT-FAT
Potatoes (*cont.*)				
Potato pancakes	1	495	113	**31**
Potato salad	½ cup	180	92	**16**
Potato sticks (*see* **SNACK FOODS**)				
Scalloped, from dry mix	1 cup	230	99	**25**
Pumpkin, cooked	1 cup	49	0	**0**
Radishes, fresh	10	7	0	**0**
	½ cup	10	0	**0**
Sauerkraut, canned	1 cup	44	0	**0**
Shallots, fresh	1 tbsp	7	0	**0**
Spinach				
fresh	1 cup	6	0	**0**
	10-oz pkg	46	0	**0**
cooked	1 cup	41	0	**0**
Spinach soufflé, made with whole milk, eggs, cheese, butter	1 cup	218	165	**64**
Squash				
summer (crookneck, zucchini)				
fresh	1 cup	26	0	**0**
cooked	1 cup	36	0	**0**
winter (acorn, butternut)				
fresh	1 squash	172	0	**0**
	1 cup	43	0	**0**
cooked	1 cup	79	0	**0**
Succotash, cooked	1 cup	222	14	**1**
Sweet potatoes				
baked in skin	1 (5 × 2″)	118	0	**0**
	½ cup mashed	103	0	**0**
boiled without skin	1 cup mashed	344	0	**0**
Tomatoes				
fresh	1	24	0	**0**
	1 cup	35	0	**0**
cooked	1 cup	60	0	**0**
canned in tomato juice	1 cup	67	0	**0**
Tomato juice, canned	1 cup	42	0	**0**
Tomato products, canned				
marinara sauce	1 cup	171	75	**11**
paste	1 tbsp	14	0	**0**
purée	1 cup	102	0	**0**

VEGETABLES AND VEGETABLE PRODUCTS

FOOD	AMOUNT	CALORIES		
		TOTAL	FAT	SAT-FAT
Tomato products, canned (cont.)				
sauce (see also **SAUCES, GRAVIES, AND DIPS**)	1 cup	74	0	0
spaghetti sauce (see **SAUCES, GRAVIES, AND DIPS**)				
Turnips, cooked	1 cup cubes	28	0	0
Vegetable juice cocktail, canned	1 cup	44	0	0
Water chestnuts, canned	1 cup	70	0	0
Yam, cooked	1 cup	158	0	0
Zucchini				
fresh	1 cup	26	0	0
cooked	1 cup	36	0	0

MISCELLANEOUS

FOOD	AMOUNT	CALORIES		
		TOTAL	FAT	SAT-FAT
Baking powder	1 tbsp	5	0	0
Carob flour	1 tsp	14	0	0
Cocoa powder	1 tsp	5	0	0
Cocoa powder	1 tbsp	14	5	0
Curry powder	1 tsp	5	0	0
Garlic powder	1 tsp	10	0	0
Gelatin, dry	1 envelope	25	0	0
Ketchup	1 tbsp	15	0	0
Mustard	1 tsp	5	0	0
Olives, green	4 medium	15	15	2
Olives, ripe	3 small or 2 large	15	15	3
Oregano	1 tsp	5	0	0
Paparika	1 tsp	5	0	0
Pickles				
dill	1 medium	5	0	0
gherkin	1	20	0	0
sweet	1	20	0	0
Vinegar	1 tbsp	0	0	0
Yeast, all types	1 tbsp	20	0	0

FOOD TABLES INDEX

This index was designed to help you find some of the harder-to-locate foods in these tables as well as those foods that appear in several different categories.

APPENDICES

THE NITTY-GRITTY OF
HOW TO KEEP A FOOD RECORD

The absolutely most effective way to lower your risk of heart disease is to eat a diet low in saturated fat. To lower your cholesterol you have to know *exactly* how much saturated fat you are eating. That is why you are keeping food records. These records are for YOUR coronary arteries and YOU, not your spouse, your mother, your brother, your doctor, your dietitian — just for you, and they must be exact and accurate. They must reflect *exactly* what you eat, not what you think you *should* have eaten. Beautiful imaginary food records have no effect on cholesterol levels. If you eat 1 cup of Häagen-Dazs ice cream, record 1 cup of Häagen-Dazs ice cream. Okay. You regret your overindulgence, but being sorry won't put the ice cream back in the carton. If you don't record what you eat, you fool only yourself, not your arteries. If you exceed your Sat-Fat Budget, your cholesterol count will be elevated whether or not you record all your sat-fat splurges. On the other hand, if you write down the 200 sat-fat calories you consumed, you can balance your sat-fat intake for the rest of the day or the next by eating less saturated fat.

Don't become frantic about your food diary. Your first records will reflect what got you into this mess in the first place. Don't feel guilty. Everyone used to wolf down hot dogs and french fries with gusto and no thought. We called whole milk pure and steak a high-protein food. Who knew? As the days and weeks progress, your records will reflect a diet lower in saturated fat and higher in complex carbohydrates. But it takes time.

> We have developed an inexpensive Passbook to help you keep track of your food intake. See the order form on the last pages of *Eater's Choice*.

KEEPING GOOD RECORDS

Time

Record What You Eat When You Eat It. Write down what you eat when you eat it. Don't fill in your record at the end of the day. You're bound to forget what you don't want to remember. Recording the time helps you see patterns in your eating. The fact that there are eight hours between your first and second entry may give you a clue as to why you were famished for lunch and gobbled down that bag of greasy potato chips.

Food and Amount

List All Foods Separately and List Amounts Accurately. Measure everything. Be accurate. Don't write down *just* "cream cheese." Write down the amount you ate as well — "cream cheese, 2 tablespoons." Don't write down *simply* "chicken breast." Write down "chicken breast with skin, batter-fried." Don't write down *merely* "roast beef sub." Ask the sandwich man how much roast beef and how much mayonnaise he gave you. (He'll know — his boss makes sure he gives everyone an exact amount.) Write down "6-inch sub roll, 4 ounces roast beef, 1 tablespoon mayonnaise." These details are important. If you eat out, ask the waiter what's in the cream sauce and how much butter is on the swordfish or rice.

Sample Food Record

	FOOD	AMOUNT		
	cream cheese	2 tbsp		
	chicken breast with skin, batter-fried	1 breast		
	Roast beef	4 oz		
	6-inch sub roll	1		
	mayonnaise	1 tbsp		

For "Hints on Measuring and Recording Foods," see page 587.

Total Calories

When people cut down on saturated fat, they often cut down on all calories. This is unhealthy. When you reduce your saturated fat intake, you must be sure to increase your intake of complex carbohydrates, fruits, and low- or nonfat dairy products. If you don't eat enough of these low-fat foods, you will miss the vitamins, minerals, and fiber they provide. You also need to eat enough calories to keep up your basal metabolic rate.

On the other hand, grossly exceeding your ideal total caloric intake indicates that you may also be overshooting your Sat-Fat Budget. You know if you are eating too many or too few total calories only if you keep track.

Your total caloric intake should hover around the number you determined on page 55. If eating more complex carbohydrates raises the total, that's okay. Fat makes fat, not complex carbohydrates.

Use the Food Tables (look under the heading "Total Calories") and labels on packages to determine the total calories of the food you have eaten. Make sure that you adjust the total calories for the amount you eat relative to the amount listed. For example, the amount listed for Cheddar cheese is 1 ounce. The total calories for 1 ounce of Cheddar cheese are 114. If you ate 3 ounces of Cheddar cheese you would record $3 \times 114 = 342$ total calories.

Sat-Fat Calories

Use the Food Tables (look under the heading "Sat-Fat Calories") and labels on packages to determine the sat-fat calories of the food you have eaten. Be sure to adjust the sat-fat calories for the amount you eat relative to the amount listed. For example, the amount listed for club steak is 1 ounce. The sat-fat calories for 1 ounce of club steak are 50. No one eats 1 ounce of meat. If you ate 5 ounces of club steak, you would record $5 \times 50 = 250$ sat-fat calories.

If you cannot find the exact food you have eaten in the Food Tables (use the Food Tables Index on page 576), find a similar food and record its sat-fat calories. For example, if you ate veal parmigiana in a restaurant, check out the veal parmigiana entries (not low-fat) in the "Frozen, Refrigerated, and Microwave Foods" section of the Food Tables.

If you ate a mixed dish such as chicken stir-fry, estimate the sat-fat calories for the individual ingredients. For example, chicken stir-fry might contain a chicken breast without skin (4 sat-fat calories), a tablespoon of corn oil (15 sat-fat calories), green pepper, onion, and garlic (0 sat-fat calories).

When saturated fat is listed on a label, it is listed in grams. There are 9 calories per gram of saturated fat. To find the number of sat-fat calories per gram, multiply by 9. For example, according to a label, 1 ounce of light cream cheese contains 4 grams of saturated fat: 4 grams × 9 calories/gram = 36 sat-fat calories. If you eat 1 ounce of the cream cheese, you would record 36 sat-fat calories. If you eat 1½ ounces, you would record 54 (1.5 × 36 = 54).

Your food record for breakfast might look like this:

	FOOD	AMOUNT	TOTAL CALORIES	SAT-FAT CALORIES	SAT-FAT SUBTOTAL
	Bran'nola	½ cup	200	4.5	
	2% milk	1 cup	121	27	
	grapefruit	½	95	0	

Sat-Fat Subtotal

You should keep a running tally of your sat-fat intake. This makes you aware of how much you have "spent" and how much you have left to spend. If, by noon, you have eaten two-thirds of your Sat-Fat Budget, you will know to budget a dinner that is low in saturated fat.

	FOOD	AMOUNT	TOTAL CALORIES	SAT-FAT CALORIES	SAT-FAT SUBTOTAL
	Bran'nola	½ cup	200	4.5	4.5
	2% milk	1 cup	121	27	31.5
	grapefruit	½	95	0	31.5

Sat-Fat Total

At the end of the day, compare your sat-fat intake for the day with your Sat-Fat Budget. Is your sat-fat consumption closer to budget than it was yesterday? Be sure to evaluate your food diary for complex carbohydrates, fruits, and dairy. Did you eat according to the recommendations in Chapter 11, "Ensuring a Balanced Diet"? Did you eat 2 to 3 fruits and 3 to 5 vegetables; 6 to 11 servings of potatoes, rice, whole-wheat bread, or cereal; 2 to 3 servings of nonfat flavored yogurt, 1% cottage cheese, or skim milk? Not only do these foods supply the vitamins, minerals, and fiber you need, they make you feel full and thus less likely to binge on high-sat-fat foods.

Get Started

Granted, keeping food records is a pain in the neck. However, the benefits greatly override the inconvenience. You'll gain insight. No longer will your elevated cholesterol level be a mystery. You'll know why your cholesterol is high, because you'll know exactly what you are eating. Those cheese and crackers you nibbled at the office cost you 150 sat-fat calories. Surprised? Is that half your Sat-Fat Budget?

You will discover where the sat-fat lurks in the foods you eat so you can make changes. You can make changes only if you know what to change. Maybe you don't even *like* cheese and crackers 150-sat-fat-calories-worth. Maybe you'd rather spend your sat-fat calories some other way. Keeping food records is worth the bother. People who keep honest and accurate food records and eat below their Sat-Fat Budget get the most cholesterol lowering (up to 33 percent).

Of course, you will not have to keep food records forever. Eventually, you will know the sat-fat calories of most of the foods you eat and will be able to make wise food choices that fit within your budget without recording your every bite.

HINTS ON MEASURING AND RECORDING FOODS

Liquids

Most Liquids. Use measuring cups to measure liquids.

Milk products, coffee whiteners, and cooking oils should be recorded in measuring-cup and -spoon amounts. Most other liquids should be recorded in fluid ounce amounts.

	FOOD	AMOUNT		
	2% Milk	1 cup		
	Half-and-half	1 tbsp		
	Coke	12 fl oz		
	Eggnog	8 fl oz		

This table of equivalent measures will help you record liquids:

1 cup = 8 fluid ounces
½ cup = 4 fluid ounces
¼ cup = 2 fluid ounces
2 tablespoons = 1 fluid ounce

Solid food

Meat. Read the meat package label or use a kitchen scale to measure the weight (in ounces) of *beef, lamb, pork, veal, poultry,* and *fish.* Record the weight of meat in ounces. Indicate whether the meat was raw or cooked when you weighed it and whether the fat is included or has been trimmed. If necessary, use the following estimates:

¼ cup meat = 1 ounce meat
Chicken breast half = 3 ounces
4 ounces raw meat without bone = 3 ounces cooked
6 ounces raw meat with bone = 3 ounces cooked

FOOD	AMOUNT		
Flank steak, meat and fat, raw	5 oz		
Salmon, baked	6 oz		

Cereals,* Cottage Cheese, Creams, Fats, Frozen Desserts, Canned Fish, Sliced Fruit, Grains, Milks, Nuts,** Pasta, Puddings (Not Canned), Rice, Salad Dressings, Sauces and Gravies, Snacks, Soups, and Vegetables. Use measuring cups and spoons to measure and record these foods.

FOOD	AMOUNT		
Bran Chex	1 oz or ⅔ cup		
Sour cream	3 tbsp		
Egg noodles, cooked	¾ cup		
Tomato soup, prepared with milk	1½ cups		
Cashews	12 nuts		

---

*If you have a scale, you may also weigh and record cereal in ounces.
**You may also weigh and record nuts in ounces or count and record the number of nuts you eat.

Fast Foods. Record by unit, piece, serving, order, or slice, except for shakes, which are measured in fluid ounces.

FOOD	AMOUNT		
McDonald's Quarter Pounder	1		
KFC (Kentucky Fried Chicken) breast	1 piece		
Jack in the Box Onion Fries	1 serving		
Long John Silver's Breaded Shrimp	1 order		
Domino's Pizza	2 slices		
Roy Rogers Chocolate Shake	11.25 fl oz		

Candy, Cheese,* Cold Cuts, Nuts, Yogurt, and Frozen Yogurt. Read the label on the package or use a scale to measure the weight (in ounces). Save packages with nutrition labeling for use later. Record weight of food in ounces or grams; 1 ounce = 28 grams.

FOOD	AMOUNT		
Swiss cheese	2 oz		
Salami, beef	0.8 oz (1 slice)		
Whitney's lemon yogurt	6 fl oz		

Bread should be recorded by slice.
Cakes and pies should be recorded by fraction of whole dessert (i.e., 1/10 cake).
Crackers and cookies should be recorded by unit (i.e., 5 crackers).
Frozen food should be recorded by package or fraction of the package you ate.
If possible, save packages with labels for future reference.

FOOD	AMOUNT		
Oatmeal bread	2 slices		
Cheesecake	1/12 cake		
Blueberry Newtons	4 cookies		
Lean Cuisine, Chicken à l'Orange	1 package		

---

*Cottage cheese and ricotta should be measured by measuring cup rather than weighed.

Here's a summary chart that lists foods and the unit used to measure them.

Summary Chart

FOOD	UNIT	EXAMPLES
Dairy/Eggs Butter Cheese, hard, soft Cheese, curd type Cream Milk Yogurt Egg	 pat, tsp/tbsp, cup oz cup tbsp cup fl oz cup 1 egg 1 egg white 1 egg yolk	 2 oz Cheddar ½ cup ricotta 1 tbsp light cream 1 cup skim 8 fl oz nonfat yogurt 1 cup low-fat yogurt
Fast Foods	unit order oz piece serving slice or fraction of whole*	1 cheeseburger 1 order fried shrimp 12-oz shake 1 chicken breast 1 serving coleslaw 3 slices, 12-inch pepperoni pizza
Fats and Oils Margarine Oils Salad dressings	 tsp, tbsp, cup tsp, tbsp, cup tbsp, cup	 2 tsp diet margarine 3 tbsp olive oil 2 tbsp Russian dressing
Fish and Shellfish	oz ¼ cup = 1 ounce 4 oz, raw = 3 oz, cooked	4 oz orange roughy
Frozen and Microwave	Depends on product	Use information on food label.
Fruits	piece cup	1 apple ½ cup applesauce

---

*Specify diameter of whole (i.e., pizza, 14-inch diameter).

FOOD	UNIT	EXAMPLES
Grains and Pasta		
Bagels	number	1 bagel
Bread	slice	2 slices rye
Cereals	cup	⅔ cup Wheatena
	oz	1 oz Cheerios
Crackers	number	2 Wheat Thins
Pasta/rice	cup	¾ cup macaroni, dry
Popcorn	cup	5½ cups, air-popped
Rolls	number	1 poppy seed roll
Meats	oz	5 oz sirloin steak
	¼ cup = 1 ounce	
	4 oz, raw (without bone)	
	= 3 oz, cooked	
	6 oz, raw (with bone)	
	= 3 oz, cooked	
Nuts and Seeds	oz	1 oz pecans
	tbsp	2 tbsp peanut butter
	number	12 cashews
	cup	½ cup sunflower seeds
Poultry	piece	½ chicken breast
	oz	3 oz white meat turkey
Sauces and Gravies	tbsp	3 tbsp mushroom gravy
	cup	½ cup cream sauce
Sausages and Cold Cuts	oz	4 oz turkey bologna
	slices	3 slices salami
	links	1 link smoked sausage
Soups	cup	1½ cups tomato soup
Sweets		
Cakes	fraction of whole	1/12 chocolate cake
Cookies, bars	unit	1 sugar cookie
Pie	fraction of whole	⅙ pumpkin pie
Sugar, jelly	tsp/tbsp	1 tsp grape jam
Vegetables	cup	½ cup spinach
	unit	1 carrot

Remember to record every detail of what you eat so you have enough information to determine the fat calories later.

From the National Institutes of Health
Adult Treatment Panel II Guidelines
National Cholesterol Education Program
(See Explanatory Notes on page 594.)

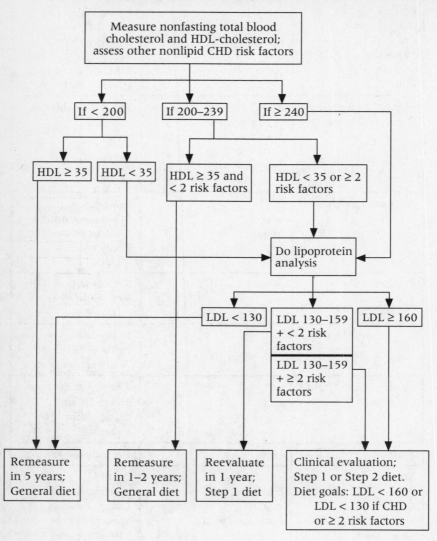

CONTINUE DIETARY TREATMENT FOR 6 MONTHS.

IF GOALS ARE NOT MET, CONSIDER DRUGS.

From the National Institutes of Health
National Cholesterol Education Program
Cholesterol Screening and Treatment Guidelines
for Children and Adolescents (Ages 2–19)
(See Explanatory Notes on page 594.)

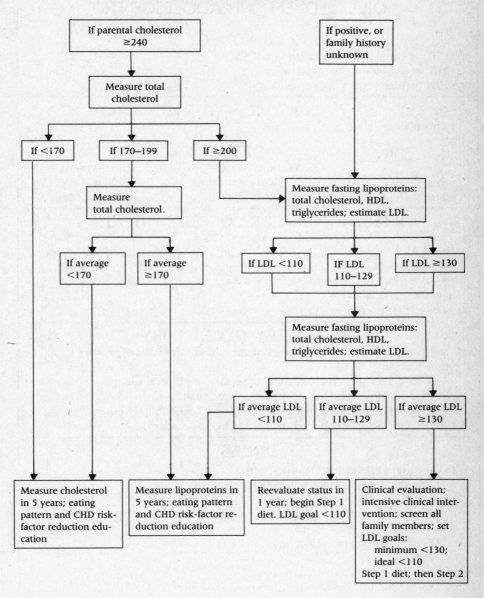

EXPLANATORY NOTES FOR ADULT TREATMENT GUIDELINES AND CHOLESTEROL SCREENING AND TREATMENT GUIDELINES FOR CHILDREN AND ADOLESCENTS

TERMINOLOGY
- CHD = coronary heart disease
- LDL = low density lipoprotein
- HDL = high density lipoprotein

LIPOPROTEIN VALUES
- All values are given in mg/dL.

DIETS

	SATURATED FAT	CHOLESTEROL
• STEP 1 DIET	<10% of calories	<300 mg/day
• STEP 2 DIET	<7% of calories	<200 mg/day

RISK FACTORS FOR CORONARY HEART DISEASE (CHD)

Positive Risk Factors: Age (men aged 45 and over; women aged 55 and over or premature menopause without estrogen replacement therapy) • High blood pressure • Diabetes mellitus • Family history of premature CHD • Low HDL <35 mg/dL • Smoking

Negative Risk Factor: High HDL ≥60 mg/dL

POSITIVE FAMILY HISTORY

Parents or grandparents, at 55 years of age or less, who have experienced one of the following:
- a documented heart attack, angina pectoris, peripheral vascular disease, cerebrovascular disease, or sudden cardiac death;
- diagnostic coronary arteriography and were found to have atherosclerosis;
- balloon angioplasty or coronary artery by-pass surgery

DRUGS

Major drugs for lowering LDL cholesterol:
- Bile acid sequestrants (cholestyramine and colestipol)
- Nicotinic acid
- HMG CoA reductase inhibitors (lovastatin, pravastatin, simvastatin)

Other drugs:
- Fibric acids (gemfibrozil)
- Probucol

Alternative or adjunct to drug therapy
- Estrogen replacement in postmenopausal women

FAT CALORIES OF EATER'S CHOICE RECIPES

	PER SERVING		
RECIPE	TOTAL CALORIES	TOTAL FAT CALORIES	SAT-FAT CALORIES
Soups			
Apple-Squash Soup	122	0	0
Avgolemono Soup	99	6	2
Barley-Vegetable Soup	100	0	0
Bean Soup with Spinach, Squash, and Tomatoes	154	8	0
Blueberry Soup	96	0	0
Broccoli Soup	99	0	0
Cantaloupe Soup	80	0	0
Carrot Soup	69	0	0
Carrot Soup des Basques	87	0	0
Cauliflower Soup	47	7	1
Chilled Strawberry Soup	90	0	0
Corn Chowder	177	23	5
Cuban Black Bean Soup	207	15	3
Cucumber Soup	78	0	0
per each walnut half	12	10	1
Gazpacho I	55	0	0
with croutons	79	1	1
Gazpacho II	53	0	0
with croutons	70	1	1
Ginger-Carrot Soup	80	6	1
Ginger Squash Soup	52	0	0
Great Black Bean Soup	227	11	1
Green Pesto Soup	53	11	1
Green Tomato Soup	66	3	2
Hot and Sour Soup	97	14	4
Lentil and Everything but the Kitchen Sink Soup	85	6	0

RECIPE	PER SERVING		
	TOTAL CALORIES	TOTAL FAT CALORIES	SAT-FAT CALORIES
Lentil Soup	141	7	1
with yogurt	148	7	1
Matzo Ball Soup	167	26	6
Mild Fish Chowder	179	18	1
Minestrone	110	8	1
Monhegan Island Fish Chowder	156	13	3
Mulligatawny Soup	114	14	2
Mushroom Soup	90	13	2
Oriental Noodle Soup	64	8	1
Peanut Butter Soup	120	67	11
Potato Soup with Leeks and Broccoli	113	16	2
Sour Cherry Soup	165	0	0
Sweet Cabbage Soup	56	1	0
Tarragon Squash Soup	122	3	1
Tomato-Rice Soup	93	0	0
Tortilla Soup	144	10	1
Vegetable Soup Provençal	58	1	0
Vegetable Soup with Spinach, Potatoes, Rice, and Corn	129	12	2
Watercress Soup	74	4	0
Zucchini Soup	80	0	0

Chicken

RECIPE			
Alex's Chinese Chicken with Onion, Mushrooms, and Zucchini	192	31	6
Apricot Chicken Divine	215	23	5
Baghdad Chicken	200	38	7
Balsamic Chicken with Potatoes and Onions	193	23	5
Bar-B-Que Chicken			
breast	173	13	4
thigh	126	24	6
Blackened Chicken	130	13	4
Cajun Chicken	196	28	2
Chicken with Apples and Onions	238	35	9
Chicken with Apricots, Sweet Potatoes, and Prunes	301	34	7
Chicken Couscous	283	24	9
Chicken Curry	164	20	5

RECIPE	PER SERVING		
	TOTAL CALORIES	TOTAL FAT CALORIES	SAT-FAT CALORIES
Chicken with Dried Fruit and Lemon	226	13	4
Chicken Fajitas	212	38	6
Chicken Kiev	175	38	6
Chicken Marrakesh	132	13	4
Chicken Nuggets Chez Goor	191	43	5
with honey-mustard sauce	211	43	5
Chicken Paprikash	152	23	5
Chicken with Rice, Tomatoes, and Artichokes	274	12	3
Chicken Smothered in Vegetables	194	23	5
Chicken Verde	187	42	8
Chinese Chicken			
breast	183	13	3
drumstick	130	19	5
thigh	134	24	5
Coq au Vin			
breast	195	35	9
drumstick	140	41	10
thigh	148	46	11
Creamy Chicken Pie	156	60	11
Cuban Chicken	252	35	7
Fifties Chicken	200	33	7
Ginger Chicken with Green Onions	172	51	9
Grilled Apricot-Ginger Chicken	191	29	6
Hunan Chicken with Onions and Red and Green Peppers	162	29	5
Indonesian Chicken with Green Beans	135	14	4
Indonesian Peanut Chicken	148	61	10
Keema Matar	249	76	13
Kung Pao Chicken with Broccoli	168	24	5
Lemon Chicken	176	13	4
Lemon-Mustard Chicken	147	33	6
Lime-Peanut-Ginger Chicken	175	64	11
Ma-Po Bean Curd	126	37	7
Mongolian Hot Pot			
sauce	69	0	0
meat and vegetables	155	25	4
broth	184	0	0
total	408	25	4
Orange-Soy Chicken	119	12	4

| RECIPE | PER SERVING | | |
	TOTAL CALORIES	TOTAL FAT CALORIES	SAT-FAT CALORIES
Peppery Chicken	172	13	4
Phyllo-Wrapped Chicken with Rice, Artichokes, and Cream Sauce	270	56	12
Pineapple Chicken	210	13	4
Sate Ajam	151	23	5
Sesame Chicken Brochettes	160	20	5
Shepherd's Chicken Chili Pie	204	15	4
Singapore Chicken	164	50	10
Szechuan Chicken with Sweet Red Pepper and Pineapple	203	21	5
Tandoori Chicken	152	13	4
Thai Chicken with Asparagus	201	42	8
Tortillas con Pollo	207	16	1
Vegetables, Chicken, and Cellophane Noodles	111	44	7

Turkey

Basic Turkey Cutlet			
cutlets made with fat	211	60	12
cutlets made without fat	158	8	4
Breaded Turkey Cutlet	228	72	11
Broccoli Baked Turkey	145	32	19
Creamy Turkey Casserole	255	49	22
Turkey with Capers			
cutlets made with fat	227	70	13
cutlets made without fat	174	18	5
Turkey Cutlets with Artichoke-Cream Sauce			
cutlets made with fat	230	67	15
cutlets made without fat	188	25	9
Turkey Mexique	146	16	4
Turkey Niçoise			
cutlets made with fat	206	55	11
cutlets made without fat	171	20	6
Turkey Roll-Ups Firenze	176	32	10
Turkey Sautéed with Onions and Almonds	200	43	8
Turkey Scaloppine Limone			
cutlets made with fat	246	70	14
cutlets made without fat	194	18	6

RECIPE	PER SERVING		
	TOTAL CALORIES	TOTAL FAT CALORIES	SAT-FAT CALORIES
Turkey Scaloppine Marsala			
cutlets made with fat	268	70	14
cutlets made without fat	216	18	6
Turkey with Snow Peas	190	26	9
Turkey with Sweet Red Pepper Sauce			
cutlets made with fat	237	48	10
cutlets made without fat	185	6	3
Turkey Véronique			
cutlets made with fat	234	60	12
cutlets made without fat	145	14	5

Fish and Shellfish

RECIPE	TOTAL CALORIES	TOTAL FAT CALORIES	SAT-FAT CALORIES
Broiled Ginger Fish	194	35	4
Broiled Monkfish with Orange Sauce	194	52	13
Cajun Fish (sole)	140	15	5
Curry Fish	283	28	5
with teaspoon of each condiment	349	41	7
Dill Fish	115	12	4
Fennel Fish	134	42	4
Fish Baked in Olive, Chili Pepper, and Tomato Sauce	150	18	5
Fish with Mushroom Sauce	254	40	8
Fish with Peppercorns, Thyme, and Mustard	70	23	5
Fish in Wine Sauce	119	12	4
Flounder Fillets Stuffed with Fennel Rice	130	22	9
Honey-Curry Scallops	140	8	4
Marinated Fish Steaks			
swordfish	241	70	17
cod	175	22	1
halibut	240	42	7
Oriental Fish Kebabs	243	51	10
Phyllo-Wrapped Fish and Mushroom Sauce	397	85	17
without sauce	342	61	12
Salmon with Cucumber-Grape Sauce			
Atlantic	202	58	17
coho	206	82	17
pink	174	86	9
Salmon Soufflé	149	32	9

| RECIPE | PER SERVING | | |
	TOTAL CALORIES	TOTAL FAT CALORIES	SAT-FAT CALORIES
Scallops Provençal	190	55	8
Scallop or Shrimp Caribbean			
scallops	170	26	3
shrimp	170	35	3
Scallop or Shrimp Creole			
scallops	177	18	6
shrimp	177	28	6
Scallop or Shrimp Curry			
scallops	187	25	7
shrimp	187	35	7
Shanghai Fish	117	12	4
Shrimp with Green Peppers	174	36	6
Spicy Shrimp Louisiana	88	28	2
Vegetables			
Acorn Squash	40	0	0
with margarine	55	15	3
Afghan Squash	25	5	1
Artichokes	26	0	0
margarine per tablespoon	90	90	18
Bouillon Potatoes	106	0	0
Braised Mushrooms Oriental	50	22	2
Broccoli and Mushrooms	51	7	1
Caraway Carrots	35	5	2
Carrots and Leeks	51	10	1
Cauliflower Sauté	47	20	3
Celery-Mushrooms	27	13	2
Chickpeas with Lemon and Herbs	170	46	5
Curried Beans	137	7	1
Curried Whipped Potatoes	168	10	1
Curried Zucchini	23	5	1
Eggplant with a Greek Influence	44	28	3
Fluffy Sweet Potatoes	118	23	8
Glazed Acorn Squash	58	0	0
Green Beans Basilico	42	13	2
Hot and Garlicky Eggplant	25	5	1
Indian Vegetables	72	7	1
Italian Mixed Vegetables	27	10	1
Keema Eggplant	86	7	1
Lentils and Potatoes	48	16	1
Muriel's Chinese Vegetables	54	9	1

RECIPE	PER SERVING		
	TOTAL CALORIES	TOTAL FAT CALORIES	SAT-FAT CALORIES
Potato Skins	66	7	1
Potatoes Lyonnaise	63	11	2
Ratatouille	32	8	2
Sesame Broccoli	50	20	3
Spaghetti Squash with Tomato Sauce	117	10	2
Spiced Sweet Potatoes	78	0	0
Spinach Oriental	30	10	1
Spinach and Tomatoes	40	9	1
Steamed Zucchini Matchsticks	17	0	0
with margarine	24	7	2
Sweet Potatoes with Oranges, Apples, and Sweet Wine	125	0	0
Sweet Vegetable Mélange	85	10	1
Vegetable Soufflé	75	22	5
Tahini Sauce	20	11	1

Pizza, Chili, Quiche, and Tortillas

Calzone	296	24	4
Chili Non Carne	117	5	1
Focaccia	113	18	3
Pawtucket Chili	105	9	1
Pissaladière	196	29	5
Pizza			
slice	116	4	1
Spinach Quiche	177	47	10
Tomato Quiche	183	63	12
Tomato Tart	173	63	8
Tortillas	90	11	0

Pasta, Rice, and Other Grains

Asparagus Pasta	253	26	4
with chicken	296	30	5
Barley Plus	150	13	3
Basic Tomato Sauce	32	5	0
Bulgur with Tomatoes and Olives	68	12	1
Dan-Dan Noodles	252	32	5
Fried Rice	154	20	4
Indian Rice	91	5	1
Lemon Rice with Spinach and Red Pepper	90	5	0

RECIPE	PER SERVING		
	TOTAL CALORIES	TOTAL FAT CALORIES	SAT-FAT CALORIES
Olive-Artichoke Rice	88	16	3
Pasta Mexicali	161	7	1
Pasta with Pesto	287	54	14
Peasant Pasta	240	41	6
Rice Pilau with Apricots and Raisins	96	11	1
Salmon Pasta Niçoise			
with salmon	378	86	19
with tuna	359	67	13
Spaghetti Sauce à la Sicilia	275	10	1
Spaghetti Touraine	165	40	5
Zesty Fresh Tomato Sauce	48	8	1

Salads

RECIPE	TOTAL CALORIES	TOTAL FAT CALORIES	SAT-FAT CALORIES
Chicken Salad with Shallots and Mushrooms	113	20	4
Coriander Chicken Salad	90	21	12
Cucumber Salad	20	0	0
Curried Tuna Salad with Pears	175	23	7
Dijon Chicken-Rice Salad	267	34	7
Eastern Spinach Salad	55	20	3
Fruit Salad with Cottage Cheese or Yogurt			
Spring or summer salad			
with cottage cheese	280	10	7
with nonfat yogurt	250	0	0
Fall or winter salad			
with cottage cheese	270	10	7
with nonfat yogurt	245	0	0
Indonesian Vegetable Salad	32	0	0
1 tablespoon dressing	43	30	5
Oriental Chicken Salad	140	29	6
Potato Salad	105	14	5
Salade Niçoise	128	43	6
Tabbouli	87	10	2
Tarragon-Raisin Chicken Salad	180	36	12

Sandwiches, Dips, and a Drink

RECIPE	TOTAL CALORIES	TOTAL FAT CALORIES	SAT-FAT CALORIES
Baba Ghanoush	12	7	1
Bagel Chips	38	2	0

| | PER SERVING | | |
RECIPE	TOTAL CALORIES	TOTAL FAT CALORIES	SAT-FAT CALORIES
Chickpea Sandwich or Dip			
sandwich	195	39	4
tablespoon	20	5	1
Creamy Ginger-Curry Dip	24	0	0
Eggplant Appetizer	38	24	5
Faux Guacamole			
per tablespoon	7	0	0
pita bread, per quarter	33	2	0
Frothy Fruit Shake	105	2	0
Ted Mummery's Turkey Barbecue	131	5	1
Yogurt Cheese			
per tablespoon	7	0	0
Breads			
Anadama Bread			
loaf	1919	257	42
slice	113	15	2
Apple Oat Bran Muffins	125	32	4
Apricot Oat Muffins	135	32	4
Banana-Carrot Muffins	195	64	11
modified	155	51	8
Bran Muffins	116	23	4
Buttermilk Herb Bread			
loaf	1842	306	80
slice	108	18	5
Buttermilk Pancakes			
total batter	495	90	6
per pancake	31	13	1
Buttermilk Waffles			
total batter	1102	107	16
per waffle	138	13	2
Cardamom Bread			
loaf	1663	255	41
slice	98	15	2
Challah			
loaf	1670	317	47
slice	70	13	2
Cinnamon Applesauce Bread			
loaf	2025	177	24
slice	119	10	1
Cinnamon French Toast	106	29	8

RECIPE	PER SERVING		
	TOTAL CALORIES	TOTAL FAT CALORIES	SAT-FAT CALORIES
Cranberry Bread			
loaf	1899	254	55
slice	112	15	3
Cumin Wheat Bread			
loaf	1814	252	35
slice	107	15	2
Focaccia Genovese			
loaf	1390	156	22
slice	116	13	2
French Bread I			
loaf	874	133	19
slice	87	13	2
French Bread II			
round loaf	942	24	4
slice	94	2	0
baguette	471	12	2
slice	52	1	0
Gingerbread Muffins	177	59	9
Ginger-Orange Bread			
loaf	1678	279	46
slice	99	16	3
Honey Whole-Wheat Bread			
loaf	2222	342	39
slice	130	17	2
Mother's Oat Bran Muffins			
with walnuts	160	49	6
without walnuts	144	36	5
Oatmeal Bread			
loaf	1630	196	31
slice	96	11	2
Onion Flat Bread			
loaf	667	56	7
slice	83	7	1
Orange Oat Muffins	110	34	4
Peanut Butter Bread			
loaf	1358	321	50
slice	78	18	3
Peppery Breadsticks	41	2	0
Pumpernickel Bread			
loaf	2273	301	39
slice	92	12	2

RECIPE	PER SERVING		
	TOTAL CALORIES	TOTAL FAT CALORIES	SAT-FAT CALORIES
Sesame Breadsticks			
total	1423	196	30
breadstick	41	6	1
Shaker Daily Loaf			
loaf	1512	117	28
slice	90	7	2
Whole-Wheat Bagels	115	23	1
Whole-Wheat Banana Raisin Bread			
loaf	2099	195	30
slice	123	11	2

Desserts

RECIPE	TOTAL CALORIES	TOTAL FAT CALORIES	SAT-FAT CALORIES
Apple Cake	220	114	13
Apple-Nut Cookies	62	25	4
without nuts	51	16	3
Apple Pandowdy	243	74	11
Applesauce Cake	250	89	14
Banana Cake	263	110	12
Carrot Cake sans Oeufs	122	40	5
Cheesecake!			
crust with margarine	120	16	4
crust without margarine	112	8	3
Chocolatey-Chocolate Cocoa Cake	273	71	13
Cinnamon Sugar Coffee Cake	299	98	20
Cinnamon Sweet Cakes	148	61	8
Cocoa Angel Food Cake	119	<1	0
Cocoa Brownies	115	54	9
Deep-Dish Pear Pie	236	61	11
Divine Buttermilk Pound Cake	175	66	13
with Mocha Frosting	225	81	18
with Walnut Glaze	199	71	14
Ginger Cake	183	63	14
with Pear Sauce	194	63	14
Glazed Cinnamon Buns	120	18	3
Graham Cracker Crust	600	186	34
Honey Graham Crackers	58	12	2
Key Lime Pie (with Graham Cracker Crust)	201	27	6
Lemon Loaf	290	142	21
without walnuts	215	76	15
Mandelbrot	46	18	2

| | PER SERVING | | |
RECIPE	TOTAL CALORIES	TOTAL FAT CALORIES	SAT-FAT CALORIES
Marble Cake	238	75	15
Meringue Shells with Fresh Strawberries and Warm Raspberry Sauce	130	0	0
Mocha Cake	140	50	10
with icing	174	61	13
Nutmeg Torte	204	54	11
Oatmeal Cookies	65	25	3
Orange Cake	180	74	15
Pears Hélène	205	23	5
Philip Wagenaar's Raisin-Ginger-Orange Cake	236	43	9
Pineapple Pound Cake	177	47	9
Pumpkin Cake	128	34	7
Spice Cake	238	96	19
with frosting	288	118	24
Strawberry-Rhubarb Pie	240	63	11
Strawberry Tart	194	35	6
Sugar Cookies	65	11	2
Tante Nancy's Apple Crumb Cake	220	60	14
The York Blueberry Cake	141	46	8

GLOSSARY

Aerobic exercise. Steady, repetitive exercise that uses the large muscles and requires a steady supply of oxygen — in contrast to exercise that requires bursts of activity separated by periods of inactivity. Examples of aerobic exercises include walking, swimming, running, and biking. Aerobic exercise burns more fat than active sports, which burn more carbohydrate.

Angina pectoris. An episode of chest pain, often caused by a temporary restriction of oxygenated blood due to narrowing of the coronary arteries supplying the heart muscle. An angina attack is not to be confused with a heart attack, which results from a severe and prolonged lack of oxygenated blood to a part of the heart.

Angiography or angiocardiography. A diagnostic method involving injection of an x-ray dye into the bloodstream. Chest x-rays taken after the injection show the inside dimensions of the heart and blood vessels outlined by the dye.

Aorta. The main trunk artery that carries oxygenated blood from the heart. Lesser arteries branching off from the aorta conduct blood to all parts of the body except the lungs.

Arteriosclerosis. A group of diseases characterized by thickening and loss of elasticity of artery walls. This may be due to an accumulation of fibrous tissue, fatty substances (lipids), and/or minerals.

Artery. A blood vessel that carries blood away from the heart to the various parts of the body. Arteries usually carry oxygenated blood, except for the pulmonary artery, which carries unoxygenated blood from the heart to the lungs for oxygenation.

Atherosclerosis. A type of arteriosclerosis in which the inner layer of the artery wall is made thick and irregular by deposits of a fatty substance. These deposits (called plaques) project above the surface of the inner layer of the artery and thus decrease the diameter of the internal channel of the vessel.

Bile acids. Breakdown products of cholesterol formed in the liver and excreted into the intestine, where they play an important role in the absorption of fats from the foods we eat.

Cholesterol. A fatlike substance found in the cell walls of all animals, including humans. Cholesterol is transported in the bloodstream. Some of it is manufactured by the body and some comes from the foods of animal origin that we eat.

A healthy level of cholesterol is below 200 mg/dL. A higher level is often associated with increased risk of coronary atherosclerosis.

Cholestyramine. A drug used to lower blood levels of cholesterol.

Chylomicrons. Largest of the lipoproteins; produced by the intestine to transport dietary fats to the adipose tissue (fat deposits).

Coronary arteries. Arteries, arising from the base of the aorta, which conduct blood to the heart muscle. These arteries, and the network of vessels branching off from them, come down over the top of the heart like a crown (corona).

Coronary atherosclerosis. Commonly called coronary heart disease. An irregular thickening of the inner layer of the walls of the coronary arteries that conduct blood to the heart muscle. The internal channels of these arteries become narrowed and the blood supply to the heart muscle is reduced.

Coronary bypass surgery. Surgery to improve the blood supply to the heart muscle when narrowed coronary arteries reduce flow of the oxygen-containing blood that is vital to the pumping heart. This reduction in blood flow causes chest pain and leads to increased risk of heart attack. Thus coronary bypass surgery involves constructing detours through which blood can bypass narrowed portions of coronary arteries to keep the heart muscle supplied. Veins or arteries taken from other parts of the body where they are not essential are grafted onto the heart to construct these detours.

Coronary heart disease. Also called coronary artery disease and ischemic heart disease. Heart ailments caused by narrowing of the coronary arteries and therefore a decreased blood supply to the heart.

Electrocardiogram (often referred to as ECG or EKG). A graphic record of the electric currents generated by the heart.

Enzyme. A protein that speeds up specific biochemical processes in the body. Enzymes are universally present in living organisms.

Fats. Also known as lipids. Fats are one of the five major classes of nutrients; the other four are proteins, carbohydrates, minerals, and vitamins. Fats in foods and in the body generally occur as triglycerides.

Heart attack. The death of a portion of heart muscle, which may result in disability or death of the individual, depending on how much of the heart is damaged. A heart attack occurs when a blockage in one of the coronary arteries prevents an adequate oxygen supply to the heart. Symptoms may be none, mild, or severe and may include chest pain (sometimes radiating to the shoulder, arm, neck, or jaw), nausea, cold sweat, and shortness of breath.

Heart disease. A general term applied to ailments of the heart or blood vessels. Some of these are present at birth (congenital) and are either inherited or are the result of environmental influences on the embryo as it develops in the womb. The majority of cases of heart disease, however, are acquired later in life, for example, through the development of atherosclerosis.

High blood cholesterol (hypercholesterolemia). An excess of a fatty substance called cholesterol in the blood, which is often associated with the premature development of atherosclerosis and therefore with increased risk of heart attack and stroke.

High blood pressure (hypertension). An unstable or persistent elevation of blood pressure above the normal range. Uncontrolled, chronic high blood pressure strains the heart, damages arteries, and creates a greater risk of heart attack, stroke, and kidney problems.

High density lipoprotein (HDL). The smallest and most dense lipoprotein, HDL removes cholesterol from LDL and cells and transports it back to the liver, where the cholesterol is broken down into bile acids and excreted into the intestine. HDL is protective against the development of heart disease; high levels of HDL are associated with low risk of heart disease.

Lifestyle. An individual's typical way of life, including diet, kinds of recreation, job, home environment, location, temperament, and smoking, drinking, and sleeping habits.

Lipid. A fatty substance.

Lipoprotein. A complex particle consisting of lipid (fat), protein, and cholesterol molecules bound together to transport lipids through the blood. Lipoproteins are classified according to their density. Four important lipoproteins are Very Low Density Lipoprotein (VLDL), Low Density Lipoprotein (LDL), High Density Lipoprotein (HDL), and chylomicrons.

Liver. A large organ in the upper right side of the abdominal cavity, which is involved in the metabolism of fats, produces bile, and performs various other metabolic functions.

Low Density Lipoprotein (LDL). LDL particles are formed by removal of triglycerides from VLDL. LDL is rich in cholesterol. High levels of LDL in the blood are associated with the premature development of atherosclerosis and an increased risk of heart attack.

Metabolism. A general term designating all chemical changes that occur to substances within the body.

Monocytes. A type of white blood cell that engulfs foreign objects. Monocytes engorged with LDL and chylomicron remnants infiltrate the arterial wall and cause thickening, known as atherosclerosis.

Monounsaturated fat. A fat chemically constituted so that it is capable of absorbing additional hydrogen but not as much hydrogen as polyunsaturated fat. These fats in the diet have recently been shown to lower blood cholesterol levels. One example of a monounsaturated fat is olive oil.

Obesity. An increase in body weight beyond physical and skeletal requirements due to an accumulation of excess fat. This puts a strain on the heart and increases the chance of developing two major heart attack risk factors: high blood pressure and diabetes.

Plaque. Also called atheroma. A deposit of fatty (and other) substances in the inner lining of the artery wall, characteristic of atherosclerosis.

Polyunsaturated fat. A fat chemically constituted so that it is capable of absorbing additional hydrogen. These fats are usually liquid oils of vegetable origin, such as corn oil or safflower oil. A diet with a high polyunsaturated fat content tends to lower the amount of cholesterol in the blood. These fats are sometimes substituted for saturated fat in a diet in an effort to lessen the hazard of fatty deposits in the blood vessels.

Saturated fat. A fat chemically constituted so that it is not capable of absorbing any more hydrogen. These are usually the solid fats of animal origin, such as the fats in milk, butter, meat, etc. A diet high in saturated fat content tends to increase the amount of cholesterol in the blood. These fats are restricted in the diet in an effort to lessen the hazard of fatty deposits in the blood vessels.

Sodium. A mineral essential to life, found in nearly all plant and animal tissue. Table salt (sodium chloride) is nearly half sodium. In some types of heart disease, the body retains an excess of sodium and water, and therefore sodium intake is restricted.

Stroke. A blocked blood supply to some part of the brain.

Triglyceride. The main type of lipid (fatty substance) found in the fat tissue of the body and also the main type of fat found in foods. Triglycerides are composed of three fat molecules attached to an alcohol molecule called glycerol. High levels of triglycerides in the blood may be associated with a greater risk of coronary atherosclerosis.

Unsaturated fat. A fat whose molecules have one or more double bonds, so that it is capable of absorbing more hydrogen. Monounsaturated fats, such as olive oil, have only one double bond (the rest are single), and recent evidence indicates that they may lower blood cholesterol levels. Polyunsaturated fats, such as corn oil and safflower oil, have two or more double bonds per molecule and tend to lower blood cholesterol.

Very low density lipoprotein (VLDL). The lightest and largest of the lipoproteins manufactured by the liver, VLDL particles carry triglycerides from the liver to muscle and fat cells throughout the body. VLDL particles are produced and released in large amounts after meals.

REFERENCES AND RESOURCES

Chapter 1

American Heart Association. *Heart Facts 1985.*

Assembly of Life Sciences, National Research Council. *Diet, Nutrition, and Cancer Committee Report on Diet, Nutrition, and Cancer.* Washington, D.C.: National Academy Press, 1982.

National Cancer Institute, U.S. Department of Health and Human Services. *Diet, Nutrition & Cancer Prevention: A Guide to Food Choices.* NIH Publication No. 85-2711. Washington, D.C.: Government Printing Office, 1984.

National Institutes of Health. *Heart Attacks.* Medicine for the Layman, NIH Publication No. 80-1803. Washington, D.C.: Government Printing Office, 1980.

Pooling Project Research Group. "Relationship of Blood Pressure, Serum Cholesterol, Smoking Habit, Relative Weight, and ECG Abnormalities to Incidence of Major Coronary Events." *Journal of Chronic Diseases* 31 (1978):201–306.

Chapter 2

Brown, M. S., and J. L. Goldstein. "How LDL Receptors Influence Cholesterol and Atherosclerosis." *Scientific American* 251 (November 1984):58–66.

Department of Health, Education, and Welfare. *A Handbook of Heart Terms.* DHEW Publication No. (NIH) 78-131. Washington, D.C.: Government Printing Office.

Department of Health, Education, and Welfare. *The Human Heart: A Living Pump.* DHEW Publication No. (NIH) 78-1058. Washington, D.C.: Government Printing Office.

Heiss, G., et al. "Lipoprotein-Cholesterol Distributions in Selected North American Populations: The Lipid Research Clinics Prevalence Study." *Circulation* 61 (1980):302.

Lipid Research Clinics Program. *The Lipid Research Clinics Population Studies Data Book, Volume 1. The Prevalence Study.* NIH Publication No. 80-1527. Washington, D.C.: Government Printing Office, 1980.

Inter-Society Commission for Heart Disease Resources. "Optimal Resources for Primary Prevention of Atherosclerotic Diseases." *Circulation* 42 (1970, revised 1972):A55–A95.

Chapter 3

Blackburn, H. "Diet and Mass Hyperlipidemia: A Public Health View." In *Nutrition, Lipids, and Coronary Heart Disease — A Global View,* edited by R. I. Levy, et al., 309–48. New York: Raven Press, 1979.

Blankenhorn, D. H., et al. "Beneficial Effects of Combined Colestipol-Niacin Therapy on Coronary Atherosclerosis and Coronary Venous Bypass Grafts." *Journal of the American Medical Association* 257 (1987):3233.

Blankenhorn, D. H., et al. "The Influence of Diet on the Appearance of New

Lesions in Human Coronary Arteries." *Journal of the American Medical Association* 263 (1990): 1646–52.

Gordon, T., et al. "High Density Lipoprotein As a Protective Factor Against Coronary Heart Disease: The Framingham Study." *American Journal of Medicine* 62 (1977):707.

Kannel, W. B., et al. "Serum Cholesterol, Lipoproteins, and the Risk of Coronary Heart Disease: The Framingham Study." *Annals of Internal Medicine* 74 (1971):1–12.

Kato, H., et al. "Epidemiologic Studies of Coronary Heart Disease and Stroke in Japanese Men Living in Japan, Hawaii, and California. Serum Lipids and Diet." *American Journal of Epidemiology* 97 (1973):372–85.

Keys, A., ed. "Coronary Heart Disease in Seven Countries." *Circulation* 41 (1970):Supplement 1.

LaRosa, J. C., et al. "The Cholesterol Facts. A Summary of the Evidence Relating Dietary Fats, Serum Cholesterol, and Coronary Heart Disease. A Joint Statement by the American Heart Association and the National Heart, Lung, and Blood Institute." *Circulation* 81 (1990):1721.

Lipid Research Clinics Program. "The Lipid Research Clinics Coronary Primary Prevention Trial Results. I: Reduction in Incidence of Coronary Heart Disease." *Journal of the American Medical Association* 251 (1984):351.

Lipid Research Clinics Program. "The Lipid Research Clinics Coronary Primary Prevention Trial Results. II: The Relationship of Reduction in Incidence of Coronary Heart Disease to Cholesterol Lowering." *Journal of the American Medical Association* 251 (1984):365.

McGill, H. C., ed. *The Geographic Pathology of Atherosclerosis.* Baltimore: Williams and Wilkins Co., 1968.

Ornish, D., et al. "Can Lifestyle Changes Reverse Coronary Heart Disease? The Lifestyle Heart Trial." *Lancet* 336 (1990):129–33.

Stamler, J. George Lyman Duff Memorial Lecture. "Lifestyles, Major Risk Factors, Proof, and Public Policy." *Circulation* 58 (1978):3.

Stamler, J. "Population Studies." In *Nutrition, Lipids, and Coronary Heart Disease — A Global View,* edited by R. I. Levy, et al., 25–88. New York: Raven Press, 1979.

Chapter 4

American Heart Association. *Eating for a Healthy Heart. Dietary Treatment of Hyperlipidemia.* AHA Publication No. 50-063-A.

American Heart Association. *Recommendations for Treatment of Hyperlipidemia in Adults.* Joint Statement of the Nutrition Committee and the Council on Arteriosclerosis. AHA Special Report No. 72-204-A, 1985.

Goor, R., et al. "Nutrient Intakes Among Selected North American Populations in the Lipid Research Clinics Prevalence Study: Composition of Fat Intake." *American Journal of Clinical Nutrition* 41 (1985):299.

"Summary of the Second Report of the National Cholesterol Education Program (NCEP) Expert Panel on Detection, Evaluation, and Treatment of High Blood Cholesterol in Adults (Adult Treatment Panel II)." *Journal of the American Medical Association* 269 (1993):3015.

Chapter 5

Anderson, J. T., F. Grande, and A. Keys. "Cholesterol-Lowering Diets: Experimental Trials and Literature Review. *Journal of the American Dietary Association* 62 (1973):133.

Dennison, D. *The DINE System: The Nutritional Plan for Better Health.* St. Louis: C. V. Mosby, 1982.

Hegsted, D. M., et al. "Quantitative Effects of Dietary Fat on Serum Cholesterol in Man. *American Journal of Clinical Nutrition* 17 (1965):281.

Keys, A., J. T. Anderson, and F. Grande. "Serum Cholesterol Response to Changes in the Diet. II: The Effect of Cholesterol in the Diet." *Metabolism* 14 (1965):759.

U.S. Department of Agriculture. *Composition of Foods.* Agriculture Handbook No. 8. Washington, D.C.: Government Printing Office, rev. December 1963.

Chapter 6

The fat tables are based on data from the following sources:

Dennison, D. *The DINE System: The Nutritional Plan for Better Health.* St. Louis: C. V. Mosby, 1982.

U.S. Department of Agriculture. *Composition of Foods.* Agriculture Handbook No. 8. Washington, D.C.: Government Printing Office, 1963.

U.S. Department of Agriculture. *Composition of Foods.* Agriculture Handbook No. 8. Washington, D.C.: Government Printing Office, sec. 1–12 rev. 1976–84.

U.S. Department of Agriculture. *Nutritive Value of Foods.* Home and Garden Bulletin No. 72. Washington, D.C.: Government Printing Office, rev. 1981.

U.S. Department of Agriculture. *Nutritive Value of American Foods in Common Units.* Agriculture Handbook No. 456. Washington, D.C.: Government Printing Office. November 1975.

Chapter 7

Block, G., et al. "Nutrient Sources in the American Diet: Quantitative Data from the NHANES II Survey. II: Macronutrients and Fats." *American Journal of Epidemiology* 122 (1985):27–40.

Chapter 8

American Heart Association. *Diet in the Healthy Child.* AHA Publication No. 72-203-A; also in *Circulation* 67 (1983):1411A.

Anderson, J. W., et al. "Hypocholesterolemic Effects of Oat Bran or Bean Intake for Hypercholesterolemic Men." *American Journal of Clinical Nutrition* 40 (1984):1146–55.

Kirby, R. W., et al. "Oat Bran Intake Selectively Lowers Serum Low-Density Lipoprotein Cholesterol Concentrations of Hypercholesterolemic Men." *American Journal of Clinical Nutrition* 34 (1981):824–29.

Liebman, B. "What Is This Thing Called Oat Bran?" and "Hot Cereals." *Nutrition Action Health Letter* 12, No. 9 (December 1985):7–11. Center for Science in the Public Interest, 1501 16th Street N.W., Washington, D.C. 20036.

Chapter 9

American Diabetes Association. "Glycemic Effects of Carbohydrates. A Policy Statement of the American Diabetes Association." *Diabetes Forecast* (May/June 1985):20–21; also in *Diabetes Care* (November/December 1984).

Case, R. B., et al. "Type A Behavior and Survival After Acute Myocardial Infarction." *New England Journal of Medicine* 312 (1985):737–41.

Food and Nutrition Board, National Research Council, National Academy of Sciences. *Recommended Dietary Allowances.* 9th edition. Washington, D.C., 1980.

Friedman, M., and R. Rosenman. *Type A Behavior and Your Heart.* New York: Alfred A. Knopf, 1974.

National Institutes of Health. *Exercise and Your Heart.* NIH Publication No. 81-1677, 1981. Available from the National Heart, Lung, and Blood Institute, Bethesda, MD 20205.

Ruberman, W., et al. "Psychosocial Influences on Mortality After Myocardial Infarction." *New England Journal of Medicine* 311 (1984):552–59.

The Sodium Content of Popular Prepared Food Items. Available from Consumer Affairs, Morton Salt Division, Morton Norwich Products, 110 Wacker Drive, Chicago, IL 60606.

U.S. Department of Agriculture. *The Sodium Content of Your Food.* Home and Garden Bulletin No. 233. Washington, D.C.: Government Printing Office.

U.S. Department of Health and Human Services. "Health Implications of Obesity." *National Institutes of Health Consensus Development Conference Statement* 5, No. 9 (1985). National Institutes of Health, Office of Medical Applications of Research, Building 1, Room 216, Bethesda, MD 20205.

U.S. Department of Health and Human Services. *Sodium: Facts for Older Citizens.* HHS Publication No. 83-2169. Available from the U.S. Food and Drug Administration, 5600 Fishers Lane, Rockville, MD 20857.

U.S. Department of Health and Human Services. "Treatment of Hypertriglyceridemia." *National Institutes of Health Consensus Development Conference Statement* 4, No. 8 (1983). National Institutes of Health, Office of Medical Applications of Research, Building 1, Room 216, Bethesda, MD 20205.

U.S. Department of Health and Human Services, Public Health Service, National Institutes of Health. *The 1984 Report of the Joint National Committee on Detection, Evaluation, and Treatment of High Blood Pressure.* NIH Publication No. 84-1088; also in *Archives of Internal Medicine* 144 (1984):1045–57.

U.S. Surgeon General. *The Health Consequences of Smoking: Cardiovascular Disease.* A Report of the Surgeon General, November 1983. Available from the Office on Smoking and Health, 5600 Fishers Lane, Parklawn Building, Room 110, Rockville, MD 20857.

Chapter 12

National Cholesterol Education Program. "Report of the Expert Panel on Blood Cholesterol Levels in Children and Adolescents."

INDEX

TABLE OF EQUIVALENT MEASURES

Volume Measures

1 gallon	4 quarts
1 quart	4 cups 2 pints
1 pint	2 cups
1 cup	8 fluid ounces 16 tablespoons
½ cup	4 fluid ounces 8 tablespoons
⅓ cup	5 tablespoons + 1 teaspoon
¼ cup	2 fluid ounces 4 tablespoons
1 tablespoon	3 teaspoons ½ fluid ounce

Weight Measures

1 pound	16 ounces 454 grams
3.5 ounces	100 grams
1 ounce	28.35 grams

Check out our website: http://www.choicediets.com

CHOOSE TO LOSE®

A Food Lover's Guide to Permanent Weight Loss
by **Dr. Ron and Nancy Goor**
Houghton Mifflin Company, Revised Edition, 1995

- ## Eat! Never be hungry!
- ## Lose weight permanently
- ## Lower your cholesterol

The GREAT news is that you have to eat to lose weight. It's not how much you eat; it's what you eat. Choose to Lose gives you the tools and skills to choose foods to make and keep you thin and healthy forever. You never feel deprived because you are enjoying **so much delicious low-fat food** and you can always fit in your high-fat favorites.

And it works!

People have lost more than 165 pounds, lowered their cholesterol and blood pressure, and normalized their blood sugar.

Available at most bookstores or use order form on next page

You will learn:

- How much fat you can eat each day (your Fat Budget) and still lose weight
- Which foods are making you fat.
- How to read food labels, order low-fat at restaurants, and modify recipes
- Why daily aerobic exercise (like walking) is essential for weight loss
- That low-fat foods taste delicious

Choose to Lose gives you:

- 50 delicious, easy, low-fat recipes with total, fat, and sat-fat calories listed
- Fat calories and sat-fat calories for over 6000 foods
- Chapter on weight control for children
- A clear explanation of how to use the new food labels and the Food Guide Pyramid to ensure you are eating a healthy, balanced diet.

(To order, see next page.)

ᴱᴬᵀᴱᴿ'S CHOICE®
POCKET COMPANIONS
Put Eater's Choice to work for you!

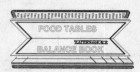

PASSBOOK

Convenient, pocket-sized passbook with vinyl cover contains
everything you need to keep track of your sat-fat intake:
- Abbreviated FOOD TABLES listing total and sat-fat calories
  for hundreds of foods
- BALANCE BOOK for keeping a two-week food record.

WORKBOOK

A step-by-step interactive companion that helps you master
the skills needed to lower your blood cholesterol.

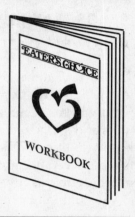

AUDIOTAPE

Ron and Nancy Goor's personal overview of the Eater's Choice
science and method. Originally $9.95 – now only $5.00.

CHOOSE TO LOSE (see preceding page)

If you need to lose weight, *Choose to Lose: A Food Lover's Guide
to Permanent Weight Loss* will show you how. You will want to
order Choose to Lose pocket companions. Call for information.

TO ORDER:

Call toll-free 1-888-897-9360 to order by credit card
or fill out and send the order form below with a check payable to Eater's Choice.

VISA MasterCard DISCOVER NOVUS [card]

SHIP TO: Print clearly or type   **ORDER FORM**

Name_____

Address _____

City_____ State _____ Zip_____

ITEM	QUANTITY	PRICE EACH	TOTAL PRICE
Eater's Choice Passbook		$ 4.50	
Eater's Choice Balance Book Refills		.75	
Eater's Choice Workbook*		9.00	
Eater's Choice book (4th edition)		15.95	
Choose to Lose book (revised edition)		13.95	
Eater's Choice Audiotape		5.00	

Send check or money order to:	5% tax (MD residents)	
Eater's Choice	Postage and Handling	2 .00
P.O. Box 2053	**TOTAL ORDER** $	
Rockville, MD 20847-2053		

*Requires Passbook. At least 2 Refills are useful.